Why Can't My Child Behave?

Why Can't She Cope?

Why Can't He Learn?

Jane Hersey

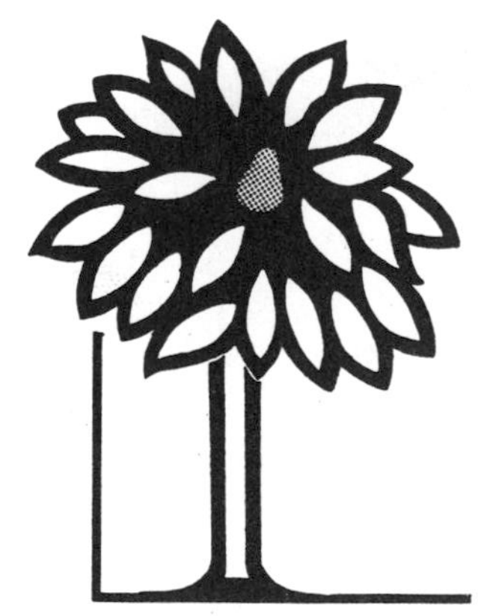

Pear Tree Press, Inc.
Alexandria, VA

DISCLAIMER

This book is presented as informational and educational material. It is not intended as medical advice, and in no way excludes the necessity for a diagnosis from a qualified health professional. Although care has been taken to ensure the accuracy of the information presented, the author and publisher cannot assume responsibility for the validity of all of the material or the consequence of it use.

Second Edition
Library of Congress Catalog Card Number: 96-92093
ISBN 0-9511050-8

Printed in the United States of America / May 1999

Hersey, Jane
Why Can't My Child Behave? Why Can't She Cope?
Why Can't He Learn? / Jane Hersey

1. Feingold diet. 2. Attention deficit/hyperactivity disorder.
3. Behavior problems in children. 4. Salicylate sensitivity.
5. Food additives.
618.92

Pear Tree Press, Inc.
Post Office Box 30146
Alexandria, VA 22310
U.S.A.

CONTENTS

PART ONE

TELL ME ABOUT YOUR CHILD 4
- Looking for answers 5
- The ages and stages of ADD/ADHD 10
- Can a diet help your child's behavior? 14
- What is the Feingold Program? 16
- Symptoms often helped 19
- Questions parents ask 21
- The first four days of Feingold 27
- Feingold – the next generation 32
- How can I gain my child's cooperation? 41
- How do I actually begin the Program? 46
- Stage One – keeping a diet diary 55

PART TWO

ADDITIVES: What are all those funny things in food? 56
- Food coloring 57
- The bug killer in the medicine cabinet 62
- Flavorings 64
- The troublesome antioxidants 67
- Five "little" food additives to consider 69
- What is corn syrup? 70
- MSG and the Feingold Program 70
- MSG and aspartame 74
- Sodium Benzoate 79
- Other additives 80
- Caffeine – more than just "coffee nerves" 82

SALICYLATES 84

FOOD, FROM BREAD TO WINE
- Breads and bakery products 92
- Candy 94
- Canned foods 96
- Cereal – snap, crackle, and … BHT? 97
- Cheese 98
- Coffee 98
- Donuts 99

Fats & oils 99
Something's fishy 100
Flour 100
Milk – looking for lowfat 101
Picnic time, pickle time 101
Rice 102
Soft drinks 102
Sugars 103
Tea 107
A sour story about vinegar 107
Wine 108

PART THREE

COPING SKILLS
"I used to hate cooking" 110
Low cholesterol diets 115
Stress has many forms – cheating 116
When Dad won't cooperate 124
Grandparents – big help or big problem 125
Parenting the Feingold teen 130
Finding a doctor 138
Emergency! Hospitalization 142
First aid help to have on hand 146
Visit the dentist but avoid the additives 146

SEASONS AND HOLIDAYS
Valentine's day 148
Enjoy a Feingold Easter 149
Suddenly it's summertime 150
Happy Halloween 154
Thanksgiving 157

YOUR CHILD IN SCHOOL 169
The sick school syndrome 179
"That kid who drives you crazy" 183
How I saved Fairfax County $62,296.00 185
Better nutrition brings up test scores 187
Edward and the KISS plan 187

SOCIAL SKILLS
Creating social skills problems 190
Asperger's syndrome 193

WHAT IS "ADD" AND HOW CAN IT BE TREATED? 194
How foods and additives affect the brain 195
EEG and foods/additives 200
ADD abroad 201
Parents under pressure 204
Better ways to help ADD children 209
Ritalin, Prozac 215
NIH panel finds inconsistencies 216
A review of the studies on stimulant medicine 224

ON THE PROGRAM AWAY FROM HOME
Steering clear of additives in your church or synagogue 227
Going to camp 231
Vacation time with restaurant food 234
The Feingold traveler abroad 242
Thinking about college 248

BABIES AND ADULTS
Predisposing babies to hyperactivity 250
"Hyperactive" adults 261

NON-FOODS
Carpeting 271
Cosmetics 272
Paint 276
Perfume – what is this stuff? 277

OTHER PROBLEMS FROM FOOD ADDITIVES AND SALICYLATES
Childhood arthritis 282
Asthma 284
Autism – the invisible prison 289
Bedwetting 307
Depression and other disorders 310
Developmental delays 320
Sensory integration therapy 320
Ear infections 324
Eye muscle disorder 327
Hives – the start of the Feingold Program 328
Nasal polyps 331
Seizure disorder – does diet play a role? 332
A good night's sleep 335
What is Tourette syndrome? 340

FOOD ALLERGIES 344

PART FOUR

THE COST TO SOCIETY
- The Kellogg Report 349
- Schools in crisis 351
- Violent behavior in children 352
- Huffing and snorting 357
- I want to help 358
- Why won't they even try the diet? 359

STUDIES ON DIET AND BEHAVIOR/LEARNING 363

COMMON ADDITIVES 381

VITAMIN C CONTENT OF FRUITS AND VEGETABLES 386

INDEX 387

Introduction

Dr. Benjamin Feingold dedicated his life to the pursuit of the relationship between what we eat and how we feel and behave afterwards. This is not a medical concern limited to children only. How we perform in school, work and at home is definitely associated with our diet. To believe that there is no correlation is foolhardy. The Feingold Association has made it possible to have a centralized location where one can go to get information, treatment and support.

The most vivid recollection I have of a patient's response occurred when I was working in my office around 12 years ago, when a mother came to see me with the cutest blond-haired, blue-eyed little two year old you have ever seen. Unfortunately her behavior was consistent with that of somebody possessed by the devil. She screamed and shrieked and was full of fright. Her mother described her as always being that way, and mom was at her wits end, crying to me about this situation. After obtaining a history and performing a physical exam I determined that this child's diet may be a strong factor in her adverse behavior so I referred them to the Feingold Association. About six weeks later mom returned with her daughter and both of them gave me hugs and kisses. It was then that I knew for certain that behavior is affected by diet. Since that time I have seen countless examples of behavioral disorders that have either been ameliorated or cured by diet.

Those of us who know children who are food sensitive are aware of their many difficulties. They have trouble in school with behavior and learning. They develop self-confidence difficulties and diminished self-esteem. They cause turmoil at home resulting in parental discord and generalized family instability.

In my opinion it is imperative to obtain a medical primary care provider who is empathetic, open minded and accepts the possibility that certain behaviors/psychological problems are related to diet. The use of stimulants in the treatment of these conditions is definitely appropriate when many factors are considered. The age of the patient, the family situation and the potential for compliance are criteria which must be weighed in determining whether a child will benefit from medication or diet. A family must not be willing to accept without a thorough neurological exam and thorough history the prescription for medication without all treatment modalities being discussed.

Based upon knowledge that I have regarding research into the value of the Feingold diet, we are approaching the dawn of a new era in the linking of foods, chemicals and behavior! We hope soon to have specific laboratory tests to determine which patient will respond to diet. This will impose serious scientific validation of Dr. Feingold's theories that are long overdue.

This effort by Jane Hersey for the Feingold Association is a labor of love and commitment. It will touch the heart of those who can relate to children whose lives were in turmoil and then became peaceful. It will give hope to those who are presently pursuing it. I am proud to be able to introduce this manuscript and to have been a part of the Feingold Association for these many years.

Jay Freed, M.D., F.A.A.P.

Dr. Freed is full attending physician in Pediatrics at St. Charles Hospital in Port Jefferson, NY, and Clinical Assistant Professor of Pediatrics at SUNY, Stony Brook. He is in practice with six other pediatricians serving central Suffolk County on Long Island. Dr. Freed practices general pediatrics with subspecialty interests in adolescent medicine and pediatric hematology.

Dear Reader,

More than twenty years ago I came upon the answer to the most difficult question I had ever faced: *Why can't my child behave?* This is the book I would have liked to have found.

Thanks to a remarkable doctor and countless volunteers, families of "impossible kids" have found answers. They helped their own children, then formed a nonprofit organization and stayed on to help others. In some cases the volunteers are adults whose parents used these techniques to help them when they were children.

It isn't possible to thank all the individuals who have given so much for two decades and more. There are doctors, researchers, journalists and counselors who have risked ridicule for refusing to see medicine as the only solution, who believed the welfare of children came first. There are countless talented volunteers who chose to donate their time when they could have enjoyed the financial benefits of a career.

I hope many of these people who have given their time and caring through the years will read this, and recognize the part they played in bringing help to families in the past as well as in the future.

But the focus of this book is not what has gone before, but what is available now, today, to help you with what is probably the most awful situation you have faced. I speak with such parents (almost always a mom) every day. You are tired and discouraged, but determined. Whether you are a successful executive or on public assistance, I hear the same words, the same doubts. Your child's behavior has shaken your confidence as a parent, and those who are supposed to be helping you have shaken your confidence as well.

Your child has probably received labels (from the neighbors as well as from professionals), but labels alone don't fix anything. There are complicated descriptions of behavior problems, and an alphabet of acronyms to go along with them. You may have told yourself that this person is a professional and must know what he/she is talking about, but deep down, it really doesn't make sense. There is blame, there are admonitions, and instructions to add to the many things you are expected to cope with. You may feel that you have been "jumping through hoops," but none of this effort really makes a difference.

This book is intended primarily to help you, but it has other purposes. Twenty years of work results in a lot of information, and this is a place to store at least some of it. Families who already know how to use diet management will enjoy having a handy reference, interested professionals will have a resource for their clients, and students writing papers may find it helpful to have the major scientific information in one place.

Although the problems of ADD (attention deficit disorder) and ADHD (attention deficit hyperactivity disorder) appear to be far more prevalent in the United States, there are many families living in other countries who do not have a support group. It is my hope that this book will be a practical guide for them.

Most of the information in this book has appeared over the past fourteen years in *Pure Facts*, the newsletter of the Association of the United States. The stories included are real. Nearly all were originally published with full names and photos. Rather than attempt to trace families with whom we have lost contact, and seek permission, I chose to include the stories, using only first names in most cases.

Although the years past have brought a great deal of information, the years to come promise so much more. Exciting things are happening in many fields related to diet and behavior. Parents, working with professionals, are finding new ways to help children with autism, seizures, and Down syndrome. There is the temptation to delay publishing this book for another six months, because even more information might be available, or because some more editing may be in order. But if you are the parent of a troubled (or troublesome) child, you won't want to wait another day! So here we go, with whatever imperfections in grammar, or typos that might have slid through.

This book is not designed to change the mind of any reader who has found the help she needs, but for those who are interested, to share what we have learned as we have helped our children.

PART ONE

Tell Me About Your Child

- ❑ Does your child get upset too easily?
- ❑ Does she seem to not hear what you are saying?
- ❑ Is his motor stuck on fast forward?
- ❑ After you have carefully explained why he cannot do something, and he seems to understand, do you turn your back only to have him repeat the behavior?
- ❑ Do you sense that she really can't help the way she behaves?
- ❑ Do all the teachers in the school know your child's name?
- ❑ Do other children avoid playing with your child?
- ❑ Does she have difficulty interacting with children her age?
- ❑ Does he always seem to be touching every person and object in his reach?
- ❑ Is she fine one minute, and out of control the next?
- ❑ Do all the games have to be played his way, with his rules?
- ❑ Does she seem to be off in her own little world?
- ❑ Can he go from here to there and lose something?
- ❑ Is homework lost, forgotten, or mutilated on a regular basis?
- ❑ Does he have a hard time understanding subtle cues, like facial expressions?
- ❑ Does she laugh too loud, or inappropriately?
- ❑ Is he really just like other kids, only much more so?

This is a sampling of some of the symptoms that can be triggered by exposure to chemicals in one's food or environment.

Looking for Answers

When you first time realize that Dr. Spock wasn't writing about your new baby, you are likely to seek someone who can help you.

If you're lucky, it will be someone who will at least lend a sympathetic ear. For most moms, unfortunately, their queries will bring blame, not sympathy. Your baby doesn't sleep? Doesn't coo? Doesn't smile and gurgle? What are YOU doing wrong? Eventually, you stop asking and stay home more than you would like, growing more certain each day that you must be the only mother in the world who is having these problems. Chances are you live a just block away from another mom who is saying the same thing to herself.

If you're especially unfortunate, you will be on the receiving end of blame from those who are supposed to be on your side, including your doctor, relatives, and perhaps even your husband.

I knew a lot about parenting before the birth of my first child, Laura. All the books I read gave roughly the same advice: provide lots of support, security, and love; notice the child when he is being good; offer positive rewards; have few rules but be consistent in upholding them; modify behavior through "natural and logical consequences;" nurture the child without pressuring him to fit your image. These are good ideas. No, actually, they're excellent ideas that generally work -- but not for the chemically sensitive child. Techniques that were successful with most of the children I had taught rolled off my daughter as though she was coated with Teflon. Laura was bright and precocious, possessing a great vocabulary and normal hearing, but my attempts to communicate with her were like reasoning with a rock. When I tried to make eye contact, her glances darted all over the room. When I asked her a question, her response -- at those times when she responded at all -- was very good, but had no relation to the question I had asked. At times I felt as though I had fallen down a rabbit hole and now lived in Wonderland.

Of all the sadness such a child brings into your life, I think the worst is that it's so hard to like them. It isn't hard to love them; that's part of the job description. But what saddened me most of all was that I found it so difficult to *like* this little girl I had wanted so much.

Laura was not always distracted and difficult. There were times when she was fine. When she was impossible, I never knew what I had done wrong, and when she was good, it was equally puzzling what I had done right! The only pattern that emerged was that she behaved better when she was sick. A bout with chicken pox produced an uncomfortable but calm and normal child. It never occurred to me that she wasn't eating much when she was sick. I let her choose what she wanted to eat and for about three days her diet was primarily 7UP and granola. It was much later that I understood that she is chemically sensitive, and that food additives were affecting her behavior.

Wishful thinking

Every new step a child takes is viewed hopefully by the parent of a chemically sensitive youngster. "She's *bound* to do better once she gets into school." "Now that he's five, he's sure to settle down." Parents search for the magical solution: a new school or day care, a new neighborhood, new therapist, new doctor, new activity, new parenting course. The list goes on and parents add to their disappointment collection. Some of these changes may be of help, but if the problem rests within the child, the symptoms follow him wherever he goes, and any improvement is still short of the mark.

Your search for answers may have taken you down many roads. Depending on whom you consult, you may have received support or blame. Parents of a chemically sensitive child rarely find what they really need: a professional who is aware of *all* the possible factors that could be triggering the child's difficulties, who will be able to select a method of treatment that is just right for your individual child, and who can recommend the best resource.

Instead, the advice parents receive usually depends much more upon the training of the advisor than on the child's symptoms. This was brought out at a major conference, "Defined Diets and Childhood Hyperactivity" (sponsored by the National Institutes of Health, 1982). There is little reason to believe things have changed since that time. If you take your child to a psychologist he will focus on the psychological aspect of the problem; visit a pediatrician who favors diet and he will refer you to the Feingold Association; see one who favors drugs and he will give you a prescription; an allergist will suggest allergy testing. What parents rarely see is that *they* are actually the ones making the diagnosis when they choose which professional to consult. In the long run, the choice is yours, and this is probably best since nobody knows your child as well as you.

Am I a bad parent?

We take years developing our self-esteem, and by the time we have it in pretty good shape, feeling we are up to almost any challenge, we welcome our little darling into the world. Suddenly, seven pounds of humanity can undo it all.

Why Can't My Child Behave?

I've never met you, but I know you are a good parent. Bad parents don't care; they don't read books on children's behavior, don't agonize over their child's problems, and don't go to the ends of the earth in search of answers.

It's easy to be a "good parent" when your baby sleeps, coos, and smiles, or when your toddler draws admiring glances from strangers. The test of a parent's ability comes from adversity, not from an obedient offspring. You may not feel lucky, but your child is. He will need all the patience and determination you can muster, and when you have turned things around and he fits in with the other children, your neighbors may not understand how hard you worked and how impressive your accomplishment. Your child probably won't understand how much of his success is due to your efforts, but you'll know, and that will be enough.

A century ago, the parents of hyperactive children would have been judged unfortunate; today they are likely to be judged guilty. When my daughter was two months old, the father of an obedient little boy -- who slept on command -- told me I needed to "train her to sleep." She's 29 years old now, and I still haven't figured out what he meant.

For the first four and a half years of my daughter's life, I questioned what was wrong with my parenting. I asked advice from virtually everyone who knew Laura, but they didn't know what to suggest. Then I decided that two well-meaning people, doing their best for four and a half years, couldn't have made *that* many mistakes. Maybe the problem lay with my daughter; maybe there was something wrong with her "chemistry," although I had no idea what that meant.

Is something wrong with my child?

Every parent's worst fear is verified when they see their child behaving in ways they know are abnormal.

By this time I was ready to accept the possibility that my child might not be normal, and even the heavy-duty labels -- emotionally disturbed, or whatever -- would have been a relief of sorts. At least it would have explained things. But there were many times when Laura behaved very normally, and she was clearly precocious: speaking early, teaching herself to read, and sounding out new words by age three-and-a-half. And I could not accept that a child could be emotionally disturbed on just Mondays, Wednesdays and Fridays.

If the year had been 1994 instead of 1974, she probably would have been given the label of "attention deficit disorder." I would have been told that my daughter had a chemical abnormality in her brain, and that it was essential she be given stimulant drugs -- which I would have gladly done.

(I would not have considered questioning my doctor.) But in 1974 there was no name for such a child. The closest term was "hyperactive," but that seemed unlikely when I lived with the slowest moving little girl this side of the Mississippi.

"Why Your Child is Hyperactive" - but mine wasn't

Many moms are silent about their agony. Not me. I complained about Laura's difficult behavior to anyone who would listen. When one friend, who had listened to a lot, handed me a copy of the book, *Why Your Child is Hyperactive*, by Ben F. Feingold, M.D., I read it -- not because I thought it applied to my child, but because I didn't want to seem unappreciative.

The book was very interesting, and some of the information was amazing, but I never recognized Laura's symptoms. My husband, Harry, read it and saw traits he had shown as a child. He also suspected that food additives could be triggering his dreadful headaches, so he began to pay more attention to what he ate.

Dr. Feingold's book describes the work that began with an adult patient's severe case of hives. After considering all the options, he prescribed a diet eliminating aspirin and other substances that contain a chemical similar to acetylsalicylic acid (the name for aspirin). Not only did the hives clear up, but the woman's behavior changed from belligerent to normal as long as she avoided certain foods and food additives. At that time, Feingold identified synthetic food dyes, artificial flavorings, and a group of foods -- primarily common fruits -- as likely offenders. A few years later he would add the antioxidant preservatives BHA, BHT and then TBHQ to the list of no-nos.

When Harry was able to identify food additives as the cause of his terrible migraine headaches it was a profound relief for us both. These headaches had started out slowly, and had gradually increased in frequency and severity until reaching the point where he was sick several times a month. At these times, all he could do was lie in a dark room for the three days or so that the attack lasted. He went from doctor to doctor in search of help, but each new doctor simply asked what pain pills he was taking, and handed him a prescription for more. Nobody ever questioned why he got the headaches in the first place.

As the headache-free time lengthened, Harry was able to identify other culprits, and he soon added MSG (monosodium glutamate) and sodium benzoate to the list.

Dabbling with this diet

I sort of used Dr. Feingold's diet with Laura, but the thought of tossing out "perfectly good" food went against the grain. I figured if I followed the diet 50%, I should see a 50% improvement.

There was no noticeable improvement, but that was fine with me. With an impossible five-year-old, a baby, plus a husband who was still sick some of the time, I didn't want to be The Happy Homemaker in some frilly white apron, cooking from scratch.

Then one day when Harry came home from work, he told me about the lunch he had eaten. When he selected a cottage cheese salad, he knew to discard the bright red cherry, but a little bit of juice from the cherry had colored the cottage cheese pink in one spot. It was just a drop or two, and he figured such a little bit wouldn't hurt, so he ate all of it. About two hours later he could feel the start of a migraine. The pain pills were strong enough to stop the headache, but it made a profound impression on him that such a tiny amount of dye could be so potent.

It made a tremendous impression on me as well. A drop or two! The next day when my daughter came downstairs for breakfast, I was careful to give her only food I believed was "pure." She had some scrambled eggs, bread and butter, and a glass of milk. I did my best with the other meals, keeping things plain and free of obvious synthetic additives.

The following morning Laura's behavior surprised and delighted me. Instead of her attention being in the next county, she was right there, hearing and responding to me. Her eyes didn't dart all over the room, but connected with mine, and her responses were reasonable. She made sense! She behaved normally, and I was amazed. Previously, when I saw normal behavior I didn't know why. Now I had something to go on.

I would later learn that this rapid 24-hour turn-around is very unusual, and that three days to three weeks is the typical response time. I don't know if our quick success was due to good fortune, or if her little body was so delighted to get real food in place of the junk that occupied our pantry that it went into fast forward!

The relief and euphoria were wonderful. We finally understood what had been going on -- and going wrong -- for more than five years. We had not been "additive-free" for more than a few days when the first infraction came our way. It was a warm spring day, and Laura was playing outside. As she passed the window I noticed she was chewing gum. Disaster alert! There could be only one source: our next door neighbor's daughter had a gum ball machine. They had been away when we began the diet, and I was not aware they had returned home, so I hadn't told them about our discovery.

Predictably, in about two hours, Laura's personality transformed from that of a child to a miniature monster. She was enraged at everything/nothing, and appeared to have a severe emotional disturbance. Our efforts to calm her went unheeded, and after it had grown dark outside, she ran out the door, shouting back that she was running away from home. (She didn't run far, fortunately.) By the following day, the effects had mostly worn off, and we resumed our new, rational lifestyle. I made a point to speak with my neighbor, and cautioned her to not give Laura *anything* edible. I doubt she really understood, but she was cooperative. That episode took place in 1975, but I have never forgotten the potential damage from one single colored gumball. I would later learn that we were exceptionally lucky. Most children would experience a three-day reaction to the same chemicals; for some unfortunate few, the reaction time could last even longer.

The Ages and Stages of ADD/ADHD

The chemically sensitive infant cries too much and sleeps too little.

He may not want to be held or cuddled, stiffening his little body in response to the affection you offer. Nothing pleases him. This little person dominates your family's life. He screams with the volume turned up to the maximum, stops taking naps long before Dr. Spock predicted, and is difficult to get to sleep at night. He seems to need less sleep than you do!

Your chemically sensitive baby may seem to have difficulty tolerating certain foods, even breast milk, and may be prone to rashes. Perhaps you had advanced notice that your baby would be a handful. Some display overactive behavior even before birth.

Carol Ann

"During the late stages of pregnancy," her dad writes, "this child was active! Sometimes in the evening our entertainment would be to watch her mother's abdomen as the baby went through a series of movements that would be the envy of most gymnasts. At times the movements were so violent that my wife would nearly be thrown out of bed."

Baby blues

Many people are aware of the connection between food additives and childhood hyperactivity, and some understand that behavioral disorders can persist into adulthood. But it is generally not recognized that food additives can produce a wide range of symptoms in people of all ages.

Perhaps the head banging, crib rocking, sleepless, screaming infant attracts less attention than the hyperactive child does because he disrupts the lives of fewer people. Furthermore, it's easy to diagnose the cause as "nervous mother." A woman who has not had a restful night's sleep in several weeks would indeed be nervous.

The previously wonderful baby becomes a terror of a toddler
The contented baby may change dramatically after he begins to eat table food, take vitamins, or discover junk food.

"Mark was such a cheerful little baby until he was about six months old and I introduced solid food. We moved at this time, and I assumed his radical change in behavior was the result of the move. I never suspected it was triggered by the foods and baby vitamins he ingested.

"His record for sleep was 3 hours. A day with my son alternated between loudness, constant motion, and short periods of sleep -- generally one or two hours. By age one he slept through the night, but woke screaming. This was his only form of communication except for one word: 'see.' When we got a puppy, Mark learned to imitate it. Looking back, it's funny to recall that my son spoke two words, one of which was 'woof.' But at the time, my husband and I didn't laugh at that, or at much of anything else, for that matter. I was with this miserably unhappy baby for 24 hours each day. Who would want to baby-sit? There were times when I thought I was cracking up, and I even daydreamed of being institutionalized -- somewhere restful and quiet!

"The few other adults I encountered weren't much help. 'You're spoiling him.' 'He certainly knows how to get his way.' Why was I made to feel so guilty? I turned to my doctor for help and received a sarcastic, 'If he's this bad at two, we'll refer you to a psychiatrist.'

"When Mark was one and a half he got a terrible case of diarrhea. (I didn't realize at the time that it was caused by cow's milk.) This went on for three months, and all the medications my doctor tried were of no help. Another doctor in the group told me to put Mark on a very restricted diet, with only three foods. Gradually the diarrhea stopped, but most astonishing was the dramatic change in Mark's behavior. Gone was the child who behaved as though he was possessed, and my sweet little boy was back. ('See, he outgrew it,' explained a relative.)

"On the Feingold diet, my two-year-old's vocabulary of one word and a bark suddenly became a torrent of words and even some short sentences. Within a week he was naming all of the letters of the alphabet."

Starting school

A tot who can manage fairly well at home may find school to be more than she can handle.

"The day she was born, the nurse warned me she was hyperactive," Lita's mother recalls. "But she was such a bright, lovable baby that we didn't even realize she was hyperactive until she started the Feingold diet at age 4.

"Lita didn't play with toys, didn't watch TV, couldn't sit at the table for a meal, and seldom slept for more than 30 minutes at a time -- even at night. But she was sweet, and I guess we just got accustomed to the level of activity.

"Developmentally, she was slow in most areas, but because she spoke in full sentences by the age of 18 months, we didn't consider the possibility of retardation.

She had done well at home and on a one-to-one basis with other children, but nursery school brought more frustration than this three-year-old could handle, so we began the search for answers.

"We followed the Feingold Diet to the best of our ability for a week, and then on Saturday I gave her a glass of H------- Punch. It made me think of a dog chasing its own tail. She chased around in circles, with no place to go; her reaction was so extreme we became fully committed to the diet that day."

Kindergarten and thence . . . or, learning to hate school

Typically, the chemically sensitive child is bright and eager to begin school. Kindergarten may be O.K., but the showdown generally comes in first grade.

Your six-year-old approaches first grade with enthusiasm and energy -- too much energy. Still, you hope this experience will be different; maybe the school can offer your child something you were not able to provide.

Now that your child is expected to sit still, listen to directions, stand in line, and finish his work, the problems become too obvious to ignore. He is doing his best but his best isn't good enough; he isn't able to keep up with the class. He begins to hear phrases that will follow him from grade to grade. Typically the child is told, "You're such a bright little boy; you could do it if you really tried." He really is trying, but he still isn't able to meet the expectation for his grade. (If he were in a wheelchair, nobody would say, "If you really tried, you could walk." But when a child is experiencing a chemical reaction, the cause is seldom understood.)

Many mothers (and some fathers) sense that their child really is unable to control his own body, but to outsiders, "all that kid needs is a good spanking." For many children, first grade is the beginning of the ego-shredding experience that will eventually turn them off to school and everything associated with it.

Even more crippling than a child's difficulty with schoolwork are his awkward social skills. He is often clumsy in his interactions with other children. He bumps into them, or pushes his chair into their desks, interrupts, misses the point of a story, laughs too loud or at the wrong time, and doesn't understand how close is too close, or where his space ends and the next person's begins. Social skills deficits are rarely addressed in school, but they a greater handicap for the child than a D on his report card. The socially awkward child is likely to grow up to be a socially awkward adult.

Chemically sensitive children often have difficulty in the use of either fine muscles or gross muscles. They may write poorly, or be the last to be chosen for a team. In either case, it is one more arena of failure for them.

Well-meaning advice . . .
or, When What You're Doing Doesn't Work, Do it Some More

As your child progresses through school and her self-esteem begins to unravel, problems are added on top of problems, and it becomes hard to recognize the causes.

Teachers, counselors, and other authority figures have told your youngster, in effect: "Do as I say and the problems will be resolved." At first, she does what they say, but things don't get better. Can you blame her for tuning you, and virtually every other adult, out?

Surviving adolescence is tough for any young person, but for the chemically sensitive teen with little reason to feel good about himself or herself, these can be dangerous years. The youngster who enters adolescence with low self-esteem is at high risk for the hazards the teen years bring, plus a lot more. Drugs or alcohol may be a form of self-medication as well as an effort to win peer acceptance. The social consequences of chemical sensitivity are found on the front page of every major newspaper. Even if self-destructive behavior is avoided, the problems can follow the chemically sensitive child into adulthood.

With a monumental amount of support and skill on the part of parents, teachers, counselors and others, some of these teens do manage to get into adulthood in reasonably good emotional and academic shape, but these are the fortunate few.

All grown-up and still hyper

The symptoms change with adulthood, but they don't go away.

"Hyperactive" or chemically sensitive adults tend to be irritable, impatient, distractible, and likely to suffer from numerous physical problems. They may be compulsive, workaholic, or prone to interrupt. There may be many lost jobs and failed relationships. They are also likely to be the parent of a hyperactive or ADD child.

When the difficult child is not your first

Just because you've raised one or more perfectly contented, well-behaved children, don't think you're likely to escape being blamed for the problems your next child is experiencing.

"By the time she was five, Carolyn had been asked to leave several day care centers. Despite the fact that my older child is a 'model' child, I felt Carolyn's behavior problems were all my fault. I knew nothing but frustration. There were times when I would lock myself in my bedroom so I wouldn't risk hurting her. Even my training as an educator, with a minor in learning disabilities, didn't help me deal with her problems or with my own distress.

"The pediatrician and psychiatrist wanted to put her on Ritalin, but I couldn't agree to that. I was on tranquilizers, but nothing was strong enough to blunt the sadness of seeing my little girl in such turmoil. She used to roll and roll on the floor in an effort to get rid of some of the frantic energy going through her little body. She was certain that God 'hated' her because he would not let her 'mind.'

"Last year Carolyn and I went to school together. My job was to try and restrain my daughter while the classroom teacher taught the other children. After six months she was asked to leave and try again next year. These days [after removing the substances which were triggering her behavior problems] I work 50 hours a week at my job while Carolyn receives rewards every week for good behavior."

Can a Diet Help Improve Your Child's Behavior?

Mothers often notice that there are times when their child's behavior seems to change after he has eaten. It could be apple juice, or jelly beans, or a bologna sandwich. It could be Halloween candy or birthday cake that seems to set him off.

You may have tried to avoid certain foods or food additives, only to find yourself bewildered as you attempt to sort out the likely trigger.

Perhaps when you go to a fast food restaurant you get her the orange drink to avoid the caffeine in cola. Within two hours of eating there you have a little terror on your hands. (The cola would probably have been a far better choice than the synthetically colored and flavored orange drink.) Have you ever thought your child might be allergic to chocolate since it seems to "turn him on?" (Most chocolate contains synthetic vanilla flavoring, called "vanillin," and this is a much more likely culprit than the caffeine, the chocolate or the sugar.) Did you ever notice, as I did, that after a few days of an illness -- and not eating much -- your child is strangely calm?

The frustrating thing is that you are operating on scant information, and trying to reach your destination with no road map. In order to identify the likely triggers for your child's behavioral outbursts, you need both information and direction, not to mention good advice and lots of support.

The good news is that you don't have to figure out your own test diet; this has already been done. There is a systematic step-by-step technique that will guide you through the process of testing your child's sensitivities. It is surprisingly easy -- kind of like a math quiz that is very easy when you know the answers! Two decades of successful experience by thousands of families have resulted in the Feingold Program.

A brief background of the Feingold Program

As early as the 1940s, allergists began to publish reports of patients who were sensitive to tartrazine (Yellow dye No. 5). The medical literature contains many references to symptoms such as hives, asthma and nasal congestion.

Doctors also found that aspirin and other substances, commonly found in some fruits and vegetables, have a chemical similarity to synthetic yellow dye. (The chemical name for aspirin is acetylsalicylic acid, and from this comes the term "salicylate," used to refer to those substances.)

Physicians later found these chemicals affect children as well as adults, and that they can trigger behavior and learning problems. The doctor who first observed this was Ben F. Feingold, M.D., Chief of Allergy at the Kaiser Permanente Medical Center in San Francisco. Dr. Feingold was both a pediatrician and an allergist, and was a pioneer in the fields of allergy and immunology. In addition to yellow dye and salicylates, he also removed other synthetic food dyes and all artificial flavorings. Dr. Feingold would later expand what he named the "K-P Diet" to exclude the preservatives BHA, BHT and TBHQ. In 1973 he reported the results of his work at the annual conference of the American Medical Association.

His research received widespread publicity, and Random House asked him to write a book parents could use to help their children. The publisher titled the book *Why Your Child is Hyperactive*. As a result of thousands of parents reading this book and using the diet Feingold outlined, volunteer support groups began to spring up around the country; they chose the name "Feingold Associations" to honor the doctor who had made such a difference in their lives. These parent associations began to share information, research brand name foods, and develop programs to make it easier for the new family to successfully use the diet. Since it covers far more than just food, the Association calls it the Feingold Program.

What is the Feingold Program?

First of all, it is a test. For several weeks, you use only foods that are free of synthetic dyes, artificial flavors and three preservatives, as well as a group of foods known as "natural salicylates." All of these acceptable foods are likely to be well tolerated. If this trial results in an improvement in your child's behavior, or in other target symptoms, then the test becomes the treatment. You simply continue to enjoy the foods and the positive change in your child. After a few weeks of success you can gradually expand the food choices, adding back natural salicylates one at a time, and watching for any return of the old behaviors. The Program is a form of the time-honored allergy elimination diet. The focus, however, is on all the foods that are allowed, not on those removed.

Your Feingold member packet

The information needed to test the Program is supplied by the Feingold Association, a non-profit organization located in the United States, with "sister" organizations in some other countries.

In the U.S., the Association researches foods to determine which brands are free of both the obvious and hidden additives. This is accomplished by sending a detailed questionnaire for each product to the manufacturer, asking about both obvious and hidden additives. If the company representative fills out the form, signs his name, and returns it, the product will be listed in *Pure Facts*. Each year, when the regional Foodlists are reprinted, the new brands are added. When a family joins the Association they receive a large package of material that includes a Foodlist for their region of the United States, as well as a handbook with step-by-step guidance, a recipe book, and phone numbers to call with any questions they may have.

The costs are kept as low as possible, thanks to the many hours of donated time from volunteers, and are a fraction of what a family could expect to pay to a commercial facility offering these services – if one existed. [Call (800) 321-3287 for current information about materials, services and fees.]

We've come a long way!

In the 1970s it was difficult to be on the Feingold diet because many foods had to be made from scratch, and eating out was risky. Today, however, the food supply has changed, and Feingold research enables members to shop at supermarkets, use many convenience foods (including candy and ice cream) and even eat at fast food restaurants. Many hard-to-find treats are available through mail order companies catering to member families. Feingold *Foodlists* include over a thousand acceptable brand name foods and non-food products.

The worst offenders

Dr. Feingold noted that a person could be sensitive or allergic to virtually anything. But he believed that of all the substances to which a person could be sensitive or allergic, there are a few groups which are the most likely offenders for those with behavior and learning problems. These are:

Food dyes (a.k.a. food colors, synthetic colors, artificial colors, coal tar dyes, FD&C Yellow No. 5, etc.)

Artificial flavorings (including "vanillin" or synthetic vanilla)

Three antioxidant preservatives: **BHA, BHT, TBHQ**

Aspirin and a group of foods which contain **"natural salicylates"** -- a naturally occurring chemical which is similar to aspirin.

Natural salicylates are:

Almonds
Apples
Apricots
All berries
Cherries
Cloves
Coffee
Cucumbers & pickles
Currants
Grapes & raisins
Nectarines
Oranges
Peaches
Peppers (bell & chili)
Plums & prunes
Tangerines
Tea
Tomato

also: Oil of Wintergreen (methyl salicylate)
Medications which contain aspirin

Although many favorite foods are removed during the first weeks of the program (Stage One), there are lots of tasty alternatives:

Non-salicylate fruits allowed:

Avocado
Banana
Breadfruit
Coconut
Date
Fig
Grapefruit
Guava
Kiwi
Kumquat
Lemon
Lime
Loquat
Mango
Melon -- all varieties
Papaya
Pear
Persimmon
Pineapple -- not fresh
Pomegranate
Star fruit

Non-salicylate vegetables allowed:

Artichoke
Asparagus
Alfalfa sprouts
Bamboo shoots
Bean sprouts
Beans - all varieties
Beets
Broccoli
Brussels sprouts
Cabbage
Carrots
Cauliflower
Celery
Chard
Collard greens
Corn
Eggplant
Kale
Kohlrabi
Lettuce
Lentils
Mushrooms
Mustard greens
Okra
Olives
Onions
Parsley
Parsnips
Peas
Potatoes
Radishes
Rhubarb
Rutabaga
Sorrel
Spinach
Squash
Sweet potatoes
Turnips
Turnip greens
Water chestnuts
Watercress
Yams

The period when salicylates are removed is called Stage One.

Most of the materials provided by the Feingold Association are directed at the family on Stage One. There are many techniques for getting around the limitations during this period, but one of the best is to use the program carefully at the start so that you will see results quickly and will be able to reintroduce these salicylates as soon as possible. The dyes, flavorings, and antioxidants are easily replaced by natural alternatives, and few people mourn their loss. But "natural salicylates" are wholesome foods, and nobody likes to have to give them up, even temporarily.

Those foods not tolerated should be kept out of the diet for awhile longer, but might eventually be tolerated.

The period when natural salicylates are reintroduced is called Stage Two.

The *Feingold Handbook* and other membership materials provide detailed information on salicylates and how to reintroduce them.

Symptoms often helped by diet management

If your child has one or more of the following symptoms they may be triggered by an adverse reaction to food additives or salicylates. Many of these symptoms may also apply to adults.

IMPATIENCE
- Low frustration tolerance
- Demands must be met immediately
- Irritable
- Cries easily or often
- Throws, breaks things

SHORT ATTENTION SPAN
- Easily distracted
- Doesn't finish projects
- Doesn't listen to whole story
- Doesn't follow directions

POOR SLEEP HABITS
- Difficult to get to bed
- Hard to fall asleep
- Restless sleeper
- Has nightmares, bad dreams

MARKED HYPERACTIVITY
- Constant motion
- Runs, does not walk
- Difficulty sitting through meals
- Wiggles legs/hands inappropriately

COMPULSIVE AGGRESSION
- Disruptive at home & school
- Doesn't respond to discipline
- Doesn't recognize danger

Compulsively repeats action
Unkind to pets
Fights with other children
Poor self-control

IMPULSIVITY
Unpredictable behavior
Makes inappropriate noises
Talks too much
Talks too loudly
Interrupts
Bites and picks nails, skin
Chews on clothing, other objects
Overreacts to touch, pain, sound, lights

FREQUENT PHYSICAL COMPLAINTS
Headaches
Hives
Stomachaches
Ear infections
Bed-wetting
Daytime wetting

NEURO-MUSCULAR INVOLVEMENT
Accident-prone
Poor muscle coordination
Poor eye-hand coordination
Difficulty writing and drawing
Dyslexia
Speech difficulties
Difficulty with playground activities
Eye-muscle disorder (nystagmus, strabismus)
Tics, some forms of seizures

Note: Always consult a physician to rule out illness.

Questions Parents Ask

Is there some type of test to determine if a diet will help my child's symptoms?

The Feingold Program is a test. If you drank a glass of orange juice each morning at 7:00, and by 8:00 am you had a stomachache, you would probably use your own elimination diet. For a week you might cut out the orange juice, and if the stomachaches disappeared you could be fairly sure that the juice was the culprit. If you wanted to try adding it back to your diet, you could test it out and see if the stomachache returned.

By removing the most likely culprits, you will be able to see if synthetic colors, flavors, certain preservatives, or salicylates are playing a part in your child's problems or in your own health problems.

How soon can I expect to see a change?

There is no way to predict exactly how long it will take, or how much of a change you will notice. For a preschool child who is not on medication, it is typical for parents to notice a significant change in a few days to a week. For a child who was previously on medicine it might take longer.

How can I be sure that a diet program will help at all?

While there are no guarantees, there is a very high probability that your child will be helped. Volunteer organizations do not even form, let alone persist for decades, unless the volunteers experience positive feedback from their work.

Your likelihood of success depends on many factors, especially how carefully you follow the program and whether your child has additional problems such as food allergies or sensitivities to substances in the environment.

If a family has the current Feingold membership materials, including a Foodlist for their area, and follows the program carefully, it is very likely that they will see an improvement. The issue is generally not *if* the program will help, but *how much* help it will provide.

Some families find that their child has additional sensitivities that go beyond the scope of the Feingold Program. Experienced volunteers can often recommend other nonprofit organizations for help in these cases.

Will my child's schoolwork be helped?

There is generally a significant improvement in schoolwork. Eliminating these additives won't teach the child math, but should enable him to pay attention so he can learn what is being taught. Behavior is likely to be the first thing to improve, with academic performance showing a more gradual but steady improvement.

My child's symptoms are so severe; how can a simple change in food make a real difference?

A switch from brand A to brand B may seem simple, but removing toxic chemical additives from a child's diet is not a simple matter. Food processing is complex, and it has taken many years for volunteers to become proficient at identifying places where additives can be hidden. What's more, companies continually come up with ways to circumvent the few labeling laws that exist. Often the laws are simply ignored.

Once the dietary changes are made, parents and professionals report even severe symptoms have shown improvement.

Is this program hard to follow?

Replacing the food in your pantry with "Feingold acceptable" is harder than using what's already there, but easier than getting through the day with a child who is aggressive, destructive and rarely sleeps.

Being selective about which foods you buy at a fast food chain is harder than ordering anything you want, but it's easier than handling that dreaded daily phone call from the school.

Using pear juice in place of apple juice (a natural salicylate) might be inconvenient, but so is washing wet sheets every morning.

Chances are, you are already under a lot of stress! This might not be the best time for you to consider making changes in your shopping and food preparation. On the other hand, if changing brands will bring about a calmer, happier household, then the sooner you begin, the sooner you will be able to enjoy the benefits. (By the way, I'm a very lazy cook, and have been happily using the Program since 1975.)

Is it expensive?

That depends on the type of food your family likes. My grocery bill went up in some areas and down in others.

Thrifty shoppers already know that the most expensive foods are the highly processed ones. Compare the cost per pound of pre-flavored oatmeal packets ($3 to $4/pound) with scooping a pound of plain rolled oats from the supermarket's bulk bin (59 cents/pound). I microwave the rolled oats, add a little sweetener or jam and end up with virtually the same breakfast (minus additives) in very little time, but at a fraction of the cost of the "convenience" product.

A major benefit was that once our family got on the Program, and my daughter's ear infections stopped, and my husband's headaches were history, the doctor's bills stopped as well. Doctors are very nice to have around, but I prefer to pay the grocer!

Is this a "health food" diet?

There are many items in a health food store that are "off limits" to the family new to the Feingold Program. Don't have blind faith that all of the foods are as healthy as claimed.

You will find lots of food in both supermarkets and health food stores that are acceptable; select those your family likes best. I buy a variety of groceries from both types of stores. My family likes nitrite-free bacon from the health food store, but we prefer the natural rocky road ice cream I buy in the discount grocery store.

Our favorite yogurt & green onion potato chips as well as cheese puffs come from the health food store. But I get pretzels at the supermarket.

Does the Program allow sugar and snack foods?

As you can see from the answers above, the program does not eliminate these, although we encourage families to use sugar in moderation, and avoid giving sweets when the child has an empty stomach. (It would be nice if we all loved lima beans more than chocolate brownies . . . or would it?) The Program doesn't tell you *what* to eat, rather it shows you how to find suitable brands of the type of food you like. I compare it to *Consumer's Reports,* which does not tell you whether or not to buy a car, but lets you know about your options.

Do I have to cook "from scratch"?

If you have access to a current Foodlist -- either from the Feingold Association in the United States or from one of the sister groups in Great Britain, Australia, New Zealand, etc. -- you should be able to use the processed foods listed. If you live in an area where there is no food research, you will probably do quite a lot of food preparation during the early days of the Program. You will be able to gradually add in processed foods, watching for any reaction.

This is not as hard as it may sound. Parents tend to learn very quickly and usually do not make the same mistake twice. This book will help you understand more about food processing and where additives may be found, and will give you practical hints for getting around the pitfalls.

Can our family still eat out at restaurants?

A child or adult is likely to be most sensitive during the early weeks of the Program. If you can avoid restaurant food for a few weeks, it will help you see good results more quickly. In the long run, it will be a lot easier.

People who are experienced on the Program can eat out at nearly any restaurant and do very well. By carefully avoiding the additives/ salicylates in the beginning, many people appear to lose much of their sensitivity. It's been many years since my family began the Program, and we can eat virtually anywhere, make educated choices and not experience a reaction.

My child is a very picky eater; how can I get her to accept new foods?

You will probably be able to find natural versions of those few foods she likes, and you may be surprised to find some of her favorites are already on the Foodlist. Stay as close as you can to the foods your child enjoys. As she becomes more reasonable, you will probably be able to gradually expand her choices.

The most important thing to keep in mind during the early weeks is not to emphasize nutrition, but to have your child accept the changes that are necessary. (Forfeit the battle to win the war.)

What happens when she's away from home and someone offers her food?

If you present the Program in a positive way and your child experiences the benefits it brings, you probably won't have to be concerned about this. It has been our experience that once they understand it, most of the children are very determined to stick to their diet. (I know you probably don't believe this. I wouldn't have either!)

How will I know which brands of food are OK to use?

The Feingold Association researches foods and publishes books listing acceptable brand name products. In many cases, a company makes several products that are acceptable and other varieties that are not. It can be pretty tricky, so follow your Foodlist carefully.

Since manufacturers change their products frequently, the Association publishes updates in their newsletter -- generally 10 times a year -- and revises all of the Foodlists each year. Please do not use an out-of-date list, since you may end up sabotaging your efforts.

Can't I just read labels and avoid the additives that way?

Much of the effort of our Product Information Committee is spent tracking down additives that are in foods but are not included in the ingredient listing.

If your child is not particularly sensitive, you might be able to see results even though you aren't always using "pure" food. If he is sensitive to small amounts of chemical additives, however, your results could be disappointing.

Any time you can eliminate synthetic colors and flavors, that's great! But please don't confuse this with the Feingold Program. (It's like Alcoholics Anonymous saying that if you skip the bourbon and vodka, then whiskey and gin are OK.)

What are food additives made from?

You might wish you hadn't asked, but here goes: Food dyes used to be made from coal tar oil (yummy!) but are now synthesized from petroleum. Petroleum is made from crude oil -- the "black gold" which pollutes the oceans when it spills.

Artificial flavorings can made from virtually anything; there are no rules. A single flavoring might be made from hundreds of different chemicals.

The preservatives BHA, BHT and TBHQ are made from petroleum.

Does the Feingold Program eliminate all additives?

No. Only those found to be the major source of learning/behavior problems are eliminated. A few others are a problem for some, but not all, of our members (MSG, sodium benzoate, nitrites, corn syrup, calcium propionate; fluoride and sulfiting agents). They are not removed, but many people choose to avoid them.

The Association recommends members avoid the use of synthetic sweeteners such as aspartame, saccharine and cyclamates.

If the additives are harmful, why doesn't the government ban them?

This is a long and complex story (spell that "$tory"). Many dyes and other additives have already been banned; it's the stubborn survivors that are causing so many problems.

What about all those pesticides?

Our family was successfully on the Feingold Program for over a decade before we had our first organic carrot. If you can easily obtain organic foods, that's great, but it isn't required. We recognize the harm that can be caused to our environment by their excessive use and that some people must avoid pesticides, but they are not specifically addressed in the Program.

Will my child have to be on this diet for the rest of his life?

As a child gets older and stays away from synthetic chemicals, he tends to develop a tolerance level. But as you become more knowledgeable about food and food additives the question may shift from "Why can't we eat imitation red cherry gelatin?" to "I can just as easily make natural cherry gelatin that tastes terrific; why would I want to eat the other stuff?"

Even the very young Feingolders catch on to the fact that the rather disgusting chemicals added to foods enable companies to save money by eliminating real ingredients from their products.

Question to ponder: If the food is fake, why can't I pay for it with Monopoly money?

Do doctors recommend the Feingold Program?

We receive many physician referrals, and some of our members are physicians using the Program for their child and/or themselves.

Most of our referrals come from doctors who have seen patients successfully use our Program. Some doctors are interested in the connection between nutrition and behavior/health, but many are not.

I've heard that scientific studies show that diet either does not help learning/behavior problems, or that it helps only a tiny fraction of children.

Feingold volunteers have heard this too! If you go back to the early studies and read what the scientists conducting the research originally reported, you would see a very different conclusion. Although none of the studies were a test of the Feingold Program as it is actually used, and most had design flaws and other mistakes, they still yielded very supportive data.

Newer studies have been more carefully designed and have yielded extremely positive results. But such information is not favorable to the many vested interests dealing with foods and food additives and their effects, so this information is not likely to be publicized. That is the topic of another book, too long to address here, but you will find a summary in the last section of this book.

Do I have to put the whole family on the Program?

No, but do you *really* want to have to cook two dinners a night?!

Why should you do double shopping, have to keep some foods separated, run the risk of using the wrong product for your Feingolder, and make him feel left out?

Take a look at the second section of this book that tells you more about food dyes and other additives; then ask yourself if you would want *any* family member to eat them.

When a child is chemically sensitive, at least one parent is also likely to be sensitive, and often the siblings are as well -- though not necessarily to the same degree. We all have the ability to tolerate negative things (stress, germs, polluted air, synthetic food additives) but our tolerance varies. Your Feingolder may be more vulnerable to certain chemicals than the rest of the family, but you can be sure they are having an effect on everyone.

I don't want to wait for my Foodlist before I get started. What can I do right now?

(If you live outside the United States, and are in a country which does not have a support group offering a list of acceptable brand name products, this information should be helpful.)

The First Four Days of Feingold

Many families of young children see a significant change in behavior after carefully following the diet for only a few days. Occasionally, an older child or an adult will also have a rapid response. This four-day sample diet is designed to help you, as well as to give an idea of some of the foods permitted, but it represents only a fraction of the items suitable for use on the Program. Although these foods are nutritious, it is not intended that they be the only foods one consumes for a prolonged time.

NON-FOOD ITEMS

Toothpaste: Tom's of Maine* Spearmint or Peppermint or Fennel
or use baking soda, or just water

Omit vitamins

Avoid products containing fragrances
Avoid products that would result in dyes on the skin

BEVERAGES
Baby food pear juice (available in large bottles)
Pure pineapple juice (dilute, if you like)
Grapefruit juice (sweeten, if you like, with granulated sugar)
Lemonade made from fresh lemons and granulated sugar
Whole milk (not low fat or skimmed)
Shake made with 1/2 cup whole milk, 1/2 cup pineapple juice, 1/2 banana; mix in blender
Water

BREAKFAST
Oatmeal (not instant); sweeten with white or brown sugar, add whole milk or non-salicylate fruit juice
French toast - homemade w/eggs, milk, real 100% maple syrup, or sprinkle with granulated or confectioners' sugar
Eggs (real, not imitation); use butter (not margarine) or Wesson* Oil for cooking
Plain Puffed Rice or Puffed Wheat, whole milk, sugar
Toast with real butter or honey

LUNCH
Peanut butter and honey sandwich (or substitute banana for the honey)
Tuna salad sandwich made with Hellmann's* or Best Foods* Mayonnaise (look for water-pack tuna which does not contain "hydrolyzed vegetable protein" and use original versions of mayonnaise, not "low-fat," "fat-free," "low cholesterol," etc.)
Leftover chicken from dinner -- sliced or made into salad; add celery, if you like
Egg salad sandwich, carrot sticks

DINNER
Roast chicken, baked potatoes w/real butter, fresh or frozen plain green vegetable (no sauces); season with salt, butter, black pepper if you like
Broiled fish fillet (season with lemon, garlic and butter if you like), salad or any vegetable except tomato, cucumber and peppers (Make a salad dressing with lemon juice and Wesson Oil)

Pork chops (broil or season w/flour and sauté in oil), sweet potato (with butter or mashed with pineapple juice), green vegetable
Ground beef patties (made with plain chopped meat), corn (on the cob or canned or frozen plain), green vegetable
[Note: for food safety, always cook hamburger well done.]

SNACK, DESSERT IDEAS
Eagle Thins* potato chips
Fresh pears
Bananas
Any melon
Whitman's* All Natural Chocolate Bar
or Baker's* Sweet Chocolate Bar, cut up (sold with baking supplies)
Haagan Dazs* vanilla or chocolate ice cream
Popcorn made from plain kernels and cooked with real butter or Wesson* oil

For breads, see the section of this book on Foods.
(The above brand name products are acceptable at press time; contact the Association to learn if they are still included in Foodlists. These brands were listed because they are generally available nationwide. Foodlists contain many other acceptable brands.)
The focus of the Program is on the many foods you can eat, not on those you cannot. By planning a few meals, with enough foods to get you through the first few days, you will see there really is a nice variety available.

The casual Feingolder: Suppose I just avoid the obvious additives by checking ingredient labels on foods -- would this help?

By all means, avoid things like food dyes and artificial flavorings whenever you can. Any harmful additive you can remove is a good idea. But you will not be able to test the Feingold Program in this way because you will still be consuming hidden additives. If you do see an improvement in your child as a result of making small changes, that's great! But if you see little or no improvement, please don't conclude that the diet won't work; you probably have a fairly sensitive child, and perhaps one who is also sensitive to natural salicylates.

Our family life is chaotic! My older kids are not easy to please, and my younger child is on a heavy dose of medicine for ADD. But I don't want to wait till life calms down, as we need help so badly. What would you suggest?

You might want to start by just eliminating the unwanted additives, and not deal with salicylates at the beginning. The good news is that this will make it much easier to implement the diet, but the drawback is that you may not see as much improvement as you would if you were on a careful Stage One (salicylate-free) diet.

If you are willing to see diet management as a long-range project, and you don't get discouraged if success comes slowly, this is a good approach to take. If your family has been using products with various additives, it may be an easier transition to focus on eliminating them first, and later give Stage One a trial.

[Note: For a child taking medication on a regular basis, and especially multiple drugs, the Feingold Association may be able to help you find them in an uncolored form. Be sure to rely on your physician's guidance if you plan to phase them out.]

Does the Feingold Program have any risks?

Dr. Feingold used the term "no harm, no risk" and while this is true, there have been a small number of children who seem to have withdrawal symptoms after they stop eating synthetic additives. In a few cases, a child will become worse before he improves, especially if he was taking multiple medicines.

Statistics - what are the chances this diet will help me?

In 1980 one of the local Feingold chapters compiled a statistical analysis of their membership. Members were sent a questionnaire, and 55% of them -- a total of 255 -- responded. They provided the following information:

The typical Feingold person is very much the same as Dr. Feingold described -- a male, between the ages of 6 and 12, who is considered by his family to be hyperactive. He has been on the Feingold Program for 6 months to 2 years, and his mother was the first to realize he had problems, usually prior to age 2. She first learned of the Program from a friend, and the whole family follows it.

There has been "great" or "much" improvement in the symptoms. Drugs had not been used to control the symptoms, and would probably not be used, even without the diet. (There is a great deal of resistance to drugs either on principle or due to previous experiences.) In addition to the various symptoms of hyperactivity identified by Dr. Feingold and others, our typical Feingold person reacts to a diet infraction by a noticeable change in his speech (rapid, loud, incoherent, and/or constant).

During her pregnancy and childbirth, his mother experienced some difficulty and/or required some procedure other than anesthesia. The child experiences a severe reaction to artificial color and flavor, and also reacts to BHT, some salicylates, and other chemicals (BHA, MSG, sodium benzoate, and sodium nitrite were specifically identified in some cases, as well as sugar).

Hyperactivity was the main reason for beginning the diet in 96% of the cases. In 43% the symptoms were apparent by the age of one year. 81% of the respondents are male, and 36% of them have blond hair; 19% are female, 41% have blond hair. 16% have been adopted.

Salicylates affect 89%, however 66% of the salicylate sensitive can tolerate some of them. 41% have food allergies, 35% have inhalant allergies, 47% are extremely sensitive to touch and 38% to noise.

49% reported "great improvement" from the diet, and 37% reported "much improvement." Only 1% reported no improvement. Of the families reporting great improvement, 77% say the whole family follows the Program and 93% use only pure foods and some salicylates. 72% of the families reporting much improvement use only pure foods and some salicylates.

Summary

In the years since these statistics were compiled, the Association's food research and information has improved significantly and the success rate seems to have increased as well.

For most children it isn't a cut-and-dried case of "the Program working" or "the Program not working." It's generally a matter of how much help the Program provides, of whether the family needs to go further to get an even better response. We rarely hear from a member who reports that they are not having *any* success.

The negative reports

Dr. Feingold's work was met with vigorous opposition by the lobbies representing the major food, chemical and pharmaceutical industries. More than two decades later little has changed.

Feingold: The Next Generation

This chapter is a tribute to "our kids" who have been following the Feingold Program for a decade or more.

This is a tribute to their parents, as well, particularly the moms who have traveled what has often proven to be a rough road, who have fought for their children and have won. It's also an acknowledgement of those who have fought just as hard, but whose kids would not stay on the diet and didn't make it -- at least as of now. Fortunately, they are in the small minority, but we salute these parents as well.

Why did our successful kids make it while others have not? We find that the parent's determination to follow the program is a crucial factor. In the sample stories we proudly present, one or both parents was an active Feingold volunteer. The successful parent gained much knowledge through work in the Association. Volunteering provided close contact with others who were also acquiring expertise.

The Feingold mom learned to speak up for herself by speaking up on her child's behalf. Many times she was called to defy the conventional wisdom because she knew her child better than anyone else -- whether it was a neighbor, teacher, doctor, or mother-in-law. "Her teachers were no help at all," notes one mother. "They thought I was a raving lunatic." Others found professionals who were sympathetic, or at least open-minded, and taught them about the diet.

Through their involvement in the Association, mothers of the children described here gained the motivation and confidence to pursue challenging careers they would not otherwise have considered. Whether it was in their Feingold work or in their personal lives, when they saw something askew, they did what was necessary to put it right. These moms learned from many sources, including their Feingold kids. Meeting the challenge of caring for their difficult child helped give them a better perspective on what's really important; it enabled them to be better parents for their other children.

The message from the veteran moms to the new members is this: There may be times when you feel like you're at war with the world, including the child you're trying to help. But don't give up; there's too much at stake, and there's a good chance that you are his best hope for the kind of happy endings you read about here.

But first, a word about the drug scene

These Feingold parents expressed gratitude that their children had been spared the disaster of drug abuse.

The common thread seems to be that our youngsters recall how it felt to be out of control, and they don't want to be in that position again. Not only do they resist taking medications of all kinds, they seem to understand that their bodies, which have been sent out of control from a colored lollypop, would be especially vulnerable to the effects of illicit drugs.

Tommy

People who know Tommy today find it very hard to believe he had been a toddler who needed constant attention, was always fussy, crying, and in "perpetual motion." He didn't sleep easily or well and had a chronic problem with rashes.

As a senior in high school he is well liked by everyone who knows him and was nominated for "best dressed," "best smile" and "best looking." An exceptional athlete with excellent motor control, he plays varsity basketball and ice hockey. His teachers like him too, and refer to Tommy as a "class leader."

Like so many Feingold successes, Tom isn't interested in experimenting with drugs. "Having to say 'no' to Hi-C in kindergarten made it easier for him to say no to the bad stuff," his mom observes. "In fact, he went into kindergarten reading labels." Tommy will be starting college in the fall, and his family is glad he won't be far from home. Not only do his parents like having him around, but (the ultimate compliment) even his sisters enjoy him!

David

"On Monday, Wednesday and Friday David took Ritalin. On Tuesday and Thursday he took Dexedrine. And on Saturday and Sunday I took Phenobarbital," recalls his mother.

She remembers how bad it was before her son went on the Feingold diet at age 7. Even after that there were problems until she realized how unusually sensitive he was to salicylates. One year she made his birthday cake with a recipe that called for a small amount of orange juice. After he had eaten a piece, David went outside to play. Cindy found her son pushing a playmate on their swing. David was 'perseverating' -- pushing and pushing, with a glazed look in his eyes. The other child held on for dear life as the swing looped all the way around the frame of the swing set.

Today David is a senior in college, majoring in psychology. He is a computer whiz, and loves working with children. "Kids are attracted to him like a magnet." He hasn't had a problem with drug abuse as have so many people his age. "David avoids all kinds of medicine, and has to be really uncomfortable before he'll even take a Tylenol."

Michael

At age 5, Michael was diagnosed as dyslexic and suffering from visual perception deficits in five areas. He was a terror to live with, and his parents were advised to place him in a school for brain-injured children. Instead, his parents began using the Feingold diet shortly after reading *Why Your Child Is Hyperactive.*

Today, Mike is a junior in college. A major in communications/ business/public relations, he is successful -- both socially and scholastically. He copes well with whatever comes his way, enjoys working with people, and is very much in control of his life.

Michael still has an abundance of energy, but channels it productively. He is involved in many sports, and in high school, had a unique technique for winning football games. Before the game, he chewed red bubble gum, which brought on the aggressive, hyper behavior that got goals. Then, he'd wear himself out in the game. "Michael didn't do drugs," his mom noted, "he did red bubble gum."

Andrea

"It all should have gone so smoothly." Andrea's mother recalled. "John and I waited over seven years for our little girl. I was a registered nurse with experience in pediatrics, and an advocate of wholesome foods. Andrea was nursed, and later fed homemade baby food -- I was a real Earth Mother! Why, then, were we worn out by this incredibly strong and active baby who scarcely ever slept?

"Some of my most vivid memories date back to the time Andrea was 18 months old -- like the time she had a bath with dyed, perfumed bubble bath powder and became wild, banging her head against the side of the tub. Or, when a small drink of red imitation punch at the coffee hour after church, she ran around biting people.

"When I put her out in the backyard to play, she'd strip off her diaper and be over the fence in no time. And more than once I saw her at the top of our neighbor's 30-foot tree! Named 'wiggle butt' by the neighbors, she could get out of just about any restraint."

This bright little girl, who spoke in sentences at 21 months, grew to be more and more frustrated. By the time she was two and a half, Andrea's temper tantrums were becoming increasingly frequent -- up to ten a day. Her parents found spanking was totally ineffective and "time-out was a joke."

While they were shopping, Andrea pulled one of her typical disappearances, but her mom delayed the search just long enough to copy down the phone number on a flier advertising a diet for hyperactive children.

The family went on the Feingold diet -- most of the way -- and saw a big improvement in their toddler. But it wasn't until they gave up the unapproved brands of cheese and crackers that they had complete success.

Her parents were astonished to find that a tiny amount of an additive could have a profound effect on their child. Andrea was 4 1/2 when they moved to a new location. She began to have episodes of severe depression, which were blamed on the move. It turned out that the culprit was the brand of milk they were now using, which had preservatives in the vitamin A fortification.

Now in ninth grade, Andrea has made her family proud of her and of her accomplishments. Last year she won the Scholastic Writing Award for the region of her state. She is making A's in advanced math, is a talented artist and loves dramatics.

Andrea has had to cut back on basketball, soccer and band in order to have time for a new interest -- jazz dancing. She is active in her church youth group and has a busy social life.

In addition to her regular classes, she teaches German to elementary aged children and has participated in the writing and filming of several videotapes for her school.

Neighbors may have called Andrea "wiggle butt," but the name her teachers use is "a joy."

Lita

"She stayed on the diet most of the time, but after she had been good for as long as she could, she would decide it was time for a 'holiday.' Then the nightmares (which we now know were actually hallucinations) would begin. Lita was terrified of them and this fear would make her want to get back on the diet. But she just couldn't handle temptation on her own; sometimes I would come into school and eat lunch with her to bolster her will power.

"Another consequence of going off her diet was a change in her school work; Lita was unable to read or write well after she had consumed the forbidden additives. Salicylates also had a severe effect on her schoolwork, and she must still be careful not to overdo them."

Lita has just learned that she has been accepted into the college of her choice. Her ambition is to study law. It may not seem feasible for a high school senior whose reading ability is only at the 8th grade level, but Lita is bright, articulate, and blessed with a great memory. She so successfully uses these talents to compensate that she has been an honor roll student throughout junior high and high school, and is receiving top grades in her honors English course.

Her maturity and ability to interact with others has brought a long list of honors and responsibilities. Lita was chosen as her school's representative by the Hugh O'Brien Youth Foundation -- an organization that identifies future leaders. At 15 she was president of her religious organization's youth chapter, and the group won many awards that year. Lita has been vice president of the regional council of B'nai Brith and is now membership chairman. For several years she represented her class in the school's student government association, is a member of the law club, and was selected to attend the Goucher College mock senate.

Derrik

For Derrik's parents, the hardest part of dealing with their 3 1/2-year-old was his sleeplessness and nightmares. Their day started at 5 am with a toddler who experienced everything with enormous intensity -- whether he was eating, playing, laughing or crying. This went on daily until about midnight.

Worn down by the activity, his mom recalls how it felt before their preschooler began the Feingold diet, "When you're in the trenches, you think you'll never make it through."

At 16, both Derrik and his parents are seeing the results of their time and patience with the diet. After trying many sports, Derrik has discovered his remarkable ability as a cyclist. The sport enables him to put his abundant energy to good use, and the rigors of training have instilled remarkable self-discipline.

Derrik's tendency to focus intently on just one thing created problems in school, but in cycling it's been a great advantage. The ultra-healthy diet required for training is not much different from the food he was accustomed to at home. And he stays away from the green sports drinks, which make him physically sick.

Today, Derrik is very healthy, with the endurance necessary to cycle 170 miles in a day.

Chris

"He was always wound tight, all helter skelter, into everything, and he wore everybody out." In addition to dealing with the problems of hyperactivity, Chris has also overcome some of the symptoms of Tourette syndrome. (The Feingold Program successfully addressed the hyperactivity, but did not help Chris' Tourette symptoms; a regimen of vitamins has been effective. Diet has helped some children with Tourette syndrome. See part three of this book for details.)

This year Chris will be graduating first in his high school class, a National Merit Commended Scholar with a better than 4.0 average. He is president of the United High School Council for the Fort Worth Independent School District.

In a letter of recommendation to Rice University, the principal of his school called him "one of the most outstanding students I have encountered in my career." He has received an early admission to Rice, but will have to make some hard choices as his interests and abilities cover so many areas: pre-law, international business, journalism and architecture.

Music has been an important part of his life, so it wasn't a surprise that he had the lead in the school's musical this year. What was a surprise was that the part also required dancing; as a preschooler Chris had been diagnosed as having gross motor disabilities.

His parents believe that his experience in traveling throughout the world with a choir group has enhanced his maturation. He holds down two part-time jobs: lawn care service and working in a gourmet grocery store. Chris especially likes the gourmet food. Having spent most of his life on the Feingold diet, his palate "knows the difference between real food and the synthetic stuff."

Michael

He was a happy, likeable child -- not defiant or hard to live with. But Michael had a great deal of trouble coping with his schoolwork. He became a real charmer, and learned to talk his way out of just about any tight spot.

His parents reluctantly tried Ritalin for a year, but couldn't stand to see their son turned into a "zombie." They learned of the Feingold diet when the support groups were first forming, and fourteen years later are profoundly grateful for the help and moral support they received. This support gave Michael the courage to stick with the diet even back then when there were so few prepared foods allowed.

His mother relates how one day his teacher gave him a cupcake. He wouldn't eat it, but kept it on his desk all day, explaining, "I just want to look at it." Today, at 21, his proud parents note that Michael is as sweet natured as ever. He takes a great deal of pride in himself and in his new career in the Navy.

Mark

Poor speech, weak motor skills, and very slow to walk -- the doctor told Mark's mother it was because she babied him.

He did not have behavior problems, but was extremely learning disabled and received remedial help for six years. Mark was dyslexic and unable to speak clearly. "I worked with him for years to get him to recognize the alphabet," his mom recalls.

Today Mark knows that his so-called developmental difficulties were triggered by BHA, BHT and salicylates, which brought about severe motion sickness. They affect his balance, hearing, and perception. (He is also very sensitive to mint flavoring.)

It is difficult for anyone to believe that Mark once had any learning problem at all. He is enrolled in advanced classes in high school, earning As and Bs. His teachers have noted he is able to store and retrieve enormous amounts of information. He also writes well. His motor skills are fine, he runs track, is very personable, and is doing well in all areas. "For us, it's a miracle," his mother relates. "But he'd lose it all if he went off the diet." Mark is aware of this and monitors what he eats. The phrase that best describes Mark is one his mother never expected to hear ten years ago as she sought help for her little boy: today Mark is "perfectly normal."

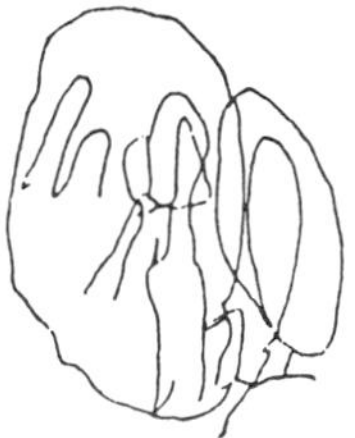

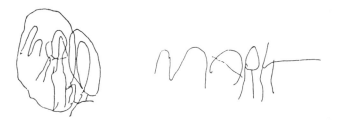

In the first handwriting sample, Mark tried to write his name just before starting the diet. The second sample was written after he had been on the Feingold Program for 5 days.

Mary Jo's Story

Our child appeared normal in every respect as an infant; there seemed to be no problems until he was about two. We began to suspect then that he was perhaps more active than most two-year-olds, but he was such a happy, bright, good-natured little ray of sunshine that we just loved him and accepted him as he was.

We did have to supervise him closely to prevent injuries, and there were still many of them. He was a regular visitor to the emergency room, and his father (a physician) stitched him up a number of times during his early years.

It was not until he was five that we began to suspect that there was something more complex than just "all boy" behavior. He exhibited most of the classical characteristics of hyperkinesis. The one characteristic not evident was a tendency to aggression. He was, in fact, rather submissive to his more dominant older brother, and was gentle and loving to his baby sister. He had lots of friends and was very popular in the neighborhood.

My attempts to get my concerns across to our pediatrician brought forth comments many parents hear in those early years of uneasiness: "He's just all boy, Mother. Let him be. You're over-anxious. Too bad you don't live on a farm where he could roam freely and not be suppressed. He'll outgrow it, etc., etc."

At age seven, when our son was in the second grade, it had become very obvious to everyone that this bright child simply could not concentrate well enough to perform normal tasks at his grade level. He read poorly and could not write. Worst of all, he began to suspect that there was "something wrong" with himself and began to experience terrible frustration at being unable to do what was expected of him. His happy, outgoing personality began to change a little, and for the first time we saw aggressive tendencies and a real spark of defiance. As the pressure increased, so did this behavior.

At this point I decided to force a showdown with our pediatrician, and Providence took a hand. I had never seen my son more "turned on" than when we arrived at the doctor's office for his exam. He explored every drawer and closet, spilled a jar of tongue blades, walked on his heels when asked to walk on his toes, wiggled and squirmed, hollered into the stethoscope, asked silly questions, and even locked himself in the bathroom accidentally (I think) when asked to produce a urine specimen. The doctor was preparing to take the door off the hinges when he was finally able to unlock it. In general, my seven-year old made a shambles of the examination room and left the pediatrician out of breath and somewhat disheveled. I made no effort to intervene and sat mute while all this went on. When we all got ourselves pulled together the pediatrician said, "(expletive deleted!!) I see what you mean. We have to do something!"

I couldn't resist saying, "Maybe you're just over-anxious. Why don't you move your office to a farm where children could have room to explore and not be suppressed?"

From that point, we obtained a psychological evaluation, and a neurological evaluation. No abnormalities could be found, but it was the consensus of opinion of all concerned that this was an "organically driven" child and a trial on Ritalin was in order.

The next year was terrible for our family. The side effects of the drug were very hard for all of us to endure. I won't dwell on this except to say that I wish I could give this year back to my son and erase it from my memory. It will always be a source of pain to me that we allowed it to take place. But the agony of that year forced me to realize that we had to find another way. I simply could not abandon my son to a lifetime of drugs, and I could not bear to see him suffer from either the frustration of being unable to control his behavior or the side effects of the drug used to control it. It was then that I began to read anything and everything I could get my hands on about hyperactivity and learning disabilities.

As I read, I picked up more and more information about the influence of nutrition and the effects of what we ingest. Eventually, I learned about Dr. Feingold's book and it opened a door of hope for us for which I will be eternally grateful.

Our son, after a few weeks on the diet, was taken off Ritalin and began to function as a calm, in-control, well behaved little boy. He was eight at the time, and he is now twelve. We have worked to remedy his "learning disabilities" which in actuality were only gaps in his knowledge that occurred while he was unable to function normally in school. We have found that he is indeed capable of learning and achieving. He brings home Bs and Cs and some As on his report card, and received satisfactory marks on behavior, citizenship, attitude, work habits, etc. He made the basketball team this year, and won third place in the Science Fair.

But the point is that he is functioning normally in a world where the demands made on him are the same as those made on the other children in our family and on others in his peer group. He is again the happy, outgoing, very gentle, very loving boy who has every reason to look forward to a full and productive life as a contributing member of society. When he was nine years old and things were once again going well in his life, he spontaneously made a poster and gave it to me. He wrote a message on it and decorated it with drawings of sailboats, seagulls, flowers, clouds and nice things. The message was "I am what God meant me to be."

How can we prove that all this happened? What proves to us that it was not just a fluke? Just the result of extra parental attention? Just the result of some variation in his development? We do feel we have proof -- we find that all the gains he has made can be reversed by dietary infraction. When our son is allowed to ingest the artificial substances, he reverts within a short time to the old behavior. We see the hyperactivity, the inability to concentrate, a certain irritability and some aggression, and most interesting of all, his handwriting deteriorates markedly. After a period of three or four days this will clear up and he again becomes the calm, controlled boy I described above. We've seen this happen over and over when we've allowed a dietary infraction to occur. He is aware when the change occurs, and will remark to us, "I feel dreamy," or "I know I am getting hyper." Frequently he will complain of headaches when he has ingested a no-no.

One of the things his father finds most interesting is that when his diet is carefully monitored and all is going well, this child who could not concentrate can beat the socks off his Phi Beta dad at chess!

How can I gain my child's cooperation?

*If you're typical of other parents trying out the Feingold Program you probably think, "My child will **never** cooperate."*

But most children do cooperate when the program is presented properly. Consider which approach is best for your family, and this begins by taking a look at your own feelings. When you read over this information, you may be thinking, "I can't believe all the disgusting things that are put in our food; what a rip-off. I'm glad there's a way to eat all the things we love without exposing the family to these additives!" Or, you may think, "What a chore; I'll have to do extra shopping to find some of these products; a loaf of bread or a quart of ice cream may cost more; I hate to think of the kids having to give up their multi-colored candies, cereal, etc. Maybe I can just change a few of the brands and get away with it."

If you see the program in a positive light, this attitude will be conveyed to your family, but if you consider it a deprivation, this will come across too, particularly if your children are older.

Spend some time reviewing your new member packet and exploring your own feelings. Think about the trade-off: short-term inconvenience may lead to long-term rewards. Consider that the hardest part of the Feingold program is likely to be the first weeks when you're getting accustomed to changing some of the brands you use. You will soon feel comfortable using the items on the Foodlist, and by that time you should be reaping rewards in the form of a much-improved child and calmer family life. If you carefully follow Stage One you might see a noticeable change in just a few days, and this is all you will need to give you the enthusiasm to continue. At that point, the effort required will seem trivial compared to the joy of seeing your child function normally. After having worked so hard at other techniques that were unsuccessful, you may find you welcome the chance to work at something that produces positive results. When selecting the right brand of potato chips, or skipping the spaghetti sauce makes such a difference, it's a small price to pay.

Substitute, don't deprive

Identify the things your child may be most reluctant to give up, and find alternatives.

* If he loves the toothpaste pump that exudes red, white and blue paste (a no-no) then substitute a snazzy cartoon character cup or toothbrush, along with one of the OK toothpastes.

* If she enjoys getting gumballs at the supermarket, let her buy one of the vending machine trinkets instead.

* If your family likes cookies made with M&M's in the dough, go ahead and make the recipe, using Stage One ingredients and the natural alternative -- Sundrops (found in many health food stores).

* If the lollypop from the bank is a treat, keep a naturally colored lollypop in your purse and trade with your child.

The very young child

The younger the child, the more control you are likely to have over her food. It may mean educating your spouse, the relatives, or day care provider, but at least you don't have to deal with school lunches. The younger the child, the easier and more effective the Feingold program is likely to be.

Pre-schoolers

For nursery school snacks, it will probably be best for you to provide them for your youngster. If the staff is not familiar with the Program they may have difficulty understanding why you are concerned about food. People who don't know your child as well as you do may look at the disruptive behaviors and assume that they are deliberate. But if you can bring about a noticeable change, if your pre-schooler changes from the terror of the sandbox to a pleasant child, the staff will have a very strong motive to support your efforts. "Feingold kids" are generally very bright, and once your pre-schooler feels the difference, he will probably be eager to keep himself on the diet.

Elementary school-aged children

The child now moves from the more casual approach of preschool to one that is structured. Your student is expected to stand in line, stay seated, pay attention, complete written work, etc. A teacher who is unfamiliar with some of the problems of chemical sensitivity may view them as lazy or defiant behaviors. Given enough frustrating experiences, a student may eventually become defiant.

Read over some of the stories in this book about children who have been helped by the Feingold program, and share them with your child. This is an excellent way of explaining that abnormal additives can create problems for normal people.

You will need to enlist your child's help as she faces the temptations ahead. School breaks and vacations are good times to begin the program since you have far more control over the food consumed. If you can make this period a fairly pure test of Stage One, you might see results before the break is over. Once she experiences the difference the program can bring about, she will have a good reason to stick with it.

If a major junk food event is coming up, talk with your child about a special toy that can be given in exchange for saying "no" to the unapproved foods. Shortly before Halloween, one mother described how she and her daughter went shopping and bought the doll her little girl had been wanting. They agreed that the doll would stay with Mom until after trick or treating was over, and then the collected candy would be exchanged for it. This worked beautifully. The evening was exciting and fun, and the child gladly handed over the candy for her new toy.

Another family has a system where their youngster can accumulate "credits" for turning down unapproved foods. When he earns a certain number, he gets to spend a small amount of money at one of the everything-costs-a-dollar stores found at many shopping malls. Eventually, the reward of just feeling and functioning better will be sufficient.

Junior high and high school

By the time he has reached the teen years, how many people have told your son he "could do it if he really tried?" How many years has he been blamed for something over which he may not have had any control? How many solutions have been tried and failed? It's no wonder both of you are discouraged!

Imagine how you would feel if you found yourself in a graduate class of quantum physics and the authority figures kept telling you, "you're really very bright. If you can't understand this it's just because you're lazy; you're not really trying."

Imagine a job where your boss belittles you in front of your colleagues, and no matter how hard you try your work never measures up. Then imagine you have no recourse; you cannot quit and find a different boss any more than your child could quit and find a different teacher. (And imagine what it must be like to be a teacher attempting to work with a child who wears one's patience thin!) In addition to all these negative experiences, add the teen's natural desire to be just like his peers. Where is his self-esteem? (*What* self-esteem?)

You know your child better than anyonc clsc. Maybc a straightforward "let's try it" approach will work; that's fine. Some families find it works best to make a contract. The child agrees to give the program a 100% effort for a set number of weeks and see if he feels/behaves any differently. If he sticks to his part of the bargain, and there is no change, Mom agrees to stop bugging him about what he eats (although she may opt to continue to buy wholesome foods). Or, the reward may be a tangible thing -- whatever fits best with your family's attitudes.

But if you suspect your teenager will see the Feingold program as just one more gimmick that won't work, just one more proof that he's a "misfit," then you may want to take an approach that is very different from what we generally suggest.

Ignore your teen

Take a closer look at the list of symptoms in the first section of this book, especially those that apply to adults. Do you see anything that sounds like symptoms *you* may have? Do you find yourself dealing with any of these: headaches, hives, asthma, impatience, distractibility, irritability, allergies, sleep disorders, or nasal congestion? Do you find you have difficulty tolerating fragrances, cigarette smoke, new carpeting or auto exhaust fumes? If any of these symptoms sound familiar, you're a candidate for the Feingold Program yourself. On the other hand, if you feel great, and are into exercise and good nutrition, then you're likely to want to incorporate many Feingold ideas into your own healthy lifestyle.

Go through the Foodlist and identify the products your family already enjoys. Perhaps the changes won't be as great as you have imagined. When you do the shopping, be sure that only Stage One products come into the house. (Pack the no-nos in a box and seal it, or give them away.) When your teen wonders what's going on you can tell him it's your own health kick -- it won't be the first time your offspring suspects Mom or Dad has really "lost it."

Be liberal about stocking up on the snacks and treats, and this "Feingold thing" may not seem like a bad idea after all. If your teen is a male, he will probably consume enormous amounts of this Stage One fare, and may find he likes it.

The goal is to see if you can notice any improvements even though he may not be following the program 100%. If your youngster is extremely sensitive, you might not see any response. While we generally discourage families from using the program less than 100%, we know that even the poorly designed studies conducted back in the 1970's showed noticeable improvements in many children. If your teen does improve, you have laid the groundwork for him to eventually make the connection. If a partial change in diet doesn't help, then your teen can't say he tried the Feingold diet, and at least you haven't soured him to the whole idea and closed the door to him considering it in the future. (Refer to the section in this book on teens.)

Negative Vibes

Many people are aware that there is such a thing as "diet" to treat behavior or learning problems; they may even have made an attempt to use one and found the experience very frustrating. The problem we encounter is the assumption that there is only one such diet, but this is not the case. Some books tell you to eliminate sugar; others have you do all your shopping in a health food store; some advocate adding vitamins and minerals; others remove foods such as milk and wheat while they toss in some vague advice about not consuming "additives." Some books tell you what menus to serve, and provide recipes, while others give a listing of which additives the authors consider undesirable.

The experienced Feingold member who has successfully used our program, and investigates other options, knows each of these techniques has validity for some people. But as an initial approach to diet management, they tend to be less comprehensive and more difficult than is necessary. It doesn't matter how good a program is if your child will not cooperate or if you cannot cope with the demands it places on you.

If your doctor is not enthusiastic about the Feingold program, he or she may believe that it is a blend of some of the other approaches named above. Or, he may have read Dr. Feingold's book, *Why Your Child is Hyperactive* and believe the diet is still difficult to follow. He may not realize the wealth of information and help which has been developed since its publication in 1975.

Contact a Feingold Association to receive information on the research supporting diet management, or share some of the scientific information in this book with your doctor. (Feel free to photocopy it.) Also, refer to the section of this book on gaining your doctor's cooperation.

Feingold volunteers have successfully helped the majority of families who have used the Program. Parents and professionals in the United States and around the world continue to volunteer their time and effort for only one reason. It works.

Candy!

Gaining your child's cooperation is an essential part of the Feingold Program, and this often translates to: candy. If your kids are accustomed to having some of the sweet stuff, this is no time to take it away. If they haven't had much of it, you will still need to know what brands are OK for those times when it's hard to avoid. (For the occasional child who is extremely sensitive to sweets, you'll have to get more creative about treats. For the rest of us, just avoid giving the child candy on an empty stomach.)

How do I actually begin the Program?

If you're the parent of an "impossible" child, and you've come this far, you're a survivor. You'll be able to survive some dietary changes too.

The first thing you'll need is that rare, precious commodity -- a little time to yourself! Read the *Feingold Handbook* for a good overview of the Program. Scan your Foodlist and see how many of the products are familiar. You may want to take a marker and highlight all the brand name foods you are already using, as well as any that look appealing to you. (Ignore the unappealing ones. If carrot juice doesn't strike your fancy, it's not something you have to drink; it just means someone once asked us to research it. That person may feel the same way about finding beer on the Foodlist!)

Explore your pantry

Go through the foods you have on hand, and compare them to the products listed in your Feingold literature. Then, using your Foodlist book, make up a shopping list of staples you want to replace. Next, plan some meals for the coming week. You'll find suggestions in your Feingold membership literature and in the *Feingold Cookbook*, but your best source is your family's preferences.

Born chef or convenience food fancier?

If you are an epicure with no budget to get in your way, and you adore cooking, tomorrow night's dinner could be: crab bisque, bibb lettuce salad with hearts of palm, Cornish game hens and chestnut stuffing, glazed tiny carrots, asparagus Hollandaise, to be followed by lemon sorbet and chocolate wafers.

But if you're more typical of the Feingold mom, dinner may be a faster, more casual one: grilled cheese sandwich and Stage One supermarket salad, with a scoop of ice cream for dessert. In other words, make life as easy as possible for yourself. Don't invite anyone over for dinner, except perhaps the kid next door. Julia Child and the relatives can wait for their invitation.

Your old standbys

See how many family favorites can be adapted to Stage One. Stuffed green peppers, baked in tomato sauce will be difficult to transform into Stage One fare, but you may find the meatloaf won't change that much by leaving out the tablespoon of ketchup and using an approved brand of cereal in place of the brand you now have.

The key to shopping and cooking during the first part of the Feingold Program is to focus on the short term. Come up with five different dinners you think the troops would like. If you can think of seven dinner ideas, so much the better. That way, there will be a different dish each night. What to do when you've reached the end of the week and run out of menus? Go back to number one and start again. Our careful research confirms that no husband ever died from eating baked chicken two times in ten days. As far as the kids are concerned, many mothers believe that taste buds don't actually develop until about age 21. Anyway, kids are notorious for wanting the same foods over and over, so don't waste your sympathy.

What now?

So we've offered reassurance and some words of encouragement, but there are still empty spaces on your legal pad waiting to be filled with something to prepare for dinner. Let's face it, grocery shopping and food preparation is not your thing; you'd rather be doing practically anything else. In that case, let's make it as easy for you as possible.

Begin by tossing out your notion of what "dinner" has to be. Maybe nobody will object to a tuna sandwich and carrot sticks. Vary the tuna salad by adding chopped hard cooked eggs. Or make chicken salad by opening a can of (approved brand) chicken in place of a can of tuna. Stick one of those toothpicks with the frilly colored cellophane into each sandwich and everyone will think they're being treated royally. You may be willing to let the kids eat their hamburgers in front of the TV occasionally. For variety, use French bread slices or pita in place of regular bread.

The sincerest form of flattery

If your offspring love the fish fillet sandwich at the local fast food dive, they might also go for your version made with approved brand fish fillet, lettuce, and approved brand ranch dressing.

Unbreaded fillet of chicken sandwiches can be imitated by marinating fillets/slices of uncooked chicken or turkey in Italian salad dressing. They cook quickly in a frying pan. Or, you can serve them as a main dish, along with thin (fast cooking) noodles. Cook the noodles according to package directions. After the meat is done, remove the fillets from the pan. Add some water to the drippings. Put the cooked noodles into the pan and toss to coat them with the drippings. Add a salad or vegetable for a meal that tastes like it took a lot of work.

Time warps

Who says breakfast can't be eaten at 6:30 p.m.? You might not mind scrambling eggs. Better yet, your spouse may claim immortality from his mushroom omelet and be willing to cook one occasionally. Pancakes, French toast, and (approved brand) frozen waffles are fair game too.

How many diets can you do at one time?

By all means, try to limit it to one! If you don't love to cook, trying to combine Feingold + gourmet is a bad idea. The same is true for Feingold + other diets.

Allergies: If you believe your child has a food allergy, or are following the advice of your doctor, you may have no other choice. But otherwise, don't try to combine your Feingold cooking with no-dairy, or no-wheat or no-sugar, etc. Life is already hard enough. Once you get into the swing of Feingold cooking you will be able to consider possible allergies, and making some more changes in the kitchen won't seem overwhelming. For now, your goal is to deal with Stage One.

Cholesterol: Here again, if you can safely put aside your concerns about limiting cholesterol for just a few weeks, do so. Once you have become comfortable with the Feingold routine, it won't seem so hard to make other adjustments. (This is the voice of Experience speaking here.)

Sugars: We're not saying that sugar is great stuff (that's the job of the confectioner's lobby). We don't even believe that other sweeteners are desirable. But your first job is to convince your child that he won't miss out on too much by cooperating with the Feingold Program. If that means more goodies than you would normally provide, but it succeeds in gaining his cooperation, it's worth losing the battle to win the war. Later, once things are going well, you can cut back on the junk food. Since you will probably be dealing with a far more cooperative child by that time, it may not be so hard.

The other meals

Breakfast is a problem if you are fond of a bowl of colored marshmallows floating in milk. But take a close look at the cereal section of your Foodlist. Not only are there a few familiar ready-to-eat products, but at least one provides as much sugar as any other kid on the block is getting for breakfast. (When you use sugary cereal, try mixing it with bland varieties. Your dentist will thank you.)

If your young'uns like hot cereal, the problem of breakfast is solved, and if you use a microwave oven to cook them in, your clean-up problems are taken care of too.

Health food stores have many varieties of ready-to-eat cereals, but you'll have to test them out as some taste different than supermarket brands. (Some taste better than mainstream brands, while others taste as good as the box they're packed in.)

Have you given serious consideration to the old time breakfast fare? Scrambled eggs, French toast, pancakes, waffles, sausage and biscuits? The French toast, pancakes and waffles can be made in quantity and frozen. (As this book goes to press, there are some varieties of familiar name brand frozen waffles in the Foodlists.)

- You can't get much quicker than bagels or toast. Spread them with cream cheese or peanut butter (or a combination of the two plus a little honey...good!)
- Melt a slice of cheese on a piece of bread...hot breakfast!
- In place of orange juice, try diluted pineapple or pear juice. (Pear juice is available in large bottles, found in the baby food section of your supermarkets. It looks and tastes like apple juice.) If your child likes grapefruit juice, that's another choice. If he doesn't like it, can you change his mind by adding some sugar?

- A breakfast shake will feed two regular sized children or one teenager. Pour the following into a blender: 1-cup whole milk, 1-cup pineapple juice, 1 banana. Whirl to blend. Serve and await the compliments. This is a thick stick-to-the-ribs kind of a drink, and contains a good selection of vitamins and protein in a glass.

Forget the five or seven different meal plans we discussed for dinner. With your kids' breakfast all you will need are two or three.

Plan a repertoire for lunches too

Remember, most kids are monotonous by nature, so don't feel guilty if you serve peanut butter sandwiches frequently. Give the impression of variety by cutting the sandwich a different way. A little deception is nothing to be ashamed of if it produces well nourished children or contributes to maternal mental health.

Check out the recipe book provided by the Association, for some more breakfast and lunch ideas.

Juggle the meals to get more variety. There's nothing inherently wrong with a child having macaroni and cheese, or a piece of pot roast at 7:00 am. We know of one child who ate baked beans for breakfast and grew up to be perfectly normal.

Leftovers from last night's dinner can travel to school in your child's lunchbox, and are a treat compared to most school lunches.

Need more help?

Still having trouble thinking of foods that are OK to use on Stage One? Lest you find yourself in a "What's left to eat?" frame of mind, we've listed some of the things that qualify for Stage One; of course, when prepared foods are listed, we are referring to the acceptable brands. Also, let your veggie-hater know that eating spinach is optional. (And notice that we've humanely left off the Brussels sprouts even though they're allowed.)

Artichokes
Asparagus
Avocado
Bagels
Bamboo shoots
Banana
Barley
Beans
Beef
Beets
Biscuits
Bread
Broccoli
Butter
Cabbage
Cake
Candy
Cantaloupe
Carrots
Cashew nuts
Celery
Cereal
Cheese
Chicken

Chinese vegetables
Chips
Chives
Chocolate
Cocoa
Coconut
Cookies
Corn
Cornmeal
Cornstarch
Crabmeat (real)
Crackers
Cream
Cream Cheese
Dates
Eggs
Eggplant
English muffins
Figs
Fish
Flour (white & whole wheat)
Garlic
Gelatin
Grains
Granola
Grapefruit
Hamburger patty
Honey
Honeydew melon
Hot dogs
Ice cream
Jam & jelly
Kiwi
Lamb
Lemon & lime
Lettuce
Lobster
Macaroni
Mango
Mayonnaise
Milk
Molasses
Muffins
Mushrooms
Mustard
Noodles
Oatmeal
Oats
Olives
Olive oil
Onions
Pancakes
Papaya
Pasta
Peanuts
Peanut butter
Pears
Peas
Pecans
Pepper (black, white)
Pie
Pineapple
Pistachio nuts
Pita bread
Pomegranate
Popcorn
Pork
Potatoes (undyed)
Pretzels
Pudding
Pumpkin
Radishes
Roast beef
Rice
Rice cakes
Rolls
Salad
Salad dressing
Salmon
Salt
Sausage
Scallions
Seafood
Seeds
Sherbet
Shortening
Shrimp
Soda
Sorbets
Soy sauce
Soup
Sour cream
Spinach
Squash
Steak
String beans
Sugar
Sweet potatoes
Syrup
Toast
Tuna
Turkey
Veal
Vegetable oil
Vinegar (white)
Waffles
Walnuts
Water chestnuts
Watercress
Watermelon
Yams
Yeast
Yogurt
Zucchini

Please be sure to refer to the current Foodlist for acceptable brand name products.

Your membership packet will also include a recipe book to help you prepare fast, salicylate-free meals, beverages and desserts. Here's a sample.

Dinner in a hurry

"Going Feingold" does not mean you have to give up the convenience you may have enjoyed from boxed dinner mixes. Here are two recipes that are easy, economical, and good tasting. They can be prepared in about 30 minutes or less from ingredients you pick up on your way home.

The shrimp dinner cooks in only one large saucepan, and the stew needs just a saucepan and large frying pan. (I hope you like them; someone's husband ate a lot of experiments so you could have them.)

Shrimp, Broccoli & Fettuccini Alfredo

This elegant dish may fool your family and friends into thinking you've gone gourmet. It's both easy and economical since it takes only a half-pound of shrimp to make 4 servings. Or you can make it with cooked diced chicken (your own or canned). If you do, skip the instructions on preparing shrimp, and add the chicken after the sauce has been cooked.

1/2 pound raw shrimp (shelled and cleaned)
2 cups broccoli florets (from the salad bar if you like)
8 ounces fettuccini or noodles
1 cup whole milk
1 - 2 Tbsp. cornstarch
1/3 cup grated Parmesan cheese
1/4 tsp. garlic salt
dash pepper
2 Tbsp. butter

1. Fill a large saucepan half full of water and add a tablespoon vegetable oil to prevent the pasta from sticking. Bring the water to a boil over high heat. While the water is heating, assemble the other ingredients and have a colander or large strainer ready.

2. When the water boils, add the pasta and stir it.
Determine how long the pasta will need to cook, and add two minutes to the cooking time since the water will cool down as you add other

ingredients. If the pasta takes 12 minutes, for example, set a timer for 14 minutes.

3. Cook the pasta on medium high heat, stirring it occasionally.
Meanwhile, measure the milk into a large measuring cup. Add the cornstarch and blend. (A small whisk works well.) Next, stir in the Parmesan cheese, garlic salt and pepper into the milk mixture.

4. When the timer indicates only 4 minutes left for the pasta to cook, add the broccoli pieces to the boiling water.
One minute before this is finished cooking, add the raw shrimp.
When the time is up, pour the pasta/broccoli/shrimp into a colander and allow the water to drain into the sink. Put the lid from the saucepan over this to keep the food warm while you make the Alfredo sauce.

5. Put the milk mixture, along with the 2 Tbsp. of butter, into the empty saucepan, and stir constantly over medium high heat. (A large whisk is good here.) As soon as the mixture thickens, remove it from the heat.

6. Add the pasta combination back into the saucepan, and gently toss it to coat it with the sauce.

Easy Beef Stew

This inexpensive meal provides a great way to use up whatever veggies, pasta, or grains you may have in the refrigerator. Choose your family's favorite ingredients, or try this version.

1 pound ground beef
1 cup (raw) macaroni or other pasta
1 can (about 15 ounces) beans - such as pinto, kidney, navy, etc.
1 can mixed vegetables, drained (or use frozen vegetables)
1 cup water
3 Tbsp. cornstarch
3 Tbsp. soy sauce
dash of garlic powder

1. Fill a medium or large saucepan half full of water; add a spoonful of vegetable oil to prevent the macaroni from sticking.

2. While the water heats up, begin cooking the ground beef in a large frying pan, breaking it up.

3. Cook the macaroni as the package directs. (If you use frozen vegetables, add them to the boiling water about three minutes before the macaroni has completed cooking.)

4. While the beef and macaroni are cooking, blend the water, cornstarch, soy sauce and garlic powder in a large measuring cup.

5. Drain the macaroni when it is cooked. Spoon off excess fat from the ground beef.

6. Add the soy sauce mixture to the beef and stir, cooking, until the gravy thickens. Add the macaroni, vegetables, and beans to the meat in the frying pan; stir.

This amount should serve at least six people.

A mom writes:

"For those of you just getting started on the Feingold program, let me share some of my feelings. I was really scared of this 'Feingold thing,' convinced that it would turn my life upside down. But it's all been so incredibly easy, and we really don't eat any differently than we did before.

"It helps that I don't mind cooking, but the big problem is that my work day is so long I have little time to do it during the week. I leave the house at 6:30 each morning, have a one hour commute, and don't return home until about 6:30 in the evening.

"I prepare many things ahead of time, and it's amazing how simple it is to do. One recipe that works very well is to coat chicken pieces with flour and seasonings in the evening. I put this in a baking pan and put it in the refrigerator. The next day when my husband comes home from work all he has to do is turn on the oven and put in the pan.

"Another easy favorite is Shish Kebab. I cut beef into large pieces and marinade it in teriyaki sauce for several hours or overnight. (Combine 1/2 cup soy sauce, 1/4 cup sugar, 2 Tbsp. vegetable oil, 1/4 tsp. ground ginger and a dash of garlic powder.) Then I put the meat on skewers, along with onions, mushrooms, etc. In the warm months we enjoy it over the grill, and other times of the year we use the oven broiler. It cooks quickly and is always a treat.

"On the weekend I cook large quantities of some of our favorites, then put portions in Ziploc bags, and freeze these. This works well for scalloped potatoes. I make a white sauce base, add some cut up mushrooms, add sliced raw potatoes and some onion. I cook this 2/3 of the way, then cool it somewhat and put portions in the Ziploc bags. Flatten them out and freeze them. The morning I plan to use it, I take one of the bags of potato out of the freezer and let it thaw. When I get home I cook it the rest of the way.

"We rearranged the family room furniture so I can see the TV with my family while I cook in quantity about every three weeks. "If you're new to the Program, hang in there – it's worth it."

Stage One -- Keeping a Diet Diary

It will be much easier to successfully use the program if you keep a diary of all the foods your child eats at the start of the program.

At least once a day, make a brief note of the behaviors you observe. This information can be valuable in the days to come; here's why. If you see uneven behavior -- good times and not-so-good, the diary can help you to pinpoint the likely culprits. On the other hand, if your child does well, then this list of the foods eaten becomes your "safe" foods. If you notice reactions later on, you can always return to this group of foods and be fairly sure you will be able to once again get these good results.

Before long you will probably be comfortable enough with the program that a diary won't be needed. If you later investigate possible food allergies, you may want to once again keep track of what is eaten and any behavioral changes that result.

Another benefit of keeping a diary for awhile is that it will help you determine how long it takes for a reaction to occur and how long the reaction is likely to last. For example, if you discover that tomatoes set your child off and the reaction lasts for a day, you may want to plan on the occasional pizza for Friday night so your child will be able to run off some of the excess energy, and be back on track for school Monday morning.

PART TWO

ADDITIVES:
What Are All Those Funny Things in Food?

The answer depends on whom you ask. The manufacturer will tell you they are "flavor enhancers" to make food taste better for you; they are "dough conditioners" to make it feel better in your mouth; they are "freshness preservers" to make sure your food is good to eat.

Critics will describe the same additives as substances that allow a company to use cheaper ingredients to create more profits and more sales, with fewer losses to them, due to food spoilage.

The manufacturer will tell you that additives have been used in foods for thousands of years, that all the chemicals he uses are legally permitted by the Food and Drug Administration, and that many have been subjected to extensive testing.

The critic will tell you what testing really involves, who pays for it, and will describe the "revolving door" between government and industry. This is the common practice of high ranking officials, policy makers, politicians and lawyers switching back and fourth between jobs in which they run government agencies, and the companies which are subject to regulation by these agencies. Such switching will bring these individuals remarkable advantage$ each time they make a move.

Critics will also tell you about some very unscientific methods often used in tests, about whistle-blowers who get fired, etc. etc.

Some elected officials have proudly described a partnership relationship between government and industry. But critics warn that the fox has been put in charge of the hen house.

All testing is not flawed; all regulating is not corrupt. In fact, there's a lot about the system that is excellent; but it's not as perfect as the consumer is led to believe, and for the chemically sensitive individual, the flaws are serious.

High tech eating

Highly processed foods -- made to look and taste like things they're not -- go through many stages of preparation and can acquire undesirable synthetic additives all along the assembly line. Labeling regulations are better than they used to be, but still too lax to include all of the additives used.

The use of additives in food is not new. Adulteration of wine goes back to the ancient civilizations in Greece and Rome, and European laws as early as the 12th century addressed the penalties for bakers and brewers who tried to increase their profit by adding unsavory ingredients. Iron filings were added to tea, and some enterprising folk collected used tea leaves, treated them with copper salts and graphite, and sold this to the unsuspecting.

Mercury, copper, and lead were used to add coloring to foods, and the unfortunate consumer sometimes didn't survive to complain. Even after the first synthetic dye was created, the earlier coloring agents continued to be used, and the practice was not outlawed in the United States until 1938.

Food Colorings

Of all the chemicals added to foods, synthetic dyes are probably the most notorious and have received the most attention.

Synthetic dyes date back to 1856 when the color mauve was first created from coal tar oil. The new hues quickly replaced fruit, vegetable, and mineral colorings that had previously been used.

By the turn of the century approximately 80 different dyes had been developed, and were used indiscriminately in foods. With the passage of the Food and Drug Act in 1906, most of them were banned. Others were created to take their place and in 1907 twenty-four were in use. In the years that have followed all but seven have been discontinued for use in foods, or banned as health hazards.

In 1960 Congress directed the Food and Drug Administration (FDA) to prove the food dyes in use at that time were safe. The agency was given two and a half years to complete the task. Meanwhile, the dyes then in use were given a "provisional" status, permitting their continued use while the testing was carried out. After the allotted time had gone by testing was still not complete, and the provisional use was extended.

When a dye is prohibited from use in foods, it does not mean it is banned from use in medicines or cosmetics. If it's unsafe to swallow a dye in food, how can it be acceptable to apply it to the skin or swallow it in the form of medicine?

Today most colorings are created from petroleum (the source for gasoline, kerosene and asphalt) but they are often still referred to as "coal tar dyes."

"Artificial coloring" -- what does it mean?

It can refer to coloring from natural sources such as turmeric, beet powder and annatto. When beet juice is added to lemonade to make it pink, the lemonade is artificially colored. Even though the beet juice is a natural product, it is not naturally occurring in lemonade. When a coloring agent of any type has been used, FDA considers the term "natural" to be misleading. Similarly, the carrot juice that farm families used to add to their butter would also be considered an "artificial" coloring.

In the United States coloring agents that are synthetic (petroleum-based) dyes are identified on their label with FD&C numbers; they are eliminated on the Feingold Program

FDA bans some uses of Red Dye No. 3

From Pure Facts: March 1990. After thirty years of hesitation, the government has begun the process of removing this cancer-causing chemical.

It won't mean the end of bright red lollypops, jelly beans and fluorescent cereal, but the recent decision concerning this notorious dye is certainly a victory for consumers. January 29 was the deadline for the most recent extension permitting certain uses for the dye Erythrosine (Red No. 3). Its continued use has long been allowed despite the fact that it has been shown to cause thyroid tumors in laboratory animals and thus may not legally be added to foods.

Feingold observers expected yet another "temporary" extension, a process that has been going on since 1962. Instead, the Food & Drug Administration, which had long tried (and failed) to ban this additive, finally succeeded to have it removed from some things. The ruling will prevent the dye from being used in some foods and in the wax coating on cheese; these represent only about 20% of the uses of the dye. (No products will be recalled and manufacturers will be allowed to use up the stock on hand.)

Curiously, although Red 3 will no longer be permitted to be added to cosmetics and drugs applied to the skin, it may still be added to ingested medicine and some foods. Red 3 is actually not found in many cosmetics. As the threat of a ban became more likely, the industry turned to other dyes. Although there are only seven synthetic colors permitted for use in foods, both the cosmetic and drug industries have many different dyes available to them. One of these, Red No. 36, was recently granted permanent approval for use in cosmetics and drugs. Like all "coal tar" dyes, it may not be added to products intended for use near the eyes.

When FDA announced the partial ban on Red 3, it also said it would begin the process of revoking the other uses of this dye. Such action could mean the end of the maraschino cherry in fruit cocktail. This prospect strikes fear into the hearts of fruit growers – those who raise peaches and pares, as well as cherries. Lobbyists claim that marketing tests indicate the removal of the bright red spots of color would result in a 20% decline in the sale of fruit cocktail. Red 3 is the only food dye that will color cherries without bleeding onto the other fruit.

When the possibility of a ban seemed likely last year, California growers enlisted one of their congressmen to block it by tucking language in an appropriations bill instructing FDA not to ban the dye without further study. Such studies would have guaranteed the dyes 4 to 5 years additional use, during which time attempts could be made to weaken the law so it would allow chemicals with "negligible risk" to be retained.

The colorful history of Red No. 3

By 1990, the third year of testing for Red No. 3 had become thirty years.

Three different FDA Commissioners tried – and failed – to have this chemical removed from the food supply.

Although Red 3 is not one of the more widely used food dyes, it has received the most attention as a possible trigger for learning and behavior problems. Dr. Herbert Levitan at the University of Maryland, found that the dye disrupted the nervous and muscular systems of test animals (*Science,* vol. 207, 28 March, 1980)

Does FDA mean "Food Dragging Administration?"

Year after year, the FDA granted additional temporary extensions to the provisionally listed dyes, and by 1985 members of Congress were exasperated. The Committee on Governmental Operations issued a report highly critical of the FDA and its parent agency, the Department of Health and Human Services. The report cites unethical governmental practices and excessive influences of the industry lobbies, particularly the Cosmetic, Toiletries and Fragrances Association and the Certified Color Manufacturers Association.

In January of 1985 the Public Citizen Health Research Group filed suit against FDA for their failure to ban ten dyes, including Red 3, which had been shown to cause cancer in laboratory animals. The Delaney Clause of the Food, Drug and Cosmetic Act states that any food additive known to cause cancer in humans or animals may not be deliberately added to foods. In October of 1987 Public Citizen won their case in the U.S. Court of

Appeals. The judges' decision affirmed that FDA was in violation of the law by permitting the continued use of Red 3.

Many years later, bright red maraschino cherries and countless other food products still contain this illegal dye.

Thyroid problems and mood swings

The case against Red 3 (Erythrosine) is based upon findings that it causes thyroid tumors in animals. Beatrice Trum Hunter, a member of the FAUS Advisory Committee, notes the dye is made of an iodine-containing compound. When it is ingested, the iodine is released in a free state. This means it can affect the thyroid system, which in turn can influence mood swings.

Another problem with Red 3 is its high "lipid solubility," or its ability to dissolve in fatty tissue. Erythrosine is fairly easily dissolved in the fatty tissues of the body, including the fatty tissues of the brain. This may account for the rapid, severe reactions so many people have to the dye.

Red 3 in combination with light

In the early 1970s researchers at West Virginia University found that one synthetic dye, Red 3, was especially damaging whit it was combined with light (photodynamic action). Dr. Feingold described the experiments on pages 118 – 119 of *Why Your Child is Hyperactive*.

Researchers at Brandeis University observed photodynamic action. They found that Red 3, in combination with light, interfered with the way nerve cells release neurotransmitters.

When Red 3 goes, where will it go?

What can a manufacturer do with approximately 300,000 pounds of the dye produced yearly? This versatile chemical has other uses. Erythrosine B is registered by the Environmental Protection Agency as a pesticide. Red 3 is not just a dye, added to the compound; it IS the pesticide. A representative at EPA told Pure Facts the chemical is an "active larvicide," sprayed on manure piles to kill fly's eggs. In order for the dye to be effective it must be exposed to sunlight.

Consumers win victory on two dyes

In December 1984, Public Citizen health Research Group petitioned the Food and Drug Administration (FDA) to ban 10 color additives because of serious safety problems including the risk of cancer.

In a major setback for the Reagan administration, the federal court of appeals in Washington, D.C., handed consumers an important victory by ruling that the FDA violated the law when it approved two color additives (Orange No. 17 and Red No. 19) that cause cancer in animals. The Court unanimously held that the FDA must abide by the Delaney Clause, which prohibits the agency from approving food additives that it has determined are animal carcinogens.

The Delaney Clause is the nation's most famous public health law, and the Reagan administration targeted it for extinction shortly after President Reagan took office in January of 1981. Almost immediately, the food industry, with the administration's support, proposed legislation that would have repealed the Delaney Clause. When Congress refused, the FDA adopted its "de minimis" policy which, loosely translated, meant that the government could ignore the Delaney Clause if it concluded that the risk of cancer was very small. The Court held that this de minimis interpretation was illegal.

FDA gives approval for blue dye

February 1988: Based upon studies of the synthetic dye FD&C Blue No. 2, the Food and Drug Administration concluded that it did not appear to cause cancer in animals. The agency has "permanently listed" this dye for use in foods, drugs and cosmetics. Food uses include: candy, frozen dairy desserts, coffee and teas, confections, and bakery goods. Blue 2 is permitted in cosmetics, but FDA regulations limit it to those not used in the area near the eyes.

The dye is manufactured through a chemical process that includes: formaldehyde, aniline, several hydrozides under ammonia pressure, and heating in the presence of sulfuric acid. As with the other FD&C dyes, each batch of Blue No. 2 must be certified to ensure it does not exceed the prescribed limit for impurities. Most of the impurities are in the form of salts and acids, but others include:

Lead – not more than 10 parts per million
Arsenic – not more than 3 parts per million
Mercury – not more than 1 part per million

As a total proportion, the coloring must be no less than 85 percent.

The problem with testing

The testing of Blue 2, as well as other food additives, raises some serous questions:

- The blue dye was tested singly, not in combination with other additives. (A consumer is unlikely to eat only Blue 2. The typical meal in the United States can contain hundreds of chemical additives.)

- The tests of this dye were carried out on animals, since clinical testing with humans is not required for additives, as it is for drugs.
- The manufacturer of the dye is responsible for hiring and paying the laboratory that conducts the testing. (The FDA reviews the procedures.)
- Food additives are not required to be tested for possible behavioral or learning effects.

The Bug-killer in the Medicine Cabinet

West Coast growers have a formidable foe in the Mediterranean and Mexican varieties of fruit fly, which can quickly destroy crops.

For years the method for dealing with this threat has been aerial spraying of the powerful chemical, malathion, but this pesticide is harmful for humans as well as bugs, and both consumer groups and organic farming advocates have encouraged the development of alternatives. One alternative being studied is to replace the malathion with an equally deadly compound -- a blend of two dyes commonly used in drugs and cosmetics. After a blend of Red dye No. 28 and Yellow 8 are fed to the fruit flies, exposure to sunlight causes the dyes to absorb light. This results in the formation of oxidizing agents in the bug's tissues within the next 12 hours and, in effect, the little critters explode!

Researchers find that the bugs will eat the dye if it is mixed with a sweetener, leading Feingold families to wonder why the growers don't simply buy up the powdered fruit drink mixes in the supermarkets, and use it in aerial spraying! Actually, the dyes permitted to be used in foods are different from those being considered as a pesticide by the Department of Agriculture, but Red No. 3, allowed in foods, has long been used as a pesticide. It, too, has a mechanism that is activated when it is exposed to light. [In his book, *Why Your Child Is Hyperactive*, Dr. Feingold described the practice of spraying Red 3 on manure piles to kill fly's eggs.]

The Red 28/Yellow 8 blend will also kill some other insects, according to *Science News* (April 15, 1995), but proponents consider it to be otherwise harmless.

FD&C dyes and D&C dyes

Dyes that go by the name of "FD&C" are allowed to be used in foods, drugs and cosmetics. Those called "D&C" are permitted only in drugs and cosmetics, but not allowed in foods. Dyes used in drugs and cosmetics are not required to meet safety standards as stringent as those used in foods, since it is assumed that the consumer is exposed to less dye in drugs and cosmetics than in foods.

Before a chemical company may receive approval to have a dye listed as "FD&C" they are required to perform extensive and costly testing. The fact that so few of the dyes are permitted in foods suggests that their manufacturers doubt the additives would receive approval.

The experience of Feingold members, as well as thousands of people who suffer reactions to FDA-approved food dyes suggests that the definition of "safety" is controversial. Allergists have reported adverse reactions to FD&C Yellow 5 for decades, but this dye is used extensively in products sold in the U.S.

Feingold families would also question the assumption that a chemical dye consumed in small quantities does not need to meet the same standards as those consumed in larger amounts.

Two other issues: unlike foods where there are many choices, consumers often do not have a choice of which medicines they can use; and since medicines are consumed by people whose health is likely to be fragile, the safety requirements should be higher, not lower, than for the general public.

Here is a sample of some of the dyes that can be found in over-the-counter medicines:
- D&C Red 7, D&C Red 22, D&C Red 27, D&C Red 28 (the red dye which kills fruit flies), D&C Red 30, D&C Red 33
- FD&C Blue 1
- FD&C Yellow 6
- D&C Yellow 10

Dyes that are permitted in foods:
- FD&C Red 3*
- FD&C Red 40
- FD&C Yellow 5
- FD&C Yellow 6
- FD&C Blue 1
- FD&C Blue 2
- FD&C Green 3

Many of the above FD&C dyes are either banned or restricted in other countries.

* Red 3 is not permitted in certain products since it has been found to cause cancerous tumors in test animals. It is prohibited for use in candies, baking mixes and the waxed coatings used on cheese. It is also not allowed to be used in cosmetics or drugs that are applied to the skin. This dye is still used in many foods, however, including the maraschino cherries in fruit cocktail.

Flavorings

Thousands of chemicals, most of them synthetic, are used to flavor foods.

There is no way for a consumer to find out what chemical flavorings are actually used in a particular food; the industry has the freedom to use virtually anything and need not declare it on the ingredient label. They are listed in general terms, such as "artificial flavorings."

Most of the chemicals used as flavorings have never undergone any safety testing, such as the ability to cause cancer or birth defects and, like other additives, they are not tested to determine if they can trigger behavioral changes.

Flavorings are used in more than just food. A representative of McCormick & Co. explained, "You can go down almost any aisle in the supermarket and, with the possible exception of produce and mops, anything you pick up will contain a flavor or a fragrance. There are places flavors appear that the average person doesn't even think about. They are even in cigarettes."

Flavor chemists use sophisticated equipment to attempt to duplicate the taste and aroma of the more expensive real foods.
In place of raspberry, they offer:

Vanillin, Ethylvanillin, Alpha-ionone, Maltol, 1-(p-hydroxyphenyl)-3-butanone, Dimethyl sulphide, 2,5-Dimethyl-N-(2-pyrazinyl-pyrrole.

Strawberry is replaced by:
Geraniol, Ethyl methyl phenyl glycidate, 2-Methyl-2-pentenoic acid, Vanillin, Ethyl pelargonate, Isoamyl acetate, Ethyl butyrate, 1-(prop-1-enyl)-3,4,5-trimethoxybenzene.

Vanilla vs. Vanillin

Have you ever wondered why your supermarket carries two such different products? There's that huge bottle of imitation vanilla at a low price, and right next to it is that tiny little bottle with the hefty price tag?

The difference seems significant until you think of how little vanilla is called for in a typical recipe -- generally about a teaspoonful.

Actually, the imitation vanilla is probably very overpriced. According to the trade publication, *Food Development*, "Fifty cents worth of vanillin is about equivalent in strength to $35 worth of vanilla. In other words, vanillin is 70 times as flavorful as vanilla on a cost basis..."

Pure vanilla extract and vanilla beans are well tolerated by Feingold members. Imitation or synthetic vanilla -- generally listed as "vanillin" -- is poorly tolerated. Some vanilla extracts contain alcohol, and may have corn syrup, but neither of these is likely to affect the typical Feingolder. If you suspect an extreme sensitivity to corn syrup, however, read the ingredient information carefully. If a product, such as ice cream, is made with only real vanilla, it can be called "vanilla ice cream." If at least half of the flavoring is from synthetic vanilla it is called "vanilla flavored." Ice cream made with only synthetic vanilla must be labeled "artificially flavored vanilla ice cream."

Imitation vanilla tends to have a more intense flavor and to stand up well under heat, and of course the cost difference is dramatic. For the manufacturer who is unaware of the harmful side effects, this could make the synthetic version seem very desirable. Dry powdered products such as pudding and cake mixes lend themselves to the use of powdered synthetic vanilla, and in white cakes and icings, colorless imitation vanilla avoids picking up a slight tint from the brown pure vanilla extract.

Tom Neuhaus, a nutritionist and biochemist, writes, "Vanilla extract, made from dried and aged vanilla beans, is a complicated mixture of many compounds. It is prepared by percolating alcohol and water over chopped beans for several days.

"Artificial vanilla flavoring is made by mixing vanillin, ethyl vanillin and a few other major components of the vanilla bean's flavor with water, alcohol and **coloring**."

In her classic book *Consumer Beware*, Beatrice Trum Hunter notes: "Other synthetics can also replace real vanilla, notably vanildene, ketone and piperonal, a well-known lice killer."

Vanilla is derived from an orchid, and is cultivated in Mexico, Indonesia, Tahiti, Brazil, and the Malagasy (formerly known as Madagascar). When the vanilla bean ripens and ferments, it develops the characteristic flavor and aroma from the compound known as "vanillin," which occurs naturally in vanilla beans. There are many other naturally occurring chemicals -- about 140 -- present in a ripe vanilla bean, but vanillin is the predominant one. When the name "vanillin" is used on ingredient labels it refers to the imitation flavoring. For practical purposes, the consumer can regard the name "vanillin" to indicate a synthetic chemical.

Because of the wide difference in the price of pure vanilla vs. the synthetic vanillin, there is an incentive for dishonest food processors to attempt to pass off the imitation product as real vanilla extract.

The biggest problem vanillin poses for the chemically sensitive person is that it is so widely used in chocolates. Feingold members used to be able to use a number of nationally available candy bars and a well-known cocoa mix. In some cases the company changed the ingredients, adding vanillin or TBHQ. Other products went off limits when a candy company was bought by a larger company, which then changed the recipe.

Consumers generally believe that expensive chocolate products use natural flavorings and inexpensive ones use synthetic, but this is not necessarily true. Check out the labels on those very expensive cookies, ice cream bars, and candies. Many contain vanillin. Then look at ingredient labels on bags of inexpensive foil wrapped chocolate holiday novelty candies. Some contain either pure vanilla or do not have any added vanilla at all.

There is no consistent rule on finding natural chocolate. Milk chocolate is more likely to have added vanilla or vanillin, and dark chocolate to be free of it, but there are exceptions. Food processing and marketing is not always logical.

Consumers have been told for many years that there is not enough natural vanilla to meet consumer demand, but the Vanilla Information Bureau in New York disputed this in correspondence to a Feingold volunteer:

"In reply to the statement that there are not enough vanilla beans in the world to meet demand, this is an old excuse from the manufacturers who are cutting costs by the use of artificial vanillin. The truth is that there is a surplus of vanilla in Madagascar (Malagasy), the main source, and that country has the potential to increase its production many, many fold. The issue is cost. Artificial vanillin is a by-product of pulp paper manufacturing (creosote) and costs a fraction of what real vanilla does."

The Vanilla Information Bureau also states that the artificial vanillin does not have the same chemical makeup as pure vanilla.

Is there really a difference?

The Feingold Program's policy of designating pure vanilla as acceptable and synthetic vanilla (vanillin) as unacceptable has brought criticism. One member wrote:

"My neighbor, who is a chemist, says that pure vanilla and synthetic vanilla are the same. I don't understand how this can be true since my little boy can eat things made with real vanilla, but has a bad reaction to foods with vanillin (synthetic vanilla)."

To get some insight into this, FAUS contacted Ruth Aranow at the Department of Chemistry of Johns Hopkins University. Dr. Aranow wrote: "I agree that the two are chemically identical. However, I doubt whether 'pure' synthetic vanillin exists. Every chemical synthesized contains some of the materials used in the synthesis.

"Just as vanilla extract contains unidentified resins of unknown toxicity and allergenicity, so too do synthetic materials contain unknown materials (i.e., reactants and other products).

"The real problem is that the nature of chemical sensitivity is not understood or even defined. But our ignorance gives us no right to either deny or affirm the existence of chemical sensitivity. There is evidence that the human eye can respond to just a few photons of light. This seems to be an extraordinary sensitivity. Until the nature of chemical sensitivity is better understood, the possibility of extraordinary sensitivity remains.

"So the question arises: If a person appears to 'react' to vanillin but not to vanilla, the sensitivity may be to components used or made in the synthesis."

The Troublesome Antioxidants

In his early work, Dr. Feingold did not remove the antioxidant preservatives BHA and BHT. (TBHQ was not then in use.) Thanks to the information provided to him by Beatrice Trum Hunter, he investigated these additives, and then removed them.

Once he eliminated the petroleum-based BHA and BHT, he found that a much greater percentage of patients experienced success.

Ms. Hunter, now a member of the FAUS Advisory Board, documented the problems caused by these preservatives in her books, *The Mirage of Safety* and *Consumer Beware*. When pregnant mice were fed BHA and BHT, it affected the brain chemistry of their offspring, resulting in approximately half the normal level of cholinesterase and serotonin. The affected mice weighed less, slept less and fought more than normal controls.

[Source: Fisherman and Cohen, "Chemical Intolerance to BHA and BHT and Vascular Response as an indicator and Monitor of Drug Intolerance." *Annals of Allergy*, Vol. 31, No. 3, March pp. 126-133.]

Human reactions to BHA and BHT vary as much as reactions to synthetic colors and flavors; and Feingold members know only too well that an "incidental" amount of a few parts per million can be sufficient to provoke a reaction, or can accumulate, thus leading to a reaction.

Many other countries either ban or restrict the use of these additives, and the state of California lists BHA as a carcinogen.

The Select Committee of the Federation of American Societies for Experimental Biology has cautioned against the additive; and the International Agency for Research on Cancer of the World Health Organization identifies it as a possible carcinogen.
[sources: *A Consumer's Dictionary of Food Additives,* by Ruth Winter, and *Safe Food*, by Center for Science in the Public Interest]

There are alternatives to BHA, BHT and TBHQ. The Henkel Corporation of LaGrange, Illinois, manufacturers an alternative product called Covi-ox by extracting tocopherols (a source of vitamin E) from vegetable oil. Henkel maintains that their natural antioxidants are as effective as BHA and BHT.

The Wysong Medical Corporation, of Midland, Michigan also has an alternative to synthetic antioxidants. Their "Oxherphol" is made from vitamin E and extracts of clove, sage and rosemary.

BHA, BHT, TBHQ and "incidental" additives

The Food and Drug Administration considers small quantities of preservatives such as sulfiting agents, BHA, BHT and TBHQ to be "incidental additives" and does not require they be listed on labels. This means we will continue to experience reactions from the many hidden additives found in vitamins, fats, packaging materials, etc.

Don't be "April Fooled" by the label:

A member writes: "Can you believe a label? Not always. When my local grocery store stopped carrying my favorite brand of yogurt, I carefully inspected the label on the local brand they now stock. The 'Natural Strawberry Lowfat Yogurt' label read OK, so I bought it. Inside the container I found a bright pink yogurt, quite different from my usual brand.

"A quick call to the dairy connected me with a very helpful lady in the lab who assured me that they did not add any colors to the yogurt. Sounds OK, doesn't it?

"Being an experienced Feingold volunteer, I knew I needed to persist, and luckily I did know the right question to ask next: 'Do the strawberries come with color already added?' A check with the lab supervisor found that my hunch was correct.

"The list of ingredients is legally correct. The label stated that the product contained strawberries. There is no requirement that they tell the consumer what may have been added to the strawberries.

"The Feingold Product Information Committee (PIC) looks into these hidden ingredients when they do product research. This incident reinforced for me how important the work of PIC is and how important it is for new members to refer to the Foodlist for acceptable brands.

"Unfortunately, a Foodlist cannot cover every occasion. The yogurt incident pales in comparison to the lemonade incident our family encountered on our vacation last summer. At a festival we attended there was a booth promoting 'fresh squeezed lemonade.' After being assured that it was freshly squeezed, we ordered some. When the cups were filled with a bright yellow liquid, I quickly asked what made the lemonade so yellow. 'It's the lemons,' replied the vendor. I persisted, but he assured me it was natural lemonade colored by lemons. After I expressed my disbelief, he explained that it was the yellow cup that made it look so yellow. He continued to insist it was natural even while his wife stood behind him shaking her head 'no' and my son was pointing out that the cups were white!

"If it doesn't look right, question it, and question again. Don't be 'April Fooled!'"

Be sure to check those labels!

Experienced Feingolders can get complacent about label reading. One member described just such an incident when she brought home a half-gallon of strawberry frozen yogurt. The family had enjoyed the same brand of peach yogurt, which was fine, and used annatto coloring. She forgot to check the ingredient label till she got home and opened it up; the strawberry contains synthetic dye!

Five "little" Food Additives to Consider

In addition to "the big five" additives eliminated on the Feingold Program (synthetic colors, synthetic flavors, BHA, BHT, and TBHQ), there are "little five" food additives. These additives are not prohibited, but are suspected of causing problems for some of our members. They are: corn syrup/sweeteners, MSG, sodium benzoate, nitrites, and calcium propionate.

What is Corn Syrup?

Glucose (or corn syrup) is made by treating cornstarch with sulfuric or hydrochloric acid. (These acids sometimes contain arsenic residue, which can add a contaminant to the glucose.) All nutritional value of the cornstarch is destroyed in this process and the product is then dark and foul smelling.

After being filtered and deodorized the end result is a clear, odorless and almost tasteless syrup which Dr. Harvey Wiley (the first Commissioner of what is now the Food and Drug Administration) worked unsuccessfully to ban from use in foods. Glucose was found to induce diabetes in test cats, and excessive use was said to have a destructive effect on the pancreas.

First marketed in 1902 under the name "glucose," the product was not well received by the public who thought it was made from glue. Changing the name to "corn syrup" transformed its image.

The ability to tolerate corn syrup (or "corn sweetener") varies with the individual; when possible it's wise to avoid it initially, and then test it out later. Since it is so widely used, avoidance is not always easy.

What is Fructose?

Fructose is the name given to the sugar that appears naturally in fruits. But the fructose that is available commercially is not extracted from fruit, as this would be too expensive.

Sucrose (granulated sugar or table sugar) is generally processed from sugar beets or cane, and it is made up of fructose and glucose. The fructose is extracted from the sugar.

High-fructose corn syrup is widely used as a sweetening agent. Corn syrup is a problem for many sensitive individuals, and sensitivity to fructose varies.

MSG and the Feingold Program

The Feingold Program does not eliminate MSG, but many are cautious of this additive... and with good reason.

The furor over MSG began with a letter published in the *New England Journal of Medicine* in 1968. It was written by a physician who found he experienced pain, weakness, numbing, and heart palpitations shortly after eating Chinese food. The condition was quickly dubbed "Chinese Restaurant Syndrome."

Studies funded by the industry have questioned the Chinese restaurant syndrome and yielded very conflicting results.

MSG and infants

Following the publication of the letter, other physicians reported a wide variety of physical symptoms that they believed could be attributed to this additive. Public pressure soon persuaded manufacturers of baby foods to remove the MSG.

While the Food & Drug Administration (FDA) has never prohibited the use of MSG in baby food, they do recommend that it not be given to children until they are neurologically mature. Diane Nixon, a Feingold volunteer, once contacted the FDA to ask them, "At what age can we consider that a child is neurologically mature?" The FDA said they didn't know.

Nobody knows exactly how MSG works.

Items found in health food stores often contain MSG in the form of an additive known as "hydrolyzed vegetable protein" (HVP) or "hydrolyzed plant protein," "autolyzed yeast," or just "yeast." According to one industry publication, HVP contains between 9 and 16 percent MSG.

Soups, gravies, and meatless dishes are particularly likely to contain MSG and/or HVP, but it can be found in foods as unlikely as chips and salad dressings.

One brand of Onion Soup is a good example of the confusion caused by the lack of labeling regulations. The front of the package prominently states, "Naturally flavored, NO MSG." But a phone call to the company disclosed that the "natural flavors" listed on the back include HVP. The company spokesman said they were changing the label to reflect the actual ingredients.

What Is MSG?

According to the Glutamate Association of the United States, MSG is "the sodium salt of glutamic acid, an amino acid and one of the important components of protein."

"Glutamate is naturally present - in 'bound' form, linked to protein and in 'free' form - in virtually all foods, including meat, fish, poultry, milk (including human milk), and many vegetables."

"Bound" and "free"

The difference between MSG in "bound" or "free" form is the crucial difference, according to food additive expert Beatrice Trum Hunter. In addressing the Feingold Association at its 11th annual Conference, Ms. Hunter explained. "It's true that glutamic acid is found in many foods, but when it's in food, it's always in a bound form. When you eat something like beef, or tomato juice or mushrooms, which have glutamic acid in them, you can handle them since it's bound to those foods.

"It's quite another matter when the glutamic acid is in the form of MSG, because then it's in a free state; in fact, it would be ineffective as a flavor intensifier if it were in a bound state. It has to be in a free state, and this makes all the difference in the world. You get it in your body in a free state, and if you're sensitive to it, you get these reactions."

How is it made?

The effects of this flavor enhancer were first noted over 2,000 years ago when Oriental cooks found that soup stock made from certain seaweeds improved the flavor of other foods.

Today, MSG is most often made from molasses that has been derived from sugar beets or sugar cane. According to George Schwartz, M.D., MSG can be made from far less savory ingredients. In his book *The Essential Update* (which followed his first publication, *In Bad Taste: The MSG Syndrome*) he writes:

"...the question has been raised as to whether some of the reactions [to MSG] may, in fact, result from a contaminant within the food-grade monosodium glutamate...MSG can even be produced from a base of motor oil or kerosene."

The many names of MSG

While most people understand MSG sensitivity, many are unaware that the popular product, Accent, is pure monosodium glutamate.

Since the industry considers MSG to be natural, and because the FDA has no regulations regarding the meaning of the word, many products labeled as "natural" contain MSG. *The Essential Update* identifies these foods as possible sources of MSG: broth, natural flavors/flavoring, malt flavoring, high flavored yeast, flavor enhancer, soybean extract, seasonings, textured soy protein, yeast extract.

MSG is no longer made in this country, but the United States imports about 80 million pounds of the white powder from Japan, and other Asian and Latin American countries.

Physical complaints

In June of 1990 the Health Hazards Evaluation Board of the U.S. Department of Health and Human Services issued a report titled, "MSG

Consumer Complaints by Reported Symptoms." Headaches were the most common reaction. A partial list of other symptoms include: nausea, diarrhea, change in heart rate, mood changes, abdominal pain, dizziness, sleep problems, numbness, and change in activity level.

Hyperactivity and psychotic symptoms from MSG

In 1978 the *New England Journal of Medicine* again published a letter from a physician who described a personal encounter with MSG. Dr. Arthur D. Coleman of the University of California Medical Center said his wife and 9-year-old son had apparently experienced psychiatric disorders as a result of eating food containing MSG.

Coleman said his wife underwent a "two-week depressive syndrome" and that his son had been in psychotherapy for hyperactivity and other problems. Coleman said his son's symptoms disappeared after he was placed on a diet free of the food additive.

How does it work?

Scientists still do not understand just how MSG functions to intensify the flavor of some foods. A popular theory is that it stimulates the taste receptors on the tongue.

Eating out

Not only should diners watch for MSG in Chinese food, but it is a popular additive in Latin American restaurants as well. Even though Japan exports MSG, you may find Japanese restaurants that do not use it.

If you suspect MSG sensitivity, speak with the manager before you eat at a restaurant. Most Chinese cooks will leave the MSG out of certain dishes if you ask, and a few advertise that they don't use any at all.

Previously prepared foods like soup and egg roll generally contain MSG, but it can be left out of main dishes that are made to order. (Feingold members should be wary of sweet & sour sauce, and pork that has been glazed with a red substance -- both generally contain dye.)

Soup - is it good food?

Not if you're sensitive to MSG. The vast majority of prepared soups contain either MSG or HVP, and many brands found in health food stores have hydrolyzed protein, or various types of yeast extracts. Soups with a meat base are the most likely to contain either MSG or one of the antioxidant preservatives that are eliminated on the Feingold Program.

If flavor enhancers are removed or reduced below a certain level, one industry representative told *Pure Facts,* the soup will lose its characteristic taste. And if the flavor in a dried mix is provided by beef or chicken fat, then the fat is subject to rancidity, thus the antioxidants such as BHA and BHT are added.

Make it

Soups take time to make but are not difficult. To replace condensed cream of mushroom soup for casseroles, make a medium or thick white sauce and add a can of chopped mushrooms (drained).

Chicken or turkey broth can be made either with the uncooked poultry or the leftover bones, skin and scraps from a roast. Put these into a large pot of water right after dinner, and simmer during the evening. Before you go to bed, drain off and refrigerate the broth. The next day, discard the fat that has solidified and freeze the broth in plastic containers. You'll always have it on hand for soups and sauces. (Your microwave oven will defrost the broth quickly.)

Excitotoxins

A comprehensive book describing the effects of both MSG and aspartame (NutraSweetTM) is *Excitotoxins, the Taste that Kills*, by Dr. Russell Blaylock.

For more detailed information on MSG sensitivity, or to order Dr. Blaylock's book, contact: NO-MSG, Post Office Box 367, Santa Fe, NM 87504, (800) 232-8674.

The Truth in Labeling Campaign has filed suit against the government for failing to adequately label MSG. TLC, P.O. Box 2532, Darien, IL 60561.

MSG and Aspartame

Dr. John W. Olney, M.D., of the Department of Psychiatry at Washington University in St. Louis, discovered many years ago that MSG had the potential to harm primate infants. He has long opposed the use of this additive, especially in foods to be consumed by children. Olney has also examined the effects of another neurotoxin, aspartame (NutraSweetTM).

As a result of "whistle-blowing" by various scientists and a deep suspicion on the part of the public, Senate hearings were held on this additive. Many doubts were raised, and it looked like the sweetener would be more tightly controlled, but this has not happened.

NutraSweetTM safety questioned by Senate committee

The following is a statement by Senator Howard M. Metzenbaum of Ohio of the Committee on Labor and Human Resources. The Senate hearing, entitled "NutraSweet: Health and Safety Concerns," was held on November 3, 1987.

It has been hailed as the most successful food additive in history. One hundred million Americans use it... it commands over $700 million in sales ... over 20 billion cans of diet soft drink containing it are sold each year.

And it seems to be in everything - cereal, kids' vitamins, cocoa, puddings, even over-the-counter drugs. There's no doubt about it. NutraSweet [aspartame] has captured the hearts and the tastebuds of the American consumer.

And why not? It tastes great, contains few calories, and doesn't cause tooth decay in children. NutraSweet is the dream-product. But for some consumers and scientists the dream may be too good to be true.

The FDA has received close to 4,000 consumer complaints ranging from seizures to headaches to mood alterations.

Studies and letters in the medical journals have warned of possible neurological and behavioral effects in humans, particularly in children and susceptible individuals.

- Dr. Richard Wurtman of MIT has warned of a potential link to seizures.
- Dr. William Pardridge of UCLA has raised concerns about excessive consumption by children.
- Dr. Louis Elsas of Emory University is worried about possible risks to pregnant women.
- Dr. Michael Mahalik at the Philadelphia College of Osteopathic Medicine warns of the possibility of brain dysfunction.
- Dr. Reuben Matalon, at the University of Illinois, has warned about potentially dangerous long-term effects on learning ability.
- Dr. Jeffery Baba, a professor of chemistry at the University of California, states that NutraSweet's decomposition products have not been adequately studied.
- Dr. Roger Coulombe, of Utah State, has cited NutraSweet's possible behavioral and neurological effects and called for new research.

In response to these concerns raised in the scientific community, we hear that NutraSweet is "the most tested food additive in history," proven safe in over 100 studies that were used for FDA approval.

What we don't hear too much about is the controversial history of a number of those much-vaunted studies: - studies which the FDA's chief legal officer once wanted investigated by a grand jury - the first such request in the agency's history.
- studies which a public board of inquiry found to be inadequate on the issue of brain tumors.
- studies which three FDA scientists called into question just weeks before a new FDA commissioner approved NutraSweet in 1981.

Any FDA approval is a scientific judgment call. We all know that. Frankly, I think there's doubt about whether they made the right call. At my request, the GAO (Government Accounting Office) investigated and said the FDA followed its approval process. But they did not evaluate the scientific controversy surrounding the tests. Today we will hear from a former FDA toxicologist who examined some of those key tests and believes there is still reason to be concerned about their credibility.

But the question before this Committee is where do we go from here? I am hopeful that this hearing will produce results. We need new, independent tests of safety. We don't need the company or non-profit institutes fronting for the company, telling us this product is safe. I hope that message comes across loud and clear here today.

We should have clear, understandable labeling that tells people how much NutraSweet is in their diet soft drink, or pudding, or cereal. We should be informed about the limits recommended for consumption.

There should be a FDA hotline for consumer complaints and mandatory reporting of such complaints by the manufacturer to the FDA.

Finally, we should learn a lesson from the NutraSweet experience. If a food additive has potential neurological or behavior effects, it should undergo human clinical testing, similar to the process a drug must undergo before it is put on the market. Only animal tests were required of NutraSweet, though at one point in the approval process, FDA scientists had recommended that NutraSweet be tested like a drug. They were overruled. I wish they hadn't been - maybe a number of questions before the Committee today would have already been answered.

These are among the issues I hope to examine at this hearing. Today we will hear from consumers who believe they have experienced severe reactions to NutraSweet, and a physician who has observed such reactions in his practice.

We will hear from scientists on both sides of the controversy and from the Commissioner of the Food and Drug Administration. We will hear from a consumer attorney who is not only concerned about NutraSweet, but also about the way research on the safety of foods is conducted in this country.

Finally, we will hear from the President of NutraSweet, Mr. Robert Shapiro. I have met Mr. Shapiro previously. In fact, we have engaged in lengthy negotiations earlier this year on getting new independent tests of safety. We haven't gotten there yet. I believe that the company was above-board and negotiated in good faith. However, we reached an impasse when it came to who would do the research. I am frank to say that the NutraSweet Company, the food and beverage industry, and their various institutes exert tremendous influence over scientific research and investigation. I want to make sure such work is genuinely independent. I do not believe that the scientists who have raised concerns about safety should be excluded from the process, and I am hopeful that the company will see fit to reopen these negotiations following this hearing.

In conclusion, let me say this. I know that diabetics and others in this country need artificial sweeteners. I want them to have them. I just want to be sure that an artificial sweetener like NutraSweet - which is being consumed by so many people in such vast amounts - is safe beyond doubt. I do not have that confidence sitting here today.

Editorial comment

Although Dr. Feingold cautioned against the use of artificial sweeteners, they were not incorporated into his list of excluded additives. Aspartame was approved for use in 1981, just a year before Dr. Feingold's death, but in the relatively short time that has elapsed, this sweetener has exploded into the marketplace.

The questions that have been raised during the recent Senate hearings are important ones. They are concerns Dr. Feingold raised about the use of synthetic colors, flavors and the antioxidants BHA, BHT and TBHQ. He often pointed out that food additives are not required to undergo the careful testing which is required for drugs. This is a point that was raised by Senator Metzenbaum and by some of those who testified at the hearing.

Feingold members will be gratified to know there are scientists and public officials who question the effects a chemical additive can have on the health, behavior and learning ability of susceptible individuals.

SCIENTISTS TESTIFY AT SENATE HEARING

Louis J. Elsas, M.D. pointed out that phenylalanine (a component of aspartame) is a neurotoxin when consumed in excess. He stated: "Normal humans do not metabolize phenylalanine as efficiently as do lower species such as rodents, and thus most of the previous studies of aspartame effects on rats are irrelevant to the question, 'Does phenylalanine excess occur with aspartame ingestion?' and if so, 'Will it adversely affect human brain function?'"

Dr. Elsas is Director, Division of Medical Genetics, Professor of Pediatrics, Emory University School of Medicine.

William M. Pardridge, M.D. expressed concern over the possibility of increased levels of phenylalanine in the blood as a result of aspartame intake. He cited a study, published in the *New England Journal of Medicine* (1983; 309:1269-1274), which showed that a five-fold increase in aspartame consumption by a pregnant woman can lower the IQ of her baby by 10 points.

Dr. Pardridge is Professor of Medicine, Division of Endocrinology and Brain Research Institute, Blood-Brain Barrier Laboratory at UCLA

M. Jacqueline Verrett, Ph.D., examined some of the studies on aspartame in her position as a biochemist/toxicologist for the FDA. She described some of the deficiencies and improper procedures: "...no protocol was written until the study was well underway; animals were not permanently tagged to avoid mix-ups; changes were introduced in some laboratory methods during the study with inadequate documentation; there was sporadic monitoring and/or inadequate reporting of food consumption and animal weights; tumors were removed and the animals returned to the study; animals were recorded as dead, but subsequent records...indicated the same animal was still alive; many animal tissues were decomposed before any postmortem examinations were performed...

"Almost any single one of these aberrations would suffice to negate a study designed to assess the safety of a food additive, and most certainly a combination of many such improper practices would, since the results are bound to be compromised."

Richard Wurtman of MIT expressed concern that the actual use of aspartame is far greater than the amount the FDA believed people would be ingesting when it approved the use of the sweetener. Since manufacturers are not required to list the amount of aspartame in a food, there is no way of knowing how much one is consuming.

He called for a change in FDA policy that would require food additives to undergo the same testing procedure that is required for drugs. This would include clinical trials on humans, not just animal studies.

It is particularly important that a substance like aspartame be carefully tested, he noted, since people do not expect a sweetener to have side effects as they would a drug. Unlike a food additive, one takes a drug for the purpose of inducing a physiological effect.

He pointed out that a drug, which is used by relatively few people, is subjected to far more careful scrutiny than a food additive, which is used by many millions.

Dr. Wurtman's recommendations included: "...that an Advisory Committee be established to recommend to the FDA standardized tests that can be used to uncover possible effects of candidate food additives on the nervous systems and/or behavior, and that such testing be required before the additive can be approved for sale."

Sodium Benzoate

Benzoates (sodium benzoate, benzoate of soda, and benzoic acid) are potential troublemakers.

The *Feingold Handbook* lists sodium benzoate as a potential problem for some people, and it may be especially so for salicylate sensitive members. (Salicylic acid is also known as "ortho hydroxy **benzoic** acid.")

Along with tartrazine (Yellow No. 5), benzoic acid was used as a challenge in the Egger study published in 1985. It was found to adversely affect most of the hyperactive children tested.

Even experienced Feingold members report they must avoid this additive. It is widely used in bottled lemon juice, soft drinks, soy sauce, pickles and many of the fruit flavored "spring waters" which have become so popular. In 1985 33.5 million gallons of these drinks were sold, and by 1991, the total had risen to 212 million gallons. Considered an "upscale" drink, with prices to match, they are really little more than an expensive soda. Most contain corn syrup, and even those claiming to be natural may be preserved with sodium benzoate.

For the rare Feingolder who is extremely sensitive to benzoates, it may be wise to remove even those that are naturally occurring, and test them out one at a time. Naturally occurring benzoates are found in:

Blueberries
Broccoli
Cauliflower
Cinnamon
Cranberries
Ginger
Green grapes
Greengage plums
Green peas
Licorice extract
Ripe olives
Spinach
Tea

Other Additives

Nitrites, fluoride, sulfur compounds and calcium propionate are troublemakers for some individuals. If you notice that your diet diary contains a pattern of reactions, consider watching for these, one at a time.

We rarely hear of phosphates being a problem, but are impressed with the detective work of one of our adult members who learned that she is very sensitive to them.

Fine tuning the Feingold Program: a member describes her sensitivity to phosphates

I was raised in a home where my mother made most of our food from natural ingredients. When I grew up and moved away from home my diet changed significantly.

My diet choices didn't catch up with me until my first pregnancy, when I suffered from exhaustion and many unexplained illnesses, as well as a worsening of psoriasis. These problems continued on and off for twelve years. I began to suspect that diet played a part when I paid closer attention to food in an effort to lose weight. I felt more energetic and positive. The earlier symptoms improved, but did not disappear.

My son also suffered from many health problems. During his first year of life he spit up constantly, had a continual runny nose, frequent ear infections, upper respiratory congestion and diarrhea. Later, he would be plagued by leg pains, vomiting, stomach pain, Tourette symptoms, bed wetting, and behavior and learning problems.

I believed there was a connection between what my son was eating and his physical and mental health. Both of us began to experiment with every diet imaginable, and found noticeable improvement by eliminating sugars and processed foods, but nothing worked consistently.

Because we were on the Feingold diet we were able to track down the other foods and chemicals we were reacting to.

By sheer accident and good luck, I came upon an article in the *Washington Post* by Marguerite Kelly. She mentioned the Feingold diet and I called that minute. Within a month our family was on the Feingold diet and from that day on, our health has steadily improved. Once we were well established on the Feingold diet we were able to readily spot other food sensitivities. Dairy, mold, yeast and fish were a problem for us, and we eliminated them. Our major success came with the accidental discovery that I could cure my psoriasis by eliminating phosphate additives from my diet! I had purchased sodium hexametaphosphate, a product that many chemically sensitive people use as a laundry whitener.

When I got the hexametaphosphate on my hands they immediately began to swell and bleed. I decided to remove phosphates from our diet on a hunch that what happened to my hands could be related to my health. Within a week I began feeling great, and my health has remained consistently good since then.

After a month on a phosphate-free diet we realized that our son's Tourette symptoms were greatly diminished, and we saw an improvement in his ability to concentrate and his overall health. I considered trying to remove all phosphates, including those which occur naturally in foods, but that's a big job, and would place a lot of restrictions on our food. We find that just eliminating the phosphate additives is sufficient, including baking powder with phosphate. We're fortunate to have a Fresh Field's market where we can buy wonderful food without the unwanted additives. It's a bit of a drive to the Annapolis (Maryland) store, but I am happy to make the trip each week and love our new way of eating. My family never lacks for anything, and both of my sons find plenty of appealing foods on hand.

There's another plus to shopping in a natural atmosphere. I used to find that when I walked through the produce department of many supermarkets I would feel sick for an hour afterward. It took years of frustration and many failures in experimenting with diet to resolve our problems. Occasionally a product like toothpaste containing phosphate will throw us off track, but since we have been on the Feingold diet it doesn't take long to isolate the offending additive.

A bit of advice for those having difficulty getting children to stay on this diet. My husband and I learned the hard way that all we could do was provide good food in the home and encourage our son to stay on his diet. We could not force him to do what he did not want to do. Through counseling we learned to be supportive and encouraging when our son maintained his diet, and to be patient and supportive when he failed.

Phosphates, used in many processed foods, were triggering the psoriasis and my son's Tourette symptoms.

Today our lives are so much different. One unanticipated side effect is that I find I am now becoming bored; since I have so much more energy I am looking for challenging things to do. But the main difference is in the quality of my son's life. He plays soccer and baseball, has earned a green belt in karate, participates in scouts and school activities, and for the first time since nursery school, he is making friends. His grades have significantly improved without our help, and teachers have positive things to say. For the most part he is a healthy, active, wonderfully normal person who is great fun to be around. Well, fun to be around most of the time -- considering he just turned 13 years old!

Caffeine -- More Than Just "Coffee Nerves"

New information on this familiar substance is pointing to its potential to cause severe behavioral reactions in susceptible individuals.

The Food and Drug Administration identifies caffeine as "a drug that stimulates the central nervous system. It can cause nervousness, irritability, anxiety, insomnia, and disturbances in heart rate and rhythm. It also seems to influence blood pressure, coronary circulation, and the secretion of gastric acids." (*FDA Consumer*, 1/88)

Andrew H. Mebane, M.D., a New Orleans psychiatrist, investigated the connection between caffeine and psychiatric disorders. One patient was a truck driver who was diagnosed as schizophrenic after doubling his intake of cola to 20 cans a day. Another psychiatrist, Michael Breslow, M.D. at the University of Arizona, suggests that caffeine can play a part in panic attacks. He notes that a single can of cola can cause a sensitive individual to experience shortness of breath, pounding heart and sweating.

Some of the effects attributed to caffeine include the ability to: reduce the body's anxiety-relieving systems, block opiate receptors that manage pain, as well as to neutralize medicines such as depressants and tranquilizers.

Caffeine occurs naturally in coffee, tea, and chocolate. While it is found in the kola nut, only about 10 percent of the caffeine in cola drinks is derived in this way. Ninety percent of the caffeine in cola drinks is deliberately added. (Some other soft drinks also contain added caffeine.) Several million pounds of caffeine are used in foods and medicines in the United States each year; it is obtained from coffee beans, treated for use in decaffeinated coffee.

Caffeine is not eliminated on the Feingold Program, and moderate amounts seem to be tolerated by most people, but very sensitive people should be aware of potential adverse effects.

Amount of Caffeine in Foods:

Item	mg. of caffeine
Coffee (5 oz cup)	115
Tea (5 oz cup)	
Brewed, major US brands	40
Brewed, imported brands	60
Instant	30
Iced (12 oz glass)	70
Cocoa beverage (5 oz cup)	4
Chocolate milk (8 oz)	5
Milk chocolate (1 oz)	6
Dark chocolate (1 oz)	20
Baker's chocolate (1 oz)	26
Cola, some soft drinks (6 oz)	15-23

What do we drink?

In 1988 Americans drank what averaged out to nearly 46 gallons of soda pop per person. Coffee, once the number one drink, was consumed at an average of 25 gallons. Beer was third at 23.6 gallons per person, and milk was fourth at 21 gallons.

Caffeine for hyperactivity?

Coffee has long been known to have a sedative effect on some hyperactive children, and was often used before Ritalin captured the market. Asked about the advisability of giving coffee to hyperactive children, Dr. Feingold responded: “It’s just another drug.”

SALICYLATES

[suh lis' uh lates]

What's Wrong with Apple Juice?

...or tangerines, or grapes, or raisins, or tomatoes, or peaches, or nectarines, or cucumbers, or almonds, or peppers?

Actually, nothing is wrong with these foods; they're wholesome and nourishing. But for someone who is "salicylate sensitive" certain foods can be terrific troublemakers.

Salicylates occur naturally in some foods, and are also found in many medicines and food additives. Aspirin is the best-known salicylate, and aspirin-sensitivity is widely recognized. It can bring on a variety of symptoms from asthmatic attacks to hives.

For many years medical journals have carried reports of adverse reactions to a variety of different substances. Much of the information came from allergists who observed physical symptoms resulting from sensitivity to food dyes, or aspirin, or some foods. Then research at the Kaiser-Permanente Medical Center in San Francisco demonstrated a link between these different substances. Even more surprising was the discovery that the same food or chemical which could bring about a case of hives in one patient could result in distractibility for another, and unprovoked anger in a third. In other words, substances that cause a reaction in one organ -- our skin -- can also affect another organ -- our brain.

What is there in an apple that is similar to a food additive or an aspirin tablet? Too little is known about salicylate-sensitivity to provide a good answer. One theory is that some foods produce their own chemicals to repel predators, and that this chemical is similar to "acetylsalicylic acid," or aspirin.

Several studies have been conducted to measure the salicylate content of various foods, with the most recent being an Australian project reported in the *Journal of the American Dietetic Association.* But food grown in Australia is not necessarily the same as food grown in North America. What's more, the salicylate content of a food is not necessarily a key to which ones are likely to trigger reactions in any particular person.

To further complicate the whole issue, a person can be extremely sensitive to one or two of the salicylate foods, and be able to tolerate the rest. It also makes a difference whether the food is fresh or processed, and salicylate content can vary among different varieties of the same fruit.

The Association collects information on salicylate sensitivity, and makes this available to professionals and the general public. Using the old fashioned technique of an elimination diet, they help people to determine if salicylates are affecting their health, behavior or ability to learn. Fortunately, there are so many non-salicylate foods to enjoy, the temporary removal of some things is not very difficult or restrictive.

What is a Salicylate-free Diet?

Salicylates -- the most puzzling part of the Feingold Program- appear to be capable of causing serious symptoms.

In his book, *Why Your Child Is Hyperactive*, Dr. Feingold described his early work with aspirin-sensitive patients at the Allergy Clinic of the Kaiser-Permanente Medical Center.

"The substance known chemically as acetylsalicylic acid is nonprescription medicine's chief do-it-all. Since the medication is used not only as pure aspirin but also in many other over-the-counter products for cold relief, headache and arthritis, adverse reactions are common. It appears to have a slowly building, accumulative effect, finally exploding into full-blown intolerance."

"Very early in the aspirin studies, we learned from a report by Dr. W.B. Shelly, in the *Journal of the American Medical Association* that a number of foods contain a natural salicylate radical that is not necessarily identical with aspirin but is closely allied in basic structure. These common foods have the potential to induce the same type of adverse reaction caused by the manufactured aspirin."

Researching the salicylates

Dr. Feingold went back to studies conducted in Germany to determine which foods contained naturally occurring salicylates. He also learned that some of the chemicals commonly used in synthetic flavorings contain a salicylate radical. These flavorings were then removed from the "salicylate-free" diet.

Some patients improved, but there were still many who did not, and this puzzled Dr. Feingold.

"Then reports by clinical investigators began appearing in medical literature with indications that tartrazine - FD&C 'Yellow 5' - could cause reactions in aspirin-sensitive patients.... I also reported the same finding from San Francisco, and we discovered the reverse was true, too: aspirin could produce adverse reactions in patients sensitive to Yellow 5. Yet, most important, aspirin and tartrazine are not structurally related."

Refining the diet

After learning this he revised the diet to remove all foods and drugs that contained Yellow 5.

"Then an observation by two London pharmacologists, Drs. John Vane and Sergio Ferreira, came to my attention." Vane and Ferreira found that "compounds with no structural relationship to aspirin could produce reactions in individuals sensitive to this drug."

"I then theorized that among several thousand synthetic chemicals in the food supply, there could be other substances potentially harmful to these particular patients. Though the compounds would in no way resemble aspirin, the chemicals had the ability to cross-react.

"On the basis of this hypothesis, I redesigned the diet once again to include all foods and all drugs that were artificially dyed; all foods and all drugs that were artificially flavored, as well as those containing nature's salicylates.... From that point on, although the responses were not 100 percent on each occasion ... we were overwhelmingly successful in patient management."

Recognizing salicylate/aspirin sensitivity

Salicylate sensitivity may be one of the least recognized and most poorly understood health problems, Feingold volunteers believe.

Professionals who understand aspirin sensitivity are likely to be unaware that natural salicylates (foods which contain a salicylate radical) can be just as troublesome as aspirin. Now that aspirin is no longer routinely given to children it is even more likely that this sensitivity would be unrecognized in the child.

In his early book, *Introduction to Clinical Allergy,* Dr. Feingold described many of the physical reactions the sensitive individual can experience from natural or synthetic salicylates. During the years that have followed, Feingold representatives and the physicians who work with them have been able to add to this body of knowledge. The most valuable source of information has been the experience of our salicylate-sensitive members. This data is now available in the revised version of the *Feingold Handbook.*

Some of the issues covered in the Handbook's section on salicylates are:

- Rating of foods from very high to very low in salicylate content
- Non-food plants and other items which contain salicylate

- Benzoate sensitivity
- Sulphur dioxide sensitivity
- Salicylate sensitivity and beta blockers
- The Australian study on salicylate content of foods
- Bibliography of medical references on salicylates

Making Sense Out of Salicylates

When it comes to salicylates, we have more questions than answers.

The information Dr. Feingold used to identify potentially troublesome foods was old in the 1960s. He found, however, that avoiding foods on this list of salicylates generally produced a good response. Today, little more is known about why certain foods can cause such severe reactions in some people, but we continue to find the original list to be a practical guide.

One theory that would explain the reactions to salicylates is that they produce their own pesticide to deter insects and other predators, and that it is this chemical which triggers reactions in some people.

The degree of sensitivity

This varies enormously among our members. Some people need not restrict salicylates at all, while others can have a profound reaction from the tiniest amount. For some, a reaction occurs in a matter of minutes, while others only react after they have eaten too many salicylates.

Those who are sensitive to salicylates are invariably affected by the synthetic additives we eliminate, and some salicylate sensitive people are also unable to tolerate much sugar.

Your ability to tolerate salicylates may vary depending upon other factors, such as exposure to allergens like pollen and ragweed. You may find that during some seasons salicylate foods are better tolerated.

Which foods are the worst offenders?

While there are too many individual differences to be able to answer with any certainty, volunteers do notice how often raisins are named. Apples are frequently mentioned as well. Many families connect diet and behavior when they see their child react to apple juice. It’s hard to know if this is because apple is a major offender or because the juice is so widely used and consumed in large amounts.

Pineapple and pear

Foods that are considered to be very low in salicylate can be troublesome for an occasional person. Fresh pineapple appears to be poorly tolerated, but in processing it changes in some way, so that canned and frozen pineapple products are usually fine. (Undiluted pineapple juice has a very strong taste. Add plenty of water so your child will enjoy it and not become tired of it.)

If you haven't tried baby food pear juice, consider adding this to your list. It is available in large bottles in the baby food section of your supermarket. Baby foods are an especially good choice for allergic or sensitive people because the companies are careful to avoid adding other fruits, as is often the case with regular juices. Products sold in health food stores frequently use salicylate fruits in juice blends, cereals, cookies, candy, and vitamins. Salicylate sensitive people should avoid rose hips and acerola berries, which are often added to natural vitamin preparations.

Are organic salicylates better tolerated?

Some people report this to be the case. If you have access to organic or homegrown fruits/vegetables raised without pesticides, these are good foods to use when you introduce salicylates. If you have reacted to a food in the past and are brave enough to try it again in organic form, you *might* be able to handle it. If your salicylate reaction is severe, however, we encourage you to avoid the food in any form.

Does salicylate sensitivity go away?

Most members (but not all) find that as they follow the Program over an extended period, their sensitivities diminish. Don't look for a change until after you have been on the Program for at least a year.

One of the best reasons for starting the Program when a child is young is so that by the time he is out on his own at the mall, he will be able to enjoy catsup and pizza along with his friends.

If you've ever thought, "a little bit of salicylate can't hurt," read this.

What can you do to help a bright child who is doing badly in school, whose grades are slipping, who drives his teacher to distraction with constant fidgeting and inability to focus?

Jerry was in fifth grade, having problems academically and getting Ds in behavior. The approaches generally recommended had all been tried: testing, counseling, behavior modification, classroom modifications, medication; but nothing was working.

He had received counseling, and by the time he was ten was seeing both a psychologist and a psychiatrist. Ritalin was tried and he had what his mother, Debra, describes as a "horrendous reaction."

In her search for answers, Debra had heard about the Feingold Program and decided to give it a try. When she told the psychiatrist this, he became very upset, urging her to forget about diet and try additional behavior-modifying drugs instead.

The family's diet was already remarkably pure. Debra cooks virtually everything from scratch and they use either homegrown or organic foods for most of their diet. It's easy to wonder what on earth the Feingold Program could offer. "Raisins and grapes." What Debra learned was that these were the two foods that were setting Jerry off. He had them often, and they were responsible for both the behavior and learning problems he had experienced for so long.

They began the Program during the second half of fifth grade, and in the last grading period Jerry's grades were all A's and B's, with a B in behavior! His academic success has continued and Jerry is now doing well in junior high school. He stays away from raisins, grapes, and the additives, but tolerates the other salicylates.

One of the biggest benefits for this bright young man was his success with karate. Jerry loved it, but was unable to advance to black belt status. In order to achieve this high level, the students must pass a test that requires them to sit on their knees, virtually motionless while each student performs. The testing period lasts for approximately four hours.

Not only did Jerry successfully complete this test and receive his black belt, but his parents have it on videotape. Friends who knew Jerry "before Feingold" didn't believe it until they saw the tape!

Salicylate sensitivity can take many forms

What had been mild asthmatic symptoms changed to violent attacks eight years ago after Sharon ate at a salad bar. Sulfites were being used liberally then, and they set her up for many other sensitivities, including reactions to salicylates.

Much of Sharon's time was being spent in a hospital, and trips to the emergency room became a weekly occurrence. She was tested for sulfite sensitivity, and despite the fact that she is highly sensitive, the tests came out negative. To make matters worse, Sharon later learned the medicine she was taking was preserved with sulfites.

Even the slightest exertion was too much for Sharon; she couldn't walk from her car to the front door without becoming exhausted. Finally, her pulmonary specialist told her, "There's nothing else I can do for you."

Eventually, a physician gave Sharon a list of foods to avoid, and she recognized they were natural salicylates. She was aware of the Feingold Association from her days as a school nurse, and called the New York office.

Combining the Feingold Program with avoidance of sulfites has enabled Sharon to lead an active, healthy life. Daily medication is still needed because the years of asthmatic attacks damaged her lungs, but with a small maintenance dose and the Feingold Program she walks 5 to 6 miles a day and leads a busy life.

After being dismissed for claiming that additives and salicylates were triggering her attacks, Sharon says, “My doctors now believe me. They listen with both ears!”

Some of the reactions she notes to salicylates are: congestion, coughing and wheezing, and swollen lips. Some salicylates are real troublemakers for her -- especially tea and fresh pineapple -- but the rest are tolerated if she doesn’t overdo them.

Sharon takes great pains to avoid sulfur in any form, including fresh shrimp and scallops washed in a sulfite solution. Corn oil and corn syrup also bring about a sulfur reaction as they are treated with this chemical. She isn’t allergic to corn, however.

Her diet is more limited than the typical Feingold member, but she’s philosophical about it. “Without the help I received, I would be wheelchair-bound and hooked up to oxygen...or dead!”

Sharon has long known about the connection between additives and behavior. As a school nurse, she kept a record of accidents and found that during the week after Halloween, the number of injuries sustained by the school children increased 300%! When she pointed this out to the administrators the reaction was...nothing.

Chris

For Chris, salicylates bring on congestion and involuntary muscular movements. Apples and oranges seem to be a particular problem, but she tolerates them better when they are cooked, rather than raw. Interestingly, aspirin and medications containing aspirin don’t bring on a reaction.

Chris has a much worse reaction from the synthetic dyes. For as long as she can remember, she suffered from night terrors, and it wasn’t until she put her son on the program and began using it herself that Chris connected her sleep disturbances with additives. If she eats something with dye, the symptoms return.

Bonnie
For most Feingolders a salicylate reaction can be uncomfortable or very annoying; for Bonnie it can be life threatening.

"My sister told me several years ago the Feingold diet would help Bonnie's behavior and school performance," Bonnie's mom, Judy, told *Pure Facts*, "but I wasn't ready to make the effort. Then when she was 11, Bonnie had a severe reaction to one Bufferin, and the allergist told us to remove all salicylates. He said one bite of the wrong food could be fatal for her."

She is 13 now, and Bonnie finds that she can do a small amount of experimenting, but the reaction is still bad enough that she doesn't have much incentive to go off the diet. Judy bought her daughter a medical bracelet, with instructions inside in case Bonnie should have a reaction and need medical care. This has been a big help in gaining understanding and acceptance from those around her. (Medical bracelets can be purchased at drug and jewelry stores.)

*****

Vitamin C and Stage One

One of the early objections raised to the Feingold diet was that the temporary removal of oranges would lead to a deficiency of vitamin C. Unbelievably, some even suggested that a few weeks without orange juice could lead to scurvy! (The critics were apparently unaware of the fact that lemons and limes -- both non-salicylates -- were commonly used in Britain to prevent scurvy.) Well, it turns out that there are plenty of good sources of vitamin C among the fruits and vegetables allowed on Stage One. In fact, in comparison to some tropical fruits, oranges aren't so impressive.

See the last section of this book for a listing of the vitamin C content of many foods.

FOODS - FROM BREAD TO WINE

Breads and Bakery Products

Breads and dairy products tend to be produced regionally, often by small companies. This makes it difficult to research all the different brands available.

Brown breads and yellow breads

Those dark, rich looking loaves may have a little secret. It is common practice for bakers to add colorings to what is essentially white bread in order to make it look like it is made with whole-wheat flour. If the first ingredient in the list is not "whole wheat flour," then it isn't really a bona fide whole-wheat loaf.

The added coloring in dark breads is likely to be caramel (probably a relatively natural ingredient, but we've been fooled before) or raisin syrup, a salicylate which would place the product in Stage Two.

The most important thing to remember with breads, as well as pastries and rolls, is to stay away from anything that is obviously yellow. Egg bread, or challah, egg bagels, even potato rolls or pastries which look like they are loaded with egg yolks almost certainly are not! Ingredient labels should note Yellow No. 5 or No. 6 if it is present, but supermarket bakery products sold from a glass display case don't come with ingredients, so keep walking past them.

Flour

Plain 'ol flour -- white, whole wheat, rye or whatever -- should not be any problem (unless you have an allergy or gluten intolerance). If you do use white flour, consider looking for unbleached; this way you will eliminate some unnecessary chemicals.

...and all those funny things added to it

Most of the odd names found on bread packages are vitamins added to fortify the refined flour. Thiamine mononitrate is not at all the same as the nitrites added to hot dogs, bacon, etc. Calcium propionate, the preservative generally added to bread, does not seem to be a problem for the majority of Feingold members.

A few people report they are unable to tolerate the small amount of corn syrup often used in bread.

Corn syrup

If the sweetener used is corn syrup, it should be listed on the ingredient label. Some Feingold members are highly sensitive to corn syrup, but do not have any problem with corn itself. In order to manufacture corn syrup, cornstarch must go through a series of chemical treatments, and we have long suspected that it picks up residues of these potent chemicals used in processing.

Even if it turns out that there is a corn syrup sensitivity, you might not pick this up in the early days of the diet. Most families identify it later when they fine tune things. But if there is a corn syrup sensitivity that you believe is quite severe, you will need to avoid even the small amount found in most bread. Corn syrup can often be avoided by using health food bread, French, pita or other non-traditional breads, as well as homemade.

Calcium propionate

Most breads and commercial bakery products contain a preservative called calcium propionate. Because it is a preservative, Feingold members routinely avoided it in the early days. The industry claims that it is a harmless substance didn't impress us; these were the same people who said dyes and flavorings are safe, and BHT somehow evaporates when a product is heated. (Then why use it in the first place?) But after many loaves, including quite a few which were preserved with calcium propionate, we have relatively few reports of children who are sensitive to this additive.

BHA, BHT, TBHQ

Preservatives can be hidden in the shortening, oil or pan grease. This will generally be one of the above antioxidants. Of course, if you like French bread, pita, and other varieties that are made without shortening, you can assume they are less likely to contain these additives.

The grease bakers use to treat the baking pans are notorious for containing TBHQ, but don't expect the baker to have this information handy. He will need to check the ingredient label found on the pan grease, or call his supplier to learn what is in it.

Once you have some experience on the Program you may want to test out breads to determine which ones you like and which are tolerated. You may want to ask the Product Information Committee to research a local brand, or you can phone the bakery and ask about hidden preservatives.

Questions for the baker

1. Do you use any synthetic coloring or artificial flavoring in the bread?
2. Does either the shortening or oil used contain BHA, BHT or TBHQ?
3. Are any of these antioxidants found in the pan grease?

The bakery around the corner

It may look like everything is made in the back by master bakers in flour-dusted white aprons, but don't bet the farm on it. Most traditional local bakeries use mixes and prepared components and simply assemble them. Bakeries which do *real* baking are found in some areas, so these would be well worth investigating once you are an old-timer with several months of successful experience behind you, but this is not recommended for the newcomer.

Health food stores & healthy markets

Just because your supermarket or bakery makes its own bread, that is no guarantee that it will be free of the unwanted additives. But if you're lucky enough to live near a well stocked health food store, or one of the attractive "healthy markets" such as Fresh Fields, Whole Foods, Wild Oats, Wellspring, etc., chances are you will find bread as pure as what you would make yourself.

Actually, it's not a bad idea. If you have serious dietary restrictions, or just love the aroma of fresh bread, consider hinting for a bread machine as a holiday gift.

Candy

In the 1970s there were quite a few brand name candies which were acceptable on the Feingold Program. As small companies were bought up by larger ones, synthetic chemicals were added and the choices narrowed.

The good news is that there are other companies that have filled the need, and there's plenty you can do at home (with very little time and effort required). At press time the Feingold *Foodlists* contain brands of candies which are natural versions of some of the old favorites: M&M's, Snickers, as well as gummy candies and bubble gum. Some natural candies are available through health food or specialty stores; others can be mail ordered.

Natural candy your kids will love

Before you dismiss the prospect of health food candy, take another look. Years ago all of the candy sold in such stores tasted like peanut butter, carob, dates, or even cardboard! They've come a long way, baby! Using newly developed sweeteners, as well as real chocolate, many of them taste as decadent as anything you'll find at the corner convenience store. One skeptical eleven-year-old sampled a natural version of one of the popular candy bars and told his mom, "This tastes too good to be good for you!" [Even the natural candies couldn't really be called "good for you," but they certainly take away any thoughts of deprivation!]

Today you can locate natural lollypops that are brightly colored, hard candies, and peppermint candies. They look like the artificial versions, but one difference is that the bright coloring is not permanent; it will gradually fade with exposure to the light. The candy you get from the bank, on the other hand, is immortal. You and I will be long gone and it will look just the same.

Diet candies, dried fruit, and old time sweets

Beware of diet candies, which usually contain all sorts of no-nos. If you use candy that is sweetened with sorbitol, don't let your child overdo it since too much sorbitol will cause diarrhea.

While it's true that most children won't be fooled into believing that dried fruits are candies, two exceptions are dried pineapple and papaya. If you can find the very sweet versions of these, that still have retained their attractive color, you'll probably agree that they are a good choice. Cut a spear of papaya into small pieces, and it will look like colorful orange gummy candy. If your family likes fruitcake during the holidays, the papaya and pineapple can be used in homemade fruitcake, in place of those dreadful dyed cherries.

In addition to the "new wave" candies, there are some old fashioned sweets that you may want to watch for, such as maple sugar and white rock candies. The section of your supermarket that stocks baking supplies generally has at least one form of sweetened chocolate which can double as candy.

If you're a chocoholic (like I am) you can make candy without the need for special equipment and expertise; all you need is some natural chocolate and a microwave oven.

Melt an acceptable brand of chocolate chips, or bar, or melting wafers in a small bowl in the microwave oven. Check the chocolate often, and stir it to see if it has melted. Chocolate chips will melt, while still holding their original shape. If you think they haven't melted yet, and keep zapping them, you'll end up with charred chocolate and a bad smell in the kitchen. (Trust me, this is the voice of experience speaking.) To thin the melted chocolate add a small amount of solid shortening, such as original Crisco [acceptable at press time; check your *Foodlist*].

This melted chocolate can be the basis for many treats:
- Dip pretzels in, and set them on a piece of waxed paper to harden.
- Coat banana pieces, strawberries (salicylate), or other fruits.
- Stir in your favorite nuts or seeds; drop by the spoonful onto waxed paper.
- Stir in puffed cereal or dried fruits as well.
- A plain cookie can be dipped to make it extra special.
- How about crackers? Even they can be dipped.

Natural peanut butter cups:

Use tiny foil baking cups (available where candy-making supplies are sold and in some craft shops). Fill the cup half way with the melted chocolate, tilting the little cup to coat the sides with chocolate. Put in a bit of peanut butter and then add more chocolate to reach the top of the cup. Allow to harden.

Chocoholics reprieve

Many people who believe they are allergic to chocolate are really reacting to the synthetic vanilla (called 'vanillin') which is used in most chocolate products.

The good news is that there are chocolates available without the cheaper imitation flavoring. Generally you're more likely to find dark chocolate to be free of any vanilla flavoring -- natural or synthetic. While this is not always the case, it's worth checking the labels of dark chocolates to be sure no vanillin is listed.

Considering the wonderful reputation Swiss chocolate enjoys, you'd think this is the perfect product for a Feingold member. Unfortunately, the Swiss have a harder time finding pure chocolate than Americans do! And be suspicious of the labels on imported chocolate products; they are likely to be less accurate than those used in the U.S.

Canned Foods

Since canning preserves foods, they generally do not contain added preservatives. An exception is the BHA or BHT added to lard that is often found in canned refried beans. So, canned peas or pineapple are probably going to be fairly pure, whereas canned soups, gravy or pasta dishes might contain unwanted additives. Even health food soups often have undesirable flavor enhancers – labeled as yeast, yeast extract or autolyzed yeast.

Cereals -- Snap, Crackle, and ... BHT?

In conducting our product information research, ready-to-eat cereals are among the most difficult foods to learn about.

It's easy enough to avoid the fluorescent sugarcoated concoctions that glare out at us from supermarket shelves. Synthetic dyes and flavorings can generally be found on the ingredient label. It's the antioxidant preservatives that cause problems for the Feingold label reader.

Despite the seemingly endless variety on the cereal aisle, there are only a few basic products. The majority of cereals are made from one of the following grains: corn, wheat, rice or oats. What appears to be a wide variety simply represents variations on a theme.

When these grains are milled, naturally occurring antioxidants are lost, and food processors replace them with synthetic ones such as BHA, BHT and TBHQ -- which are prohibited on the Feingold Program. In a conversation with an executive of a major cereal company, *Pure Facts* learned that the need for antioxidants depends in part, upon which type of grain is used. In the milling of wheat, for example, it is fairly easy to separate out the germ. This is the portion that is highest in nutrients, but it also is richest in oil, making it vulnerable to spoilage (oxidation). When oat grains are milled it's difficult to remove the germ. Consequently, the oils are released, natural preserving agents are lost, and the flour is more susceptible to spoilage.

In some products, BHA or BHT is added directly to the foods, but many cereal manufacturers prefer to treat the packaging (the inside of the bag containing the cereal). This allows the chemical to slowly migrate into the cereal. The use of antioxidants raises interesting issues. Manufacturers see them in a positive light - protecting the food from spoilage. Some consumers counter that the antioxidants are added to protect the manufacturer. By prolonging the shelf life of cereal, the company does not lose money through spoilage.

The health food cereals

If you're on Stage One the biggest problem will be avoiding salicylates, both those added as fruit pieces, and salicylate juices used as a sweetener. Another impression to reconsider is that health food cereal will cost more than supermarket brands, but this isn't necessarily so.

Much too sweet!

Consider mixing types of cereals to provide variety or reduce the amount of sweetener your child ingests. Add some sweet cereal to some bland flakes or puffs, and you may just hit on a winning combination.

Breakfast isn't just cereal

See the section on beginning the program, and check *The Feingold Handbook* for a wide variety of breakfast ideas. Anything nourishing and edible is fair game for the day's first meal.

Cheese

Most white cheeses are acceptable. Ingredients should read: milk, enzymes, salt, calcium chloride.

Pizza Cheese

The labeling of cheese products gets especially confusing in frozen pizza. If you buy a "cheese" pizza with imitation cheese, it must say "imitation cheese" on the front of the package along with the name. But if you buy a sausage pizza, mushroom pizza, etc., and it contains imitation cheese, this information may be hidden in the fine print of the ingredient label.

Coffee

Since coffee is a salicylate, it is not included in the first phase of the Feingold Program (Stage One). The good news is that if you are using the Program primarily to help a child, you don't need to give up your favorite brew. For the salicylate-sensitive adult, it would be best to try to get along without it for a little while. There are grain-based drinks that some people consider an acceptable substitute. Others will be satisfied with hot chocolate. If it's the caffeine that is missing from your life, there are other "delivery systems" – bottled water with caffeine added and those little white pills we all tried in college when we needed to stay awake and study for an exam.

If you just can't face the world without that java, don't give up on the whole thing. Go ahead and have your coffee, but avoid all of the other salicylates and the no-no additives. Your results might not be as good, but your nerves will handle it all better.

Make it Yourself -- Donuts!

"My boys always wanted donuts 'with holes' instead of the drop donuts I made. We have no natural donuts here, and it was such a chore to make them from scratch."

Feingold mom, Gayle Cloud continues, "Now I make them from frozen dinner rolls so we can have donuts any time."

- Defrost as many as needed. (You can defrost them in a minute or so by using the microwave oven.)
- Flatten the dough with a rolling pin or by hand, then cut with a donut cutter.
- Allow them to rise until they have nearly doubled in size, about 30 minutes or so, depending on the room temperature.
- Fry them in hot fat (365 degrees) until they are light brown on both sides. Drain on a rack. Coat each with powdered sugar or frost tops with a glaze.

By the way, don't forget to fry the "holes" too!

Other inventive Feingold moms have reported they use an acceptable brand of ready-to-bake biscuits (found in the refrigerator section of the supermarket) to make doughnuts. Cut out a center hole and fry in oil.

Fats & Oils

Animal fat- lard, beef fat, chicken fat- These generally are preserved with BHA or BHT, so if you see them on ingredient labels you can assume there is a hidden antioxidant.

Butter- although it often contains added color, the source of the coloring is generally annatto or carotene, which are well tolerated.

Oils that are used in commercially prepared products often contain BHA or BHT, and sometimes TBHQ. But it is not hard to find oils and shortenings in the supermarket that are free of these additives.

Frying oils used in restaurants- The major chains have switched from an oil that was preserved with proply gallate (which was well tolerated) to oils with TBHQ. This signaled the end of fries and chicken nuggets for Feingold kids.

Margarine- Oddly enough, it isn't the coloring that is likely to keep that supermarket margarine out of your shopping cart, but the artificial flavoring. Typically, margarines are colored with an acceptable substance. Health food stores and markets often have natural alternatives.

Pan sprays, pan grease- More manufacturers are bringing out pan sprays that are free of synthetic antioxidants, so you might be able to find several acceptable brands.

Commercial bakeries have a choice between pan grease with and without BHT. They don't always make the best choice!

Shortening- Here again, you can find suitable choices in the supermarket, but manufacturers often opt for the version with additives.

Something's Fishy

Many Americans are eating "surimi," Japanese fish paste, and most of them probably don't know it.

Surimi can be disguised as various highly priced seafoods at a fraction of the cost. A blend of inexpensive white fish and additives is the material that forms the growing number of shellfish analogs (imitations). In some cases real crabmeat, shrimp or lobster are incorporated into the mixture, which is glued together with egg white and starch before being molded and dyed. Surimi enthusiasts do not believe the future of this product is limited to seafood. They envision surimi-based cold cuts, pasta, eggs, and ice cream.

Synthetically colored/flavored seafood presents a particular problem for Feingold members. Served in a salad, hot dish, or on display at the fish counter, it generally carries no ingredient label. The average consumer would have no way of knowing he is eating a low-priced fish paste with crabmeat flavoring ... whatever that is!

Flour

Plain flours are allowed on the Feingold Program. This includes white, rye, whole wheat, as well as all the varieties made from different grains (and even from vegetables). Nutritionally, whole wheat is preferred over white, and unbleached is more desirable than bleached; but all of them are acceptable.

Milk - Looking for Lowfat

It generally comes as a shock to health-conscious families that the lowfat milk they use contains hidden preservatives in the vitamin A palmitate.

The added BHA, BHT or TBHQ is not required to be listed since the Food and Drug Administration considers it to be an unimportant "incidental" additive. The reactions it triggers are far from incidental, however, especially when it is consumed daily.

Unlike cereals or potato chips, researching milk is far more difficult. There are thousands of dairies in this country, and this industry has traditionally been exempted from the same labeling laws that apply to other food suppliers. Dairymen are not accustomed to listing which of the various additives are used in their product.

The FAUS Product Information Committee researches lowfat milks to identify those free of the preservatives. As a result of this work, and the awareness it brought, some major vitamin suppliers are switching to vitamin E as a preservative. To locate suitable brands of lowfat milks check your Foodlist and watch for updates in the Feingold newsletters.

Picnic Time, Pickle Time

Searching for the perfect, additive free pickle can be discouraging for someone wishing to avoid Yellow No. 5.

One of our adult members wrote to a pickle company in North Carolina, asking why they did not offer products free of yellow dye. She received this response:

"*Our pickle recipes are based upon a product mix found in homemade-old-fashioned pickles. Many of the ingredients used in the old days would be extremely expensive if used today. Therefore, we use safe, approved, and cost effective alternatives. This allows us to sell our product at reasonable competitive prices.*"

In other words, they use an old fashioned recipe, but don't use the ingredients in the recipe. (?)

Let's take a look at some of the "extremely expensive" ingredients to which they refer. Pat Palmer shared her grandmother's recipe that she uses today. Here are her recipe's "extremely expensive" ingredients: unwaxed cucumbers, onions, garlic, dill seeds or fresh dill, Heinz white vinegar, water, and kosher salt. It's hard to imagine being able to make a dill pickle without any of these (inexpensive) ingredients. What ingredient would the pickle company leave out?

The letter further explained that they use yellow dye. *"FD&C Yellow #5 has undergone years of extensive testing and has been shown to be safe. It does cause an asthmatic reaction in a very small percentage of the population. However, many foods, such as chocolate or even milk can cause such a reaction in some people."*

The adult member who inquired has found that the "safe" FD&C Yellow #5 triggered major health problems that had caused her frequent hospitalizations.

"FD&C Yellow #5 is the best available agent for stabilizing color in pickles. It prevents the fluorescent lights in grocery stores from bleaching the natural color of our cucumbers. Without it, our products would look very pale and unappetizing, so much so that consumers would not buy them."

Health food stores use fluorescent lights as well, but find that their dye-free pickles hold up fine.

Rice

Any supermarket will have a variety of good choices. Plain white or brown rice are fine, but there are also quick cooking versions that are free of the unwanted additives. Where you find the questionable ingredients will be in the pilafs and flavored rice mixes. Even health food stores carry rice mixes with disguised MSG.

Soft Drinks

One of the common misconceptions about the Feingold Program is that it banishes all sodas. Most families limit their child's consumption at home, but allow occasional treats when they are away from home. Let's face it, when you're at the mall, there may be few choices.

Veteran Feingolders have tolerated regular Coca Cola and Pepsi Cola (not diet colas) for years. You won't find these products on the Foodlists because the companies will not fill out our detailed inquiry forms, (secrecy is very big in the cola industry) but they do appear in the Fast Food pamphlet the Association compiles. Regular (not cherry flavored or diet) 7UP has also been a mainstay for many Feingold families.

Soft drinks are generally labeled clearly, so you can be on the lookout for things like imitation vanilla flavoring in root beer. Of course, if the beverage is a day-glo color, you know not to even bother scanning the label.

There are many delicious health food sodas now on the market, but the main issue with them will be salicylate-based sweeteners (white grape juice, etc.) For the family on Stage Two, there's a world of delicious flavors.

New sweeteners are being developed, including low calorie products, that *might* prove to be well tolerated; as this book goes to press, it is still too early to know. Please check future issues of *Pure Facts*.

The Feingold Program and Sugars

When a colleague asked Dr. Feingold why he didn't add sugar to the list of forbidden substances he quipped, "I think I've already bitten off more than I can chew!"

Many people assume the Feingold Program forbids sugar; others criticize it because it permits sugar. But for most families the reality is somewhere in between. Soft drinks are an occasional treat, not an everyday beverage. Desserts are served only after a nourishing meal. And servings of candy are small and rather infrequent.

The majority of children who begin the Feingold Program are accustomed to highly sweetened foods. Gaining and keeping their cooperation is essential for success on the diet. After the child's behavior improves and he feels better in general, he will be more receptive to learning about good nutrition.

Elimination of several categories of synthetic additives is the primary focus of the Feingold Program. However, there are ways to cut back on sugar intake without making major changes in the family's lifestyle.

- The sugar in most recipes can be reduced by one quarter to one third with no noticeable change.
- If an extremely sweet dessert is served, make the portions small.
- Timing is important. Sweets on an empty stomach can bring about a not-so-sweet behavioral reaction. But the same treat eaten after a nourishing meal may cause no problem at all.
- Whipped cream, sweetened with a little confectioner's sugar, makes a good frosting. Cream cheese frosting is a good choice. Like the whipped cream, it doesn't require much sugar, but the cream cheese frosting will keep much longer.
- A sprinkle of powdered sugar makes a cake look like it has been frosted; eventually the family may become accustomed to doing without the frosting altogether.

- Bananas, dates, and coconut juice are some sources of natural sweetening; and applesauce or pear sauce doesn't need sugar to taste delicious.
- Each time you make an apple or pear pie, try reducing the sugar a bit. You may find it much more flavorful.
- Sugar may be better tolerated if you combine it with a protein source, such as peanut butter, nuts, seeds, cheese. For example, the cream cheese and eggs in a cheesecake help to balance the sugar content.

Can sugar cause hyperactivity?

"My little boy became hyperactive after eating a candy bar," the father wrote to a psychologist whose syndicated column appears in many newspapers. The columnist's response was that "recent studies indicate sugar doesn't cause hyperactivity." This reflects the common misconception that candy bars and sugar are the same.

"Candy" and "Sugar"

In our culture, these two words are frequently used interchangeably, but there is an enormous difference between them.

While sugar is a fairly simple substance, candy is generally composed of many compounds, both natural and synthetic. In addition to sugar, some candies contain synthetic dyes, artificial flavorings and one or more of the antioxidant preservatives eliminated by the Feingold Program. Glazes, gums, emulsifiers, etc. are often used as well.

To equate "sugar" with "candy" is like saying a string bean is the same as vegetable soup.

Studies on sugar and hyperactivity

The double blind British study by Egger and colleagues indicated that only 16% of the hyperactive children tested reacted to sugar. In addition, thc parents of several other children in the study felt their child reacted to sugar when he ate a great deal of it. The experience of Feingold volunteers supports these findings. When too many sweets are consumed, the parents report their child's behavior changes for the worse. A few children are very sensitive to sugar and/or other sweeteners, but most can tolerate them in moderation.

A study conducted at Children's Hospital in Washington, DC supported another Feingold observation -- sugars seem to be tolerated by most children if they are eaten after a nourishing meal.

Some studies claim to demonstrate that there is no link at all between sugar and hyperactive behavior. One that is widely quoted was conducted by Mark L. Wolraich at the University of Iowa. (Funding was provided by the Sugar Associates, Inc., and the National Institutes of Health.)

Feingold members will readily see some of the serious flaws in the design of this study:

- The hyperactive children being tested were taken off behavior-modifying drugs only 24 hours before the beginning of the study. (Dr. Feingold observed that it could take as long as 30-40 days for a child to be free of the effects of the drugs.)
- The control drinks were sweetened with aspartame (NutraSweetTM) which has been linked with neurological disorders, and could affect behavior.
- The drink given to the subjects was KOOL AIDTM, containing two of the additives found by Feingold members to be capable of triggering severe behavioral reactions: synthetic dyes and artificial flavorings.

1994 sugar study

A later study from the University of Iowa was published in the *New England Journal of Medicine.* Following a press conference, the study was covered in newspapers and on TV news throughout the United States. The stories were taken from the press release given out to reporters, and it does not appear that any of those reporters read the actual study.

Background: In 1989 researchers at the University of Iowa, under the direction of Dr. Wolraich, announced they would be initiating a major study to investigate how food ingredients, including synthetic dyes, preservatives, aspartame (NutraSweetTM), and sugar affect a child's behavior and school performance.

The study design had been changed when the conclusion was finally published in 1994. Synthetic dyes and preservatives were no longer important factors and the study became a test of sugar and aspartame.

Area newspapers originally reported that the research would include 80 children and last for 16 weeks, but the researchers had difficulty finding 80 families to participate. It was later announced that the study would last just 9 weeks and be composed of 24 children diagnosed as having attention deficit disorder with hyperactivity (ADHD), and an equal number with no such symptoms. The final study contained only 5 hyperactive children.

The $600,000 project was to be sponsored by the Institute of Child Health and Human Development of the National Institutes of Health, with funding help from the International Life Sciences Institute. The ILSI is composed of the major food, pharmaceutical and additive industries, including the Sugar Association and manufacturers of synthetic sweeteners.

Although many newspapers reported the study as eliminating "artificial color or additives" this was not the case. The authors wrote, "all the diets were *essentially* free of additives..." [emphasis added]. Then in the study they wrote that additives were "kept to a minimum." This is a far cry from the Feingold Program, but it's interesting that the researchers knew these chemicals could affect the children.

The quantity of sugar given to the children when they were being challenged was surprisingly small, and it was given throughout the day, not in one dose.

The most important result of the study did not make any news reports. The researchers wrote, "...behavior ratings and test scores generally improved during the dietary periods, as compared with the base-line values." In other words, the biggest dietary change was the removal of many synthetic additives. When the children were eating fewer additives their behavior and learning improved.

What Dr. Feingold recommended

Dr. Feingold noted: "The quantity of any sugar that causes hyperactivity will vary from child to child." He advised parents to keep a diet diary to determine their child's tolerance. He also recommended parents avoid giving sugars on an empty stomach when they are more rapidly absorbed. He did not single out any type of sweetener (such as honey, fructose, raw sugar, maple syrup, etc.) as more desirable than another, and believed that most people consume too many of these.

The many different sugars

Not only does the quantity of sugars tolerated vary from one Feingold member to the next, the type of sugars varies as well. Many successfully use white granulated or confectioner's sugar, while others do best with honey. The salicylate-sensitive member may be likely to have problems with one or more varieties of honeys.

Other sweeteners

Corn sweeteners and corn syrup are widely used in foods because they are less expensive than sugar. Unfortunately, they cause problems for many Feingold members, especially those who are new to the Program. Since these people can generally tolerate corn in other forms, it is not believed to be an allergic reaction.

Food chemists are working on the development of several new synthetic sweeteners: acesulfame K, sucrolose, alitame and Lactitol. Abbott Laboratories, who manufactures cyclamate, has petitioned the Food & Drug Administration to allow them to once again market this sweetener. Cyclamate was banned in 1970 after tests showed a mixture of cyclamate and saccharine caused cancer in laboratory animals.

Dr. Feingold felt that in the absence of studies that could demonstrate the safety of synthetic sweeteners, chemically sensitive individuals should avoid them.

Sucanat

This is made from dehydrated sugar cane juice. It looks somewhat like brown sugar, but provides a taste to baked goods, which is similar to white sugar. It is available in health food stores, and is used as a sweetener in many natural products.

Tea

The issue here is not that tea is likely to contain additives, but that it is a natural salicylate. However, teas can be made from various plants, and if you miss that steaming brew, a mint or chamomile version would be worth trying; some salicylate sensitive people tolerate these.

When you are ready to move on to begin reintroducing salicylates, there are many teas, and even some instant ones, that should be suitable.

A Sour Story about Vinegar

At a local Feingold board meeting, a dish was served which contained white vinegar. Three of the chemically sensitive adults attending developed severe headaches late that evening and were laid-up for the entire next day.

Unwilling to attribute the reactions to bad cooking, the hostess came up with the following item by Beatrice Trum Hunter:

"White vinegar is made from grain based alcohol.... Some of the white vinegar is made from alcohol derived from natural gas or petroleum derivatives. However, vinegar manufacturers need not label the source of the alcohol...and consumers cannot know the source. The Vinegar Institute, an association of vinegar manufacturers, questions whether there is actually a valid distinction between grain based or petroleum-based white vinegar. An official of the Institute was quoted as saying 'If you go back far enough, petroleum is natural too.'"

These sensitive adults had been successfully using Heinz white vinegar, which lists grains as the source of their product. The vinegar used in the dish served at the board meeting was a store brand with little information listed.

Wine

Feingold adults on Stage Two may find it difficult to obtain information on ingredients in wine. Like all alcoholic beverages, wines are under the jurisdiction of the Bureau of Alcohol, Tobacco & Firearms, and are not subject to the same labeling regulations as other food products.

Consumer groups have fought for many years to persuade the government to require ingredient labeling on alcoholic beverages.

On several occasions, mandatory labeling has been announced, only to be squelched by industry influence. In one memorable case the alcoholic beverage industry managed to have the judicial proceedings moved to Bourbon County, Kentucky. Guess which side won!

Although wines may legally contain synthetic dyes, artificial flavorings and anti-oxidant preservatives, it is unlikely that they are used. The additives most likely to be a problem are sulfiting agents, which function as a preservative in many wines. Sulfites occur naturally as the wine ferments. Federal law requires wines to state "contains sulfites," but only if there are more than 10 parts per million. Amounts below that are assumed to be safe, even for sulfite sensitive people. Wines bottled prior to 1987 are not covered by the regulation, and should be avoided by the sulfite-sensitive. Feingold members who are asthmatic are advised to avoid sulfites, but other members might not be affected.

Of the 500 million gallons of wine sold in the United States each year, about one percent is made from organically grown grapes. The amount of acreage being converted to organic farming is growing quickly, and organic, low sulfite and no-sulfite wines are becoming increasingly easy to find.

The Feingold Program does not require one eat organic foods, nor does it eliminate sulfites, but many members prefer to avoid pesticides and preservatives whenever possible. If a winery goes to the expense of using organic grapes, and goes to the trouble of avoiding/reducing sulfites, there's a good chance the wine will be free of unnecessary additives. If you have access to a natural food supermarket, you might find the wine you want there. But don't overlook the traditional places where wine is sold; many carry a small selection of organic or no-sulfite brands.

PIC research on wines

The FAUS Product Information Committee (PIC) is not conducting research on organic wines. There are too many varieties available, and they change every year. If you are on Stage Two and find you are able to tolerate grape juice, you may be ready to try out some wine.

A sulfite-free or low-sulfite organic wine would be a good choice. Test it as you would any salicylate.

Best choices for Feingolders

Since it is not possible to obtain accurate information about alcoholic beverages, Feingold adults should use caution. Products that appear on a Feingold Foodlist would be the best choice since this means the manufacturer provided detailed information on the product.

Members report that, as a rule, they tolerate the imported beers and wines better than domestic U.S. brands. Vodka appears to be the best tolerated of the hard liquors.

Dr. Feingold's comments on children and alcohol

"We know that alcoholic beverages are extremely important factors influencing the behavior of not only adolescents but even for children as low as the 7th, 8th and 9th grades of school. I feel what happens is this: The violent, uncontrollable behavior of the adolescent or preadolescent following a single drink cannot be attributed to the alcohol alone but to the additives present in practically all alcoholic beverages. Most people are not aware that alcoholic beverages... are loaded with various additive chemicals, of which we have absolutely no knowledge."

Ben F. Feingold, M.D. in an address before the New York State Assembly Standing Committee on Child Care - May 1981.

PART THREE

COPING SKILLS

"I Used to Hate Cooking"

When Sharon took an aptitude test in college, cooking wasn't even on the chart. In fact, she recalls, this skill was two inches of it.

But as the mother of three young children she feels different about the time spent in her kitchen. With children, unanticipated events have a way of popping up, and a treat is often required. Sharon has the option of packing the kids in the car, unloading them at the store to hunt for something decent, reloading kids into the car and unpacking them again at the house. That comes to a minimum of 30 minutes on a good day. The alternative is a mere 10 minutes or so, whipping up a pan of brownies, and the taste of homemade can't be compared.

Now that Sharon is doing more cooking, she has decided to view it as an interesting challenge, rather than as an unpleasant obligation. An investment in some good equipment makes cooking much easier, and pays off in lower grocery bills. Then, as long as she's putting the effort into preparing the food, she generally opts for really nourishing ingredients such as whole grains and fresh vegetables. Another money-saving use of Sharon's newly developed skills is giving home baked goods as gifts.

Her family appreciates her efforts. She is becoming known for a delicious but decadent pecan cheesecake -- a departure from the family's generally healthy diet. The children much prefer her pizza, with the hand tossed crust, to anything commercially available. And every Saturday morning they ask for a homemade coffeecake. Sharon says that it takes only about ten minutes to put it together (longer when the children help).

The family likes the fact that they are spending less money on food these days, and has some extra funds to use in other ways. Typically, this family has noticed an improvement in their health. Trips to the doctor's office have been reduced; this is an extra bonus, in addition to other benefits, such as happier children.

Sharon has not developed a love for cooking, but as long as she's doing it she sees no reason to be dreary about the whole thing.

"I still hate to cook"

Nancy was worried about how she was going to manage the Feingold Program, but things had gotten pretty bad and she didn't see any alternative.

Her 4-year-old, Krissy, could change in a flash from calm and sweet to out-of-control. She was extremely destructive in preschool, throwing books and toys, talking back to her teacher, not listening, and generally doing what she wanted, instead of what the rest of the class was doing. It was only a matter of time before she would be expelled. The pediatrician said "It's just a phase," but Nancy knew better and worried for her daughter's future.

At the beginning she found the Feingold Program somewhat confusing, but now that she has been using it for about a year, Nancy says she doesn't even think about it. There are so few changes in the way they eat, that it was hard for Nancy to identify them. Then she recalled: toothpaste, fruit snacks, chewing gum, and children's vitamins were the major changes.

"Krissy likes to eat the same things over and over," her mom recalled, "she ate fish sticks for five weeks!" Now she's on a "waffle kick" and likes them for breakfast, so Nancy buys a brand on her Foodlist, along with approved syrup and juice. Lunch is typically peanut butter sandwiches or cheese sticks, same as always. The major change in dinner is the switch from margarine to butter. A typical dinner for the family is baked chicken or fish, a baked potato, plus canned or frozen vegetables.

Krissy likes being able to choose her own snacks, and Nancy takes her to a health food store where there are so many choices. If they're out shopping, she keeps a snack bar in her purse in case Krissy gets hungry.

When they go out to a restaurant, nobody orders dessert (unless they know it's natural) to support Krissy. The whole family follows the same diet, and Nancy says they all feel better.

Krissy responded to the diet in about five days, and the people who knew her a year ago are impressed at the change. The staff at the preschool has been very supportive, and lets Nancy know when a food event comes up. If another mom will be bringing in cookies or cupcakes, Nancy phones and asks her to use pure vanilla and real butter. None of the mothers have been offended by the request. Nancy does some baking, but generally has no trouble finding prepared treats. In fact, she has to watch that she doesn't overdo the holiday candy.

For Nancy, the Feingold Program translates to reading labels in the supermarket. Krissy is not terribly sensitive, and now that she has been on the program for a year, she is able to expand her diet quite a bit. Nancy would much rather read some labels and bake cookies occasionally than deal with the behavior that kept the family in turmoil. "I used to go to bed crying every night," Nancy recalls, "I never would have survived to this point." She also recalls the anguish her child must have felt for behavior over which she really had no control.

Mulling over what additional changes she would like to see in her five-year-old, the only one Nancy could come up with is, "I'd like to get her to clean her room."

Nancy will never love to cook, but she loves the calm, sweet daughter she now has, and feels, "It's just crazy not to use the diet."

Another way to look at your role of chief cook and bottle washer

After dealing with our everyday challenge of maintaining some order in our homes while trying to keep everybody happy, we rarely have time to stop and think how lucky we are. Yes, we have children who are chemically-sensitive; and dealing with reactions is a burden; and you feel like screaming if you have to supply safe substitutes for birthday party junk one more time this month.

But wait! Remember back, if you can, to how things were before you became aware of all the problems that your child's former diet caused. We tend to forget the frustration we felt at not being able to get any answers to our child's problem, the embarrassment it caused to bring him or her to a friend's home or the hurt that you felt when you thought that you must be doing something wrong. Remember how you felt when there were no birthday party invitations for your child.

Take a moment to think back on those times. If you see an improvement, be very thankful that you found a solution -- it may be one that we have to work at times, but for many of us, we are very thankful that it is there.

The Feingold Program on a tight budget

One mom has found a way to feed her family well, and she relies on food stamps.

Cynthia D. has two children, Jeremy, age 4 and Daniel, a 13-year-old with an appetite that doesn't quit. They follow the Feingold Program and eat well on food stamps totaling $244 a month.

Meat is a big part of any food budget, and the Ds eat a lot of it, especially during the cold months. Cynthia buys economy packages of chicken, pork, etc. she repackages it and freezes the food in smaller portions.

Some foods can be bought in larger size or in quantity when they are on sale, and will keep for a long time. When sugar, oatmeal and chocolate chips go on sale, Cynthia stocks up. Some canned foods are most economical for the family to buy in large size, and when canned vegetables go on sale, a big supply goes into the pantry.

Now that the Ds have been on the Feingold Program for over a year, Cynthia has a good idea of her children's sensitivities, and can do some experimenting. She has found many store brand products the boys can tolerate. They are as much as half the price of the name brands, and taste as good.

By watching the newspaper ads and clipping coupons, Cynthia is able to trim even more off the weekly grocery bill. Turkey sales make this food even more economical. The extra meat is frozen and leftovers become turkey sandwiches or casseroles.

If she runs low on a food, Cynthia has learned to get creative. Four eggs fed six hungry people one morning by making a version of fried rice. She fried some bacon, removed it and sautéed leftover rice and spring onion slices, added soy sauce and scrambled in the eggs. The bacon topped off this delicious breakfast for six.

Her casseroles often combine any type of pasta, meat or fish, chopped broccoli or other vegetable, held together with shredded cheese and topped with cracker crumbs or crushed Fritos and some more cheese.

Cheese is a frequent guest at the dinner table, and Cynthia says her boys will eat any vegetable if it has her homemade cheese sauce on top. She makes a white sauce, and adds shredded cheese -- whatever she has on hand. Cook it, stirring, only long enough to melt the cheese, and serve right away. This is a good beginning to homemade nacho dip for tortilla chips. Cynthia adds chili and seasonings to the cheese.

The Ds no longer buy the frozen hot pockets now that they use a sandwich maker that seals food between two slices of bread. Some favorite combinations are cheese and broccoli with either chicken or beef, and hamburger/onion pizza (Stage Two).

Pasta salads are popular during the hot weather months, and Cynthia serves a dip for cut up raw vegetables. She keeps a bowl of fruit in the refrigerator and a supply of toothpicks nearby for the boys to help themselves. Cynthia makes up her own mixes for cocoa and biscuits. Each is kept in its own large canister with directions for use taped on the outside.

She bakes two batches of cookies each week, and the boys have their own supply of treats; they have learned how to make a bag of Mom's cookies last for the week. They are free to eat their treats when they wish, as long as it's not before a meal. Sometimes she makes homemade custard or a cake. Commercial treats are also offered, but the boys love their mom's cooking and don't feel deprived.

Of course, cooking from scratch takes more time, and since she is a single mom and enrolled as a student, Cynthia doesn't have much time to spare. But she feels it comes down to what she needs to do in order to care for her children. Daniel is doing well in school now, and has been mainstreamed out of special classes since he has been on the Feingold Program. He likes getting good grades and having better handwriting.

As for Jeremy, Cynthia finds it a lot easier to prepare food than to deal with her youngest when he's had synthetic chemicals. He's a sweet natured little boy unless he goes off the diet. Then the Ds are in for 3 to 4 days of whining, foot stamping and general pitching of fits. You can tell when he gets something off the diet, Cynthia notes, you can't handle him.

She has helped some of her neighbors succeed with the Feingold Program as well. One friend's little girl acts retarded when she eats an apple, or food with the prohibited additives. Cynthia was gratified to hear her friend say, "My children are nice! They're not hateful anymore!"

Saving money on food

The Ds use techniques any family would use to keep their food budget in bounds. The most expensive food in a supermarket is generally that which is highly processed, so preparing some things from scratch fits right in with the Feingold Program.

Every stage of commercial food processing offers an opportunity for more synthetic chemicals to be added, so when you do the processing in your kitchen, you have control over the final product.

Sometimes a natural product is actually less expensive that the synthetic. In one supermarket the same size box of junk chocolate chip granola bars cost more than twice the price of the natural version! Or check out real bacon bits compared to those little disasters found at salad bars. The difference in cost is small, but the difference in the contents is enormous.

Even if cost is not a concern, you may find there are some things you will want to make from scratch, since it isn't easy to find acceptable prepared products. Making breadcrumbs in a blender or food processor is quick and easy. Cookies and salad dressings don't take much effort, and your family will probably prefer your homemade versions.

Low Cholesterol Diets & Feingold

It really isn't hard to combine a low cholesterol diet with the Feingold Program.

There are some margarines on our list of approved brand name foods; generally they are available in health food stores. At press time, Feingold *Foodlists* note that Butter Buds, a natural butter flavor may be used on Stage I; Molly McButter is acceptable for Stage II.

But for reducing cholesterol, margarine is not necessarily the best choice. Barbara Hoffstein, R.D., points out the margarine in stick form uses oil which has been hydrogenated, and the process of hydrogenation causes the oil to become "saturated." It is these saturated fats you should be avoiding on a cholesterol-reducing diet. Hardened fats are not significantly better than butter.

Instead, use oil in your baking and cooking whenever possible. The best choice for sautéing is olive oil, which appears to help reduce cholesterol. A small pat of butter added to the olive oil will give some of the flavor you want without adding very much cholesterol.

As with many diets, you should concentrate on gradually improving your choices, not making drastic changes. A small amount of butter on those foods that cry out for the real thing - corn on the cob, perhaps -- will keep you from feeling deprived.

In the same way, you may find it hard to give up whole milk on your cereal, but not care if you use an approved brand of skimmed milk in baking or in sauces. If you use lowfat or skimmed milk, stick with a brand that has been researched by FAUS and is free of BHT in the vitamin A fortification.

"Better Butter"

This is a good alternative to either butter or margarine. You won't need to add the salt if it is to be used in cooking.

2 sticks (1/2 pound) butter, at room temperature
1/2 cup approved brand vegetable oil
1/4 teaspoon salt

Combine in blender or food processor. Pour the mixture into a plastic container and store it in the refrigerator. Once it is chilled, the mixture will become semi-hardened. You can use it in recipes or spread it on toast, etc. It will spread easily even when it is cold. (For a delicious creamy spread, blend in 1/2-cup honey and omit the salt.)

In place of butter, there are other delicious spreads to consider.

The best peanut butter

On a low cholesterol diet, stick with the "natural" peanut butters and those made up fresh at your supermarket or health food store. They contain just ground up peanuts. While there are well-known brands on our Foodlists, these generally contain added hardened (saturated) fats.

Dairy products

Cream cheese can be used if it is done sparingly. Any cheese made from skimmed milk is good for those watching their cholesterol intake. Select cottage cheese, low-fat mozzarella, etc.

Low fat yogurt can be substituted for sour cream in dips and as a topping for baked potatoes.

The heart of a low-cholesterol diet is a variety of delicious and nourishing choices such as fruits, salads, vegetables, pastas, poultry, fish and whole grains. All of these fit in perfectly with the Feingold Program. Bon appetit!

[Note: Brand name products listed in this book are acceptable for use on the Feingold Program at the time of printing; products can change at any time.]

Stress Has Many Forms

There's an enormous variation among "Feingold children," but if you were to name one characteristic that all of them share it is that they are especially sensitive to stress.

Our body must work harder when it is coping with chemicals in food or in our environment, but it can have an equally difficult time dealing with emotional stresses.

The child who moves from a familiar neighborhood, or must adjust to a new baby in the family, who doesn't get along with his teacher, or needs eyeglasses, is facing a stressful situation.

So if you have a Feingold child who is having behavior problems or a reaction of another type, look first at his diet. If you can't find the answer there, then look to other sources of stress. Don't assume that "the diet isn't working anymore." If it has worked before, it doesn't suddenly cease to be effective. Additives are a major source of stress, but they are not the only source.

What good is being on a diet if you can't cheat?

When our family was new to the program my "Feingold kid" was very conscientious about avoiding all of the no-no's, but she liked to offer her little sister the vending machine junk, or junk food she had been given. I went along with it for quite awhile, and then one day when she saw a gumball machine and wanted to get one for Karen, it occurred to me how contradictory my message had been. I told Laura that I didn't give her synthetic chemicals because they were bad for her, and because I loved and cared about her. Then I'd turn around and let the baby have them!

I had fallen victim to the advertising propaganda that assaults us every day. Inferior products with harmful ingredients are presented as "fun foods;" in fact the less a product has to be proud of, the more loudly and persistently it is promoted. We're accustomed to being cynical about cigarette advertising (the Marlboro Man is shown on his horse, not in the hospital dying of cancer, as was the case). Healthy young people are "alive with pleasure" and we never see the underweight babies who will later be born to mothers who smoke, or their asthmatic children.

How do you feel about it?

Some days it seems that we have no influence over our child's perceptions, but deep down we know that we do. The way you feel about unallowed foods is important, and will come across loud and clear to your family. Even if your child is very careful about sticking to his diet, as most children are, if you see it as a deprivation it will wear away at his resolve. One of our volunteers years ago coined a favorite phrase, "Love is not a lollypop."

Home is probably the only place your child will be able to avoid being faced with chemicals at every turn. He needs to have this oasis where he doesn't have to read labels or question what goes into his mouth. Advertisements and our society in general bombard us with food additives, but it's up to us to decide what is best for our kids. Your neighbors may think your family is on a special diet, but once you have reintroduced the natural salicylates, look at what your "special diet" really is. If you eat food and your neighbor eats petrol, then who is really on a special diet?

There will probably come a time when your child wants to experiment with going off the diet, but that decision should be his alone. Cheating on the diet and experiencing the consequences is generally an unpleasant event, but one which has a valuable lesson on making informed choices. If the choice to cheat and suffer the results is yours, not your child's, there aren't any positive results. Without your resolve to back him up, his determination to continue on his diet may be badly damaged.

The young child typically is very careful to stay on his diet, often to the amazement of adults. Don't be complacent about this determination. Even the most disciplined six-year-old can start to feel restless about the diet by the time he is seven or eight. If you have kept your home (and your child) "clean" of the chemicals, then you have built up a good foundation in two ways. First, the child's system will be pretty well cleaned out, and later infractions might not have a serious effect. Second, he has a clear, unambiguous message that certain additives are not OK for him, and that everyone else would be better off without them too. It will be much easier for your child to bounce back from a reaction, decide it wasn't worth it, and return to his diet. If Mom gives off an ambiguous message about the importance of his diet, it will be much harder for him to return to it. Most children, especially young ones, do better with clear-cut choices of: OK or not OK. In other words, you need to be a rock; your child needs a stable anchor in this stormy world.

Planned cheats

If, despite your best efforts, you find that your child has a great deal of trouble sticking to the program, you might want to consider a technique some parents have found useful. This works best for the child who has been successfully on the program for more than a year.

When there's a party, an overnight camping trip, or other special event coming up, the parent and Feingold child discuss the food likely to be served, and what she would most like to have. If the child agrees to pass up any bright colors, she will be avoiding major potential offenders. In fact, most people are better off drinking colas than synthetically colored "fruit" drinks.

The parents make it clear that the youngster will still be held responsible for her behavior. Some children will find that even with an occasional deviation from the diet, they can keep their behavior under control. Here the key word is "occasional." Constant infractions would return the family to their pre-diet difficulties.

A child who has not eaten synthetic additives for a considerable length of time might find she can eat even the dye with no apparent reaction. It appears that one gets "cleaned out," and it may take a little while for the chemicals to once again accumulate before the symptoms re-appear. And as a child grows and her body weight increases, her tolerance may increase.

Caution: Please remember that these suggestions are directed to the parents of the child who shows strong resistance to his diet. If your child is cooperative, deliberate infractions can open a Pandora's box of problems. When the parent sees cheating as a positive or "fun" experience, it can seriously damage the child's commitment to the program.

Consequences of cheating

"My eleven-year-old daughter does well as long as she stays on the diet. When she cheats the headaches and asthma often return, and she becomes defiant.

"We've talked about this, and she knows she should not eat some of those things her friends are having. We do well during the week, but on the weekend when she's out with other girls she finds it hard to resist, then she comes home and we end up in a war of words. I've told her that if she wants to eat those things, I shouldn't have to put up with it, and she is to stay in her room while she is having a reaction, although I insist she come out long enough to set the table since I feel she needs to know that she is expected to do her chores.

"Recently, this happened and she went to her room, as was expected of her. Later that evening, my husband went in to say goodnight and found her lying on top of the bed, reading. He suggested she change into her pajamas, get into bed, and read there. She really lost it, screaming at him that she went to her room as she had agreed, and that he should leave her alone, etc. It was really extreme, and she felt terrible the next morning. What do you suggest?"

Another Mom's advice

Actually, I agree with your daughter! Your husband's gesture was a caring one, and of course her reaction was inappropriate, but it's not surprising for someone in the throes of a reaction. A chemically sensitive person simply is not capable of functioning normally when they are experiencing a reaction, and whether they are 11 or 41, they are much better off if they are left alone. As soon as you step into the picture, you become enmeshed in the problem, and not only are you needlessly bruised by it, but the individual's anger gets directed in the wrong place. She needs to spend the time by herself, knowing any unhappiness that has occurred is hers alone. Your daughter understands the consequences of her choice. You wisely discussed the appropriate steps for her to take when she chooses to go off her diet, and she was keeping her part of the agreement. Both of you are right on the mark!

Where I disagree is in you and your husband using appropriate parenting techniques under the wrong circumstances. In other words, your wish that she do her chores, and his suggestion of getting ready for bed are fine for a child who is functioning normally, but the sensitive individual having a reaction is just not capable of behaving reasonably. If you like, think of it as trying to deal with someone who has consumed too much alcohol or been exposed to mind-altering drugs; it doesn't matter how good your parenting techniques are, they won't work for the person who is incapable of controlling their own body.

You and your husband didn't eat that Twinkie, so why should your evening be ruined? As long as the reaction does not pose a danger -- such as an asthmatic attack or other health consequence that your child can't handle on her own -- as long as she is old enough to not need your supervision, your best course of action is to stay away.

You have done a very good job of implementing the Feingold program in your home -- congratulations! Your daughter knows that some additives have a negative effect, that she feels and acts better when she avoids them, and that there is a price to pay when she chooses to go off her diet. Now, at age 11, she has to be given the choice of benefiting from this knowledge, or of ignoring it and paying the price (isolation), but she needs to really be by herself as long as there is no danger to her.

Continue to follow the diet, as I know you will. Home needs to be a refuge, a place where all the food is "safe." She may have to choose the wrong foods many times, but I believe she will ultimately decide that the price of cheating is too high, and that it's preferable to say "no" to her friends rather than suffer the consequences. As hard as it is to watch our children make the wrong decisions, it is essential for them to make mistakes as long as such a mistake does not cause irreparable harm. Mistakes are important teaching tools, and in a few years when you look back, you'll probably see that events such as this played an important part in your child's development into a responsible young adult.

Nathan and Stephen

Sweetarts, watermelon candy, bubble gum -- so mouthwatering, so tempting, and so forbidden to my special little boys, ages 6 and 7.

After returning from a birthday party toting a bag of "feisty" foods (our special word for non-Feingold foods), the boys began wondering out loud what these feisty foods tasted like.

I have tried to let my boys know that we have healthier alternatives to the feisty foods, and that, because I can not be with them all of the time, they must be relied upon to turn down unacceptable foods on their own.

Giving them this responsibility for their own feelings of well being has been one of our greatest assets on the Program, and they are very proud of their Feingold diet.

However, realizing how very important it was to them to taste and experiment, we agreed to a supervised taste test under the condition that they controlled their behavior. They were absolutely certain, of course, that such delicious, mouthwatering treats would have no effect on them. I reserved judgement.

Behaviorally they were just fine. Good as gold. The same candies that would have spelled disaster four years ago did not appear, at first, to cause any change. Insidiously, however, the effects of the additives made themselves known.

Every Friday, the boys' camp counselor would send home a note relating the week's activities. Each child would sign his or her name to the note. Two days after the taste test, I received the camp reports. When I got the note, I said, "Nathan, you didn't sign your name."

"Yes I did. Here it is," he replied.

Nathan had signed his name backwards, but could not recognize it as out of the ordinary.

It was only several days later that he looked at his name again and said, "Why did I write my name backwards?" I pointed out to him that, while I was very proud of his behavior, the "feisties" can affect us in other ways and interfere with our ability to think straight. While Steven's handwriting and behavior were not affected, he could not add and subtract (something he is normally a whiz at) and he again started to walk sideways (crab-like is about the only way to describe it).

Because it was summertime, I took the chance and it was a wonderful affirmation of how positively effective the Feingold Program is in so many little ways. It also showed me how insidiously the additives can affect the brain without the marked change in behavior that we have been accustomed to look for. Strangest of all, while the additives were in their systems, they could not recognize their inability to perform simple tasks.

Consumer's rights?

Our new car must state estimated gas mileage; our clothing must tell us what the fabric is made of; pillows carry little tags warning of arrest if they are removed before sale. But what about the food we eat? Unfortunately, when it comes to food additives, the consumer has no rights. But isn't it more important to know what goes into our bodies than to be told the content of our shirt or our sofa cushion?

When Dad Won't Cooperate

New Feingold moms often report that their greatest problem is not in winning the cooperation of their child, but in convincing their husband to go along with the diet. We have no foolproof answers, but here are a few suggestions.

Many dads feel very defensive about their child ("There's nothing wrong with *my* kid" syndrome). Attending an introductory meeting if there is one in your area, or looking at the FAUS video tape can be valuable, as he will see the problem rests not with his child but with the child's diet. If your physician is receptive to the Feingold Program, his or her recommendation may convince a reluctant spouse to give it a try.

Plan to have plenty of safe treats on hand at the beginning. While we don't really advocate junk food, even "natural" junk food, winning your family's cooperation is vital; you can work on improving nutrition later.

Make as many "little" changes in the shopping list as you can. Someone may notice if you change the brand of bread, but who cares what brand of vegetable oil you use?

Don't take away Dad's coffee, beer, or other grown-up beverages that the children don't care about anyway. And remind sports-loving dads that improved coordination frequently results from an additive-free diet.

If all else fails, you can challenge your reluctant relative to prove that the Feingold Program does NOT work. See if he will agree to strictly support your efforts for a set time (2 or 3 weeks minimum, but the longer the better). Be sure to follow your *Foodlist* to the letter!

Check your new member information for the name of a volunteer. Don't be shy about calling someone for help, or even just moral support.

Dealing with Dad - a note to new Feingold moms

You have a right to feel disappointed and hurt if your husband is uncooperative about changing foods. Unfortunately, this response is not unusual. These dads usually come around once the child's improvement is clear to them, although it sometimes requires a figurative sledgehammer to get them to see the difference. But if a child's problems "aren't that bad" it can be especially hard for Dad to acknowledge that a problem exists.

But you know your child needs help, and want to test out the Feingold Program. What can you do if your spouse is like this one? He likes his jellybeans and his familiar brand of chips. He refuses to confine them to work, and doesn't hesitate to eat them in front of his child. He expects you to buy his favorite junk foods and has no intention of being inconvenienced by the needs of his child. He will not agree to speak with a counselor or doctor, will not read the Feingold literature or look at a videotape.

What can you do?

Since Junior's reaction to additives is not drastic, arranging for Dad to be responsible for him after a jellybean episode would not accomplish much. The sad truth is that if this describes your husband, then you have two little boys. One is age seven and the other is thirty-two, going on six. How would you deal with a situation where the welfare of one of your children was being harmed by the selfishness of the other?

Some men feel very threatened by the suggestion that there could be "something wrong with my kid." The problem is most likely to come up when the child in question is a son, especially the first-born. Dad may say, "That's just the way I was when was a kid," and he's probably right!

Most married couples have leverage with each other; when one feels very strongly on an issue, the other cooperates. In the family where Dad dictates everything, there's little a mother can do beside take a hard look her life and ask herself if this is how she wants to spend it and if there is a way to bring about some balance. The problem is not about diet but about a troubled relationship, and diet is simply the current battleground. The same kind of counseling that would be used for other problems in the marriage would be suitable, especially if the counselor understands the value of a diet that reduces synthetic additives.

When her child's welfare is at stake, a normally submissive woman can find a strength she didn't know she had; this may be the first time she has taken a firm stand, and her husband is understandably perplexed. The outcome can be a real rift, or it can be a more equitable partnership. But if your spouse is not a control freak you may need to ask yourself just how strongly you feel, then put your foot down and request/insist on a trial period of 4 to 6 weeks of cooperation, after which you can both evaluate your child's progress.

Behind the successful Feingold youngster there is generally a determined Mom, so you probably hold the key to your child's future. If you are married to a Daddy who rolls up his sleeves and pitches in to help, give him a hug and tell him how wonderful he is.

Divorce and the Feingold Diet

You have your child on the diet, but your "ex" insists on filling him up with junk food. What can you do?

This is a true story of one Feingold mother (who we will call Joan Smith) and how she resolved what is becoming an increasingly common problem.

"It shouldn't have come as such a surprise to me to learn that Tim was hyperactive," Joan reflected, "both his father and I had some of the symptoms as children, so our son got a double dose."

"My idea of hyperactivity was some kind of off-the-walls-and-ceiling behavior. Since I grew up with this condition I thought Tim was normal. But every time we had spaghetti for dinner, I noticed the next morning that I couldn't even get him dressed." When she discovered her son was learning disabled, Joan tried to discuss it with her husband. "He turned his back to me and stared at the wall. He confused 'learning disabled' with 'retarded,' and neither he nor his family could accept the possibility of this child being less than perfect.

"The basic issue was one of a power struggle - my right to have an independent thought, or the possibility that I could be right." The chances of saving the marriage seemed slim, but Joan was determined to do all she could to help her child.

With great reluctance she began using Ritalin. Initially, the drug caused tremors, but after the shaking subsided, Tim responded beautifully to the Ritalin. In fact, his behavior changed so markedly that even his 3 and 4-year-old classmates noticed how different he was. This confirmed for her that Tim's diagnosis of attention deficit disorder was correct.

"I was scared of the Ritalin," Joan told *Pure Facts*, and opted for the diet, "which didn't suppress Tim's perky personality." With the behavior under control, she set to work finding help for her son's learning disabilities. "It took him a whole year to learn the number seven, but now, thanks to the help of a great resource teacher, he is almost completely mainstreamed. He's in the highest math class in 5th grade and is doing 6th grade reading."

This same determination enabled Joan to win a court ruling in favor of the diet. "You can't be wishy washy about this," she warned. "You have to make up your mind you're going to do it. Life is not always nice, and being aggressive is sometimes the only way to get what you want."

The biggest obstacle Joan found was her mother-in-law, who often cared for Tim and his sister on the weekends. Grandmother would give the children food not permitted on Tim's diet and say, "Don't tell your mother about this."

With the help of her attorney and a letter from a pediatrician who believes in the diet, Joan was able to demonstrate that Tim needs the Feingold Program and that his father's actions were undermining the child's diet. Her ex-husband and in-laws are now fairly cooperative, and since the children are older, they know which foods are acceptable.

Their father has even acknowledged the difference and once when Tim went off the diet his father brought him back early!

Here are some of Joan's suggestions on how to go about winning your case:

1. Be sure of your determination; this will take time, effort and persistence.

2. Shop for a good lawyer if you don't already have one.

3. Keep a diet diary, noting what was eaten and reactions which occurred afterward, including the dates. If possible, include dated notes from the teacher.

4. Obtain written statements from as many professionals as possible -- such as a pediatrician, psychologist, principal, etc.

5. Have Feingold literature available, and explain that the program means simply eating a wide variety of wholesome foods. But don't try to teach the judge the fine points of the diet.

Grandparents -- Big Help or Big Problem

Your parents and in-laws can be a terrific ally or the source of a lot of aggravation.

Most of our mail comes from parents of troubled children, but a close second are concerned grandparents. A typical letter reads, "My daughter and I are beside ourselves concerning my grand-daughter. She is only 8 months old and driving us up the wall. She sleeps very little, is on the go all day, and has been in a walker since 3 1/2 months old. She is very smart for her age, but very strong willed.

"As young as she is, she has temper tantrums when she can't do things or can't have her own way. Can you help us?"

There are many ways grandparents can, and do, help.

- Contact the Association and ask that information be sent to your grandchild's parents. Or, provide a gift membership, as many grandparents do. One woman wrote, "I'm ordering two memberships, one for my daughter and one for myself since I am around our grandson quite a bit. I want to be able to help as much as possible."

- Consider using the Feingold Program for yourself as well. It appears that the tendency to be chemically sensitive may be inherited, so you might find you feel much better after you have removed certain synthetic chemicals from your diet.

- Once your grandchildren have become established on the Program, you may find you will welcome their visits. It will be important for you to have "Feingold-acceptable" foods in your home.

- If you have a good relationship with the child's parents, and live nearby, you can be helpful to the family getting started on the Program. Do you have a little extra time to hunt down that special product that's hard to find? Would you be willing to ask the local grocer to carry it, or would you write a letter to a manufacturer? Would you baby-sit while Mom makes her first trip to the grocery store with her new Foodlist?

- If the mother simply hasn't the time to bake cupcakes for the class party, can you volunteer? (Has anyone ever been the "Room Grandmother"?)

How many other grandparents do you know who are deeply troubled about children they love? You can be the one to make a difference, by telling them about the help available.

At war with my Mother-in-law

Holiday family gatherings should be warm and wonderful, but in some families they can be very stressful.

One member described the typical holiday scene: "We arrive to find my mother-in-law has prepared an elaborate meal. She's a very good cook, but there's nothing my daughter can eat. We end up angry at each other, with lots of hurt feelings, and my husband caught in between." The member had already provided her mother-in-law with information on the Feingold Program, but none of it was being absorbed. The following is a recommendation for anyone dealing with a similar situation.

Recognize that your mother-in-law just doesn't understand the Feingold Program; assume she is not being malicious, and try to put yourself in her place. What do you think her motives are, and how do you think she feels when this happens? Consider this scenario: She wants to feel needed. (Who doesn't?) She expresses her love by the hours and effort spent in the kitchen. She is saying, "Notice me. Value me as a person and as an important member of our family. Look at how lovely this meal is. Look at how much I care." Then consider how you would feel if something you had labored over was rejected.

You can turn an adversary into a powerful ally by finding ways to make her needs and yours complimentary. For example, consider the probability that she has extra time and loves to cook, whereas you don't have much time or desire. If your mother-in-law loves to cook, begin by calling her and asking for her advice and help with a recipe. Let her know you think she is a good cook and that you value her opinion. If she lives close enough, call her another time and ask her if she would be willing to bake cookies for the school open house, or cupcakes for the class party. Insist that you will supply all of the ingredients, and bring the flour, shortening, pure vanilla, etc. to her house. By this time there should be enough good will beginning to blossom that she should be agreeable to using the ingredients you have supplied.

Get back to her each time, and let her know how much she helped you, how successful the class party was, etc. If she is at your home, ask her to prepare some of the food (with your Feingold-safe ingredients). She should gradually begin to see that Feingold cooking is not so much different from what she is accustomed to. Once she feels secure that you value her advice, she may become more open to asking for your suggestions on ingredients.

The main point of this family feud is recognizing that your mother-in-law wants to feel needed and loved, and that you can show her how to gain this approval.

Not everyone understands

One mom recalls, "My mother was willing to cooperate with Mark's diet, but couldn't understand what it was all about. She hadn't had problems with us, and I reminded her that we ate from the garden and she made everything from scratch. Then it made sense to her.

"My mother-in-law was a different story. She's a member of the 'just a little bit won't hurt' school of thought, and would sneak treats to Mark without my knowledge. I told her that if she expected to see her grandson she wouldn't do that anymore. 'Furthermore,' I told her, 'if you do it again, I'll bring him back here and you can keep him for two days while he gets over his reaction.' I have found you must put your child's welfare first, even if it means someone's feelings get hurt. She never really understood, but she cooperated after that."

Many parents announce to the relatives as they arrive for the holiday gathering, "Whoever turns him on gets to take him home and keep him for three days while he bounces off the walls of YOUR home." It's proven to be very effective!

The good old days

Another approach for a reluctant Grandma or Grandpa is the "good old days" technique. Since the older generation typically likes to look back with nostalgia at their childhood, and describe how much better things were then, this is a time to remind them that - at least as far as additives are concerned – they're absolutely right! Ask them, "What color was your toothpaste? Did you drink orange colored sugar water for breakfast? Were there dyed marshmallows floating in your cereal? If your mother made you take vitamins, what were they like? How did medicine taste? Did your teachers hand out candy?"

Ask them "What sort of food did their school cafeteria serve? What sort of discipline problems did a teacher face? How does that compare with classrooms today? Did children respect authority figures in those days? Do they respect them now?"

Your parents did eat foods with synthetic dyes and flavorings. There were pink hearts on Valentine's Day, jelly beans at Easter, candy corn at Halloween and candy canes at Christmas. But they were not consuming petroleum-based chemicals every day, day in and day out. Every household product was not saturated with fragrances. Offices and schools didn't have tightly sealed buildings. (When things got "stuffy" teachers opened the windows.) Classrooms didn't have carpeting, and the powerful chemicals used in their manufacture. Desks were made of wood, not laminated fiberboard treated with formaldehyde. Scented crayons, markers and stickers didn't exist, and nine year old girls didn't wear cologne to class.

If they still get on your case that your parenting is to blame, tell them that you probably are doing a very good job since you had better parents than they did! Maybe the changes in the chemicals we are all exposed to have something to do with your child's difficulties.

(Note: If your parents grew up in the 1960s or later, then you need to go back to the days of your grandparents to find the scene described above.)

The child who's "not that bad"

Most people believe that the child who has severe problems will be the hardest to help, but this generally isn't the case.

When a youngster's behavior is extreme, when learning or health problems are too obvious to be ignored, everyone's efforts are spent in seeking answers, not in denying a problem exists.

If diet makes a significant difference, if the response is dramatic, then relatives, teachers, neighbors -- and just about everyone else who comes in contact with the child -- will do what they can to cooperate. What's even more important is that the youngster himself has a terrific motivation to stick closely to his diet, and most of them do.

The belief that it's harder to help a child with an extreme behavioral reaction is based on what generally is the false assumption that the child's behavior is due to some physical or chemical abnormality. But the child who goes out of control when he drinks a glass of synthetic "fruit punch" is likely to be different from the next child only in the degree of his sensitivity.

It's very hard to hear someone say, "I thought about the Feingold Program, but my child's not that bad." Volunteers have long puzzled over a way to respond to a statement like this. Thus far we're speechless.

Parenting the Feingold Teen

It's quite possible to successfully raise a difficult child. All it requires is that you be twice as good at it as most other parents.

On the other hand, children who do not live on chemically laden junk food are often the calmest, nicest kids on the block. But Feingold parents know that their young Dr. Jekyll has a flip side. Dealing with the Feingold teen when s/he is off the diet merely takes the wisdom of Solomon and the patience of Job.

We hope that these suggestions, as well as those found in the *Feingold Handbook*, will help to keep your teenager on the program and will be of assistance to you if s/he should go off it.

Each family is different and each child a unique challenge, but there are some common experiences we all share. Our parents of teens have said their major concern is to help their child internalize the decision to stay on the Program.

If you have been following the Feingold Program for many years, you know this comes long before adolescence. The preschooler who visits the next door neighbor's without Mom at his side needs to be able to say "no," and they generally are very good at it.

Make the program a family affair

Now that you know about food additives, about how harmful and unnecessary many are, it shouldn't be hard for you to banish those that are excluded from our diet. (Since most of them are petroleum derivatives, you aren't missing much!) If your spouse simply can't do without a favorite junk food, ask him/her to get it at the office vending machine, not in the home. And don't waste any sympathy on the siblings who miss their fluorescent cereals. They will probably get plenty of their old favorites at a friend's house, the nearby convenience store, or the school cafeteria.

The family is your child's primary support group. Discuss how each of you is supported by the others. Chances are, other family members are experiencing benefits from the diet as well; your food selections are then a part of your family's value system. Discuss the diet just as you would speak of other ethical and moral attitudes.

Yes, your child is different

In a society where Dr. Feingold estimated 80% of the food found in a supermarket contains one or more of the prohibited additives, the person who eliminates them is different. But then, the rock star is different; so is the Olympic medallist or the Rhodes Scholar.

Actually, the purpose of the Program is to produce a normal range of behavior. By eating food that may be somewhat different from his peers, your teen's behavior should be much less "different."

For the youngster who must avoid some or all of the salicylates, this difference is more similar to a person with a food allergy. It's a real bummer having to skip the ketchup; but it's also hard avoiding gluten or taking insulin shots every day, or communicating only in sign language. Life deals us a tough hand sometimes. Your sympathy will be welcome, but be careful that it doesn't cross over into pity. You're not "depriving your poor child" of anything except some serious problems.

Don't make the diet more different than necessary

Of course you'd like to see your teen enjoy whole wheat bread and brown rice; it also would be nice if she hated candy, but let's not set our expectations too high.

Gaining and keeping a child's cooperation is the most fundamental requirement. If this means a candy bar at the movies or burgers, and a soft drink at the mall, then focus on steering your teen toward the less junky of the junk foods. If he has been on the Program for a few years, an occasional cheat may be tolerated.

Be sure there are lots of acceptable foods in the house, and encourage any signs of interest your children have in cooking or food preparation. And don't forget to check out the UnTomato Sauce in your FAUS cookbook – it's great for pizza.

The consequences of going off the diet -- or: "Placebo effect, where are you when we need you?"

If the effectiveness of the Feingold Program were the result of placebo effect, as critics like to believe, there would be no consequence for cheating. Unfortunately, infractions and reactions are a hard fact of life for the Feingold member of any age.

For the teen with several years of experience on the program, it should be fairly clear what form a reaction takes. If it means a loss of coordination, the athletically inclined has a strong motivation to stick to his diet. If schoolwork is affected, the student who wants to make good grades has this incentive.

For many Feingold youngsters, a reaction shows up mostly as pain-in-the-neck behavior. (This is the best motivation for the rest of the family to support adherence to the Program!)

Whatever the consequences of an infraction, most Feingold members come to the conclusion that their child needs to experience the result of a deliberate mistake. Talk it over with her, but wait until the reactions subsides; few people of any age are able to recognize it when they are in the midst of experiencing a reaction.

The rebellion years

As your teen undergoes the difficult task of separating from you, he will probably seek out a way to rebel. If you're lucky, he will be satisfied with rebelling in a limited area. Do what you can to prevent that area from being food.

Someone once suggested that whoever came up with the idea of long hair deserved a Nobel Prize for peace. If your teen makes a statement with a mane which is shaggy, shorn, or multi-colored, and if this is the extent of the rebellion, consider yourself fortunate. Hair will grow out. Black nail polish doesn't last forever. Ask yourself if your teen's latest personal statement will inflict permanent damage, and if the answer is "no" try to live with it. Even when the rebellion is directed at food, stick to your guns, and keep your refrigerator Feingold-safe.

Positive rebellion

There are some things you can do to encourage your teen's positive rebellion. In seeking an area he can call his own, your child may outdo you in the healthy food department. You know enough not to preach nutrition to him; but don't be irritated if he preaches it to you, or scolds you for eating too much sugar. Admit you're imperfect. (You may as well; if you try to disguise that fact, your youngster will work diligently until he uncovers it.)

In other words, give your teen a niche that can be hers alone. It's O.K. if she's wiser than you in some areas. Admit you're a fallible human and admire her strength.

One mom relates, "My kids love to hear about how 'Poor Ole Mom' messed up again. They like feeling a bit superior, and it seems to help defuse their desire to rebel." "I haven't been the mother of a teen before," another writes, "I tell my kids I'm still new at the job and they'll have to be patient while I learn the ropes."

A classic trait of teenagers has always been a delight in uncovering the folly of the older generation. In many cases their disrespect is well deserved. The older generation produces, promotes, protects and profits from additive-laden food. Contact FAUS for a copy of their "Food

Additive Quiz" to stimulate some thought about practices of the older generation -- practices deserving of adolescent indignation.

Maybe this type of information will encourage your young person to become involved in our work; there are those who think it's a form of rebellion!

Try to be aware of what's normal and acceptable behavior for the age

There are many good books and seminars on the issue of dealing with teens. We need to remember that what is true for the young child is just as true for the teen: diet is not always the reason for a behavior problem. Don't hesitate to seek professional help if your family is faced with issues you are unable to resolve. Be sure to screen the counselor first, and find out how he/she feels about the Feingold Program. The last thing you need is someone who thinks the diet is causing the problem.

Fringe benefits

Look for an added reason for your teen to stick to the diet (you hit the ball better, avoid headaches, and have clearer skin).

Life isn't always fair

Life is a series of problems, much as we would like to think otherwise. Show your teenager that since it's virtually impossible to avoid them, what's important is how he or she responds to them. Diet restrictions are a problem for anyone, but dealing successfully with this problem yields great benefits.

In the final analysis, the best you can do for your children, whether they "need" the Feingold Program or not, is to teach them about foods. You may think they don't hear you, and they may go through periods where they seem determined to eat all the wrong things, but they have heard you. When their own welfare becomes important to them, the information will be there.

The deaf ear

A good way to be sure your child or teen hears what you have to say is to avoid speaking directly to them. Discuss this with your spouse in advance, then when the family is together, perhaps at dinner, tell your partner about something you read in the paper or the Feingold newsletter. Or talk about a TV show on the hazards of pesticides, food additives, or whatever. If your children think you aren't talking to them they're more likely to listen.

Incidentally, this also works in families where everyone but Dad is concerned about foods and food additives. Discuss the subject with your children at the dinner table, and your reluctant spouse is more likely to absorb the information.

The "clumsy" driver

The drunk driver is not the only roadway hazard.

The National Highway Traffic Safety Administration points to two groups of [non-drinking] drivers as having the highest risk of accidents: those over 75 years of age, and those under 25. In the case of the older driver, there may be a diminishing of eye-hand-brain coordination, and slower reaction time. (Medication may also be a factor.)

"In the case of the young drivers," notes Richard Restak, M.D., "their road accidents are merely the most conspicuous aspect of the hyperactivity, attention difficulties and learning problems that are present within this age group. Popular opinion to the contrary, these conditions are not limited to children and adolescents."

The clumsy person is accident prone both in the car and out. Some of the symptoms which create potential hazards are: poor eye-hand coordination, a slower reaction time, impaired ability to anticipate changes in the environment, inattention or day dreaming, a disturbance in judgement.

"He or she acts too fast or not fast enough," Dr. Restak continues, "steps on the accelerator when the intention is to put on the brake; slips the gear into reverse instead of forward; comes to a full stop when the sign merely indicates 'yield.' In all cases, the response is almost but not quite appropriate to the situation."

Alcohol

Other researchers note that the young driver who consumes one or two drinks may test out to have blood alcohol levels below the legal limit, but still be impaired. The inexperience of the young driver, along with a relatively low tolerance for alcohol is a deadly combination, according to the Addiction Research Foundation of Toronto.

Dr. Feingold noted that a young person's reaction to alcoholic beverages may not be just from the alcohol alone, but also from the many synthetic additives which may be found in them.

One member writes: "Our son had to give up driving after three accidents. When at home he had no accidents, but out on his own in his apartment, off Feingold food, he had three accidents within a short time. The insurance went up and no one really wants to insure him."

My Ordinary Kid

By Annette Miller

You'd never pick him out of a roomful of kids as being different. Today he's just an ordinary kid, and that's what I always wanted.

From day one, Billy was a hyper, cranky, angry child who was always moving, scarcely slept and had a very short fuse. He really was off-the-wall -- literally our "bouncing baby."

Even as a baby, his room consisted of a mattress on the floor since he had demolished all of the furnishings. Nothing could confine Billy. As soon as the men completed installing the fence surrounding our yard, my toddler climbed over it and was on his way. At the tender age of 2 1/2 he was known to take off and visit his grandmother who lived nearly a mile away.

The evaluation for Billy and his future was very pessimistic. He was diagnosed as having autistic characteristics and a developmental delay. Although he was clearly very bright, he couldn't sit still long enough to learn. All this took place before Billy's third birthday.

I was up early every morning, and happened to see Vickie Gelardi on TV. She described a child who fit my son to a 'T,' but all the while she was seated next to a calm, well-behaved little boy. At first I didn't understand that the boy she was describing was the same child beside her, now successfully on the Feingold diet.

With Vickie's help and the support of the local Feingold chapter, Billy's behavior changed dramatically in ten days. This was back in 1975, and being on the diet was a lot different than it is today. We made everything from scratch because we really didn't know that much about additives -- especially the hidden ones. We didn't understand what questions to ask manufacturers, particularly about antioxidant preservatives hidden in the oils, the vitamins or the packaging materials.

I later learned that BHA and BHT were major offenders for Billy, as were all petroleum-based additives. The fumes from petro-chemicals were just as bad as those ingested, and his worst times in school turned out to be when the building was treated with insecticides each month. (Once we tracked down the cause, the principal tried to schedule this for Friday afternoons.)

While the diet made a world of difference for Billy, he still had many problems. His eye-hand coordination was very poor and it was extremely hard for him to write and to copy words from the blackboard or from a book. Paperwork is still difficult, and he looks forward to graduating from high school this spring. Bill has a real talent for aircraft maintenance and design and will receive further training in a F.A.A. approved program.

With the help of our doctor we were able to add back all of the salicylates and foods to which he was allergic, and just eliminate the synthetic additives; Billy then gave his full cooperation. If he went to a birthday party, he would bring home all the food he was given and trade it for acceptable foods. The same was true at Halloween; he would give me everything he had collected, in exchange for the allowed treats. If I had his willpower, I'd be a size 5!

At 16, Bill is the easiest of my three kids to get along with. He's a funny, bright, witty young man who likes people and they like him as well. He is very sensitive to the feelings of others. Bill is wonderful with children, even babies, and has such strong feelings of empathy -- especially for the kid who doesn't fit in.

Having been on the diet for so many years, Bill knows how much he can cheat, and when he needs to get back to the "safe" foods. At the mall or movie, he chooses the junk food that is not likely to have petrochemicals and it isn't hard to fit in with the group.

So many people have seen the changes in Bill as he grew up, and understand the help the Feingold Program can provide. I get calls from out of nowhere. People tell me our pediatrician referred them to me, or the school nurse, or one of his former teachers, principals, etc.

In addition to his interest in engines, Bill has discovered another skill -- pistol shooting. (They use air pistols, and he is extremely safety-conscious.) I didn't really think much of it until I learned that after only about a year of shooting, he was invited to participate in the Junior Olympic Championships held in Colorado. Out of 77 marksmen, Bill came in 13th. His hand-eye coordination must have improved an awful lot!

Michael's Best Year

My 14-year-old son has been on the Feingold diet for one year, the best year of his life!

I remember seeing Dr. Feingold on the Phil Donahue Show in 1973. I couldn't understand why anyone would resist the idea that added colors, flavors and BHT, BHA, and TBHQ would change a person's behavior. Additives are synthetic chemicals and are like drugs in your system. Why then, did I wait 13 years to put my son on the diet? I didn't know ALL of the facets of a person's life that would be affected. He never was "hyperactive" as the word implies, though I found out he did have certain learning deficits.

Michael had a difficult time adjusting to junior high school. He could not get himself organized enough to remember homework assignments given early in the day. He worried constantly about getting to class on time and, if he did remember his assignments, book, and lunch money, he worried about remembering to turn the work in after he had done it. After nearly failing seventh grade, his ego was almost non-existent.

Then a very dear friend told me about the same problems her son had sleeping, remembering, and worrying. I read her Feingold literature several times, thinking of all the nights I sat up with Michael, trying to get him to sleep. That very afternoon we put the popsicles down the drain and made real lemonade pops. After only a few days he began to stop worrying so much and began smiling again! He would go to bed and fall right to sleep -- a restful sleep.

I've decided every child deserves the right and the opportunity to be the best person possible. The best place to start is to remove all the colors, flavors and the 3 preservatives from the day care centers and the school cafeterias. I plan to go back to school and earn a degree in nutrition, promoting the Feingold diet. It's not fair to see children fed red gelatin for lunch and later see them being reprimanded for a behavior problem, or see them so depressed about zeroes on forgotten assignments that they are certain the world would be better if they were not around.

My son has just finished his eighth grade year. Now he has two of the most important things possible to start high school: PRIDE AND SELF-CONFIDENCE. His grades this year were above average, As and Bs. His intelligence has always been there. It was just "colored and flavored" and preserved too much!

Finding a Doctor

Like most Feingold children, Dottie's son is seldom sick. But she wanted a pediatrician who would support them in following the Feingold Program.

Several neighbors recommended a young doctor in the area who had been practicing for about a year. Dottie called his office and asked if he was sympathetic toward the Program. After checking with the physician, the receptionist said he knew a little about it and was neither "for" nor "against" it. Having been president of the Indiana Feingold Association, Dottie had come to believe that an open-minded attitude such as this was very desirable.

She made an appointment for the entire family to consult with the doctor; and meanwhile mailed him a packet of literature prepared by the Association. When Dottie and her husband later met with the doctor it was obvious he had read the material and would cooperate with them in following the program.

"My husband doesn't charge for consultations in his line of work," Dottie told *Pure Facts,* "and we were favorably impressed that the doctor did not charge us for this initial visit." Her child has not needed to see the pediatrician often, Dottie reports, but on those few occasions, it has been so nice to have a doctor who will work with you.

Why doesn't my child's doctor support the Feingold Program?

While many doctors do support the Program, and refer patients to us, others brush off a parent's desire to try this technique. Some do not even acknowledge a child's obvious improvement. Why?

Most of us don't welcome change. We have our own familiar ways of looking at the world; we have a framework with slots where all the bits and pieces of things we hear and see fit in. We want it to make sense, just as we want a jigsaw puzzle to come out as a finished picture.

When something comes along that doesn't fit in neatly, we have the difficult choice of either rebuilding the framework or discarding the new data. We may feel uncomfortable that we have rejected reasonable information, but this discomfort is balanced by the relief that we don't have to dismantle any part of our old belief system. Just about everyone shares these traits to some degree. But for your doctor, there are other factors that may predispose him or her to resist the concept that diet can influence behavior. The young man or woman who graduates from medical school has become proficient in the practice of "medicine" -- notice how the same word is used to denote both the profession and the drugs it employs. Doctors are taught to identify and treat diseases and disorders. This is their framework, or paradigm. If one looks at the symptoms of learning/behavior problems as a disease or disorder (i.e., attention deficit *disorder*) then it is not surprising so many physicians reach for the prescription pad.

The Kellogg Report (discussed in the chapter on social costs) describes the problems inherent in the training given to physicians. The authors of this major study are highly critical of what they consider to be the outdated approach of medical schools. They call for a new medical paradigm, a new frame of reference, which recognizes our individual differences and health requirements, and which looks at the total lifestyle of the patient when diagnosing illness.

But don't consider skepticism to be a negative attribute; we want those who impact upon our wellbeing to be cautious. Your doctor may have read some of the negative information on our program that is generated by the industry lobbies, and may not be aware of the supportive information in medical journals.

Dr. Feingold predicted that it would take many years before the diet/behavior connection gained recognition. This has always been true in medicine. Major developments we now take for granted were first greeted with ridicule, and only incorporated into the mainstream years later. Mrs. Jane Heimlich, author of *What Your Doctor Won't Tell You,* notes that for years the Red Cross laughed at her husband's anti-choking "Heimlich maneuver." Not too many years ago, only hippies ate yogurt, only your grandmother talked about fiber (roughage), and who dared suggest that certain nutrients in foods could help prevent cancer?

The Harvard School of Public Health investigated the lag between the discovery of a new method of treatment, and the length of time it takes before its publication in medical journals and textbooks makes it available to the physician. The time is believed to be a decade or more. The study estimated as many as 25,000 lives could be lost each year as a result of this time lag.

An additional problem is that support groups tend to have a hard time gaining acceptance. Alcoholics Anonymous and La Leche League fought long and difficult battles for recognition from the medical community. Like the Feingold Program, these groups had the support of individual physicians, but they did not enjoy the confidence of the establishment for many years.

Your doctor

But how does this translate into your dealing with your doctor or your child's pediatrician?

At a conference in Towson, Maryland, a panel of supportive professionals suggested some ways to find a doctor who will work with parents as they use the Feingold Program.

"When I speak with other doctors, the first thing I mention is studies," said Richard Carlton, M.D., a psychiatrist practicing in New York City. "I refer to 'this study in the *Lancet*, that study in the *Journal of Pediatrics*'...that automatically commands their respect. I think the Association should provide a summary for all members -- something they can bring to the doctors. In this summary, have absolutely no anecdotes; there's nothing that turns off the medical profession more than anecdotes. It's almost like waving a red flag at them."

Note: The Feingold Association now has professional packets available for doctors, teachers and counselors.

Paul Lavin, Ph.D., a psychologist and Assistant Professor of Psychology at Towson University, recommended parents take an assertive stand. "If the pediatrician does not have any enthusiasm about the diet, the kid is going to pick up on it and feel that it's not important. Just like kids pick up on the differences between parents -- one parent is easy and the other is tough, they will go with the weak link in the chain.

"I think you need to tell the physician where you're coming from up front in terms of the diet. And you need to ask the physician directly what his point of view is with relation to the use of diet. I think you need to take an assertive position. Tell the pediatrician...what the evidence [to support the Feingold Program] is and then ask some very direct questions and make a selection." [Dr. Lavin is the author of *Parenting the Overactive Child, Alternatives to Drug Therapy.*]

Jay Freed, M.D. practices pediatrics on Long Island, and is Clinical Assistant Professor of Pediatrics, SUNY, Stony Brook. He offered the following suggestions: "I think that if the pediatrician is not familiar with the Program there's no reason why you can't present literature to [him or her]. Bring Dr. Feingold's book or any literature that you have about it and educate him. And if he's totally closed minded about it, then leave. If he's receptive to it, have him read it, get back to him in a month and find out what he thinks. Ask 'Do you think we can have a relationship based on what I presented to you?' If he says 'Yes, I'd like to work with you and try' -- great. If he says 'this is ridiculous,' well, 'have a nice day.'"

To sum up the advice from doctors and parents we suggest you:

- contact the Association for appropriate literature, or photocopy information on the studies at the end of this book.
- ask the doctor to read it.
- go back and ask him/her if you will receive their support.
- be sure you feel comfortable in discussing any of your concerns with the physician. This applies not only to the Feingold Program, but to all health matters. Don't forget that you are the consumer paying for a service, and this is your right.

Here are some of the criticisms you are likely to encounter:
"The Feingold Program hasn't been scientifically proven." This is true, since it has never been scientifically tested! There are numerous studies listed in the last section of this book which provide supportive information, but so far none has been a study of the Feingold Program as we use it in our homes.

"Only 1% of the children succeed." Ask to see the evidence. Where are the scientific studies that demonstrate this? There are none.

"It works because of placebo effect." (because you expect it to) Several of the studies -- particularly the most recent -- were designed to control for placebo effect. They found that this was not a factor.

"It's too difficult, restrictive, expensive, etc."

1. Nothing is as difficult as dealing with a troubled child.
2. A program that lets you eat at McDonald's can't be called restrictive.
3. The most expensive foods are the very highly processed ones, so grocery bills generally go down. What a family can save on doctor's bills and medicine will buy a *lot* of groceries!

Planning for your child's hospital stay

If you know in advance of a hospital stay, there is a lot you can do to help it run smoothly. You can request assistance from various professionals, especially your primary care physician, the hospital dietitian, and the nurses who will be caring for your child. The Feingold Association's membership packet contains detailed suggestions on gaining cooperation, as well as ways to avoid synthetic colorings and flavorings in medicines. Even when the stay is unplanned, as in the story that follows, you do much to avoid potential problems.

Emergency!

A week ago our 5-year-old son ran into a storm door and ended up with glass lodged in his chest and temple.

We took Kyle to an emergency clinic where the doctor did what he could, and then transferred him to the hospital by ambulance. The doctor in the hospital's emergency room worked on him for several hours then sent him to surgery to remove the rest of the glass. (A piece had lodged between his heart and left lung.) After surgery he had I.V.s in his arm and a tube in his chest. Through this whole ordeal in two emergency rooms, with doctors sticking needles into him and sewing up the wounds, he was very calm. We were with him the entire time until surgery and no one could believe how brave and calm he was. In fact, Kyle took the whole thing much better than Mom and Dad did!

He had never been in the hospital before so this was a whole new experience, and we know that he never would have been so calm if he had not been on the Feingold Program. After the surgery the doctors and nurses were interested in the diet and tried to be helpful, although none of them knew anything about it.

It's a stressful experience having a child in the hospital without adding to these problems. And when he has to be kept in bed and quiet, hooked up to tubes, you don't want him reacting to the wrong foods.

Today we returned to the doctor to have the stitches removed (there were quite a few). Kyle just lay there and let the doctor remove all of those stitches without even a squeak. It could have been a much more unpleasant experience if we had an uncontrollable child on our hands. As you can tell, we're very proud of our son, and grateful for the Feingold diet.

How can I find out the ingredients in medicine?

There are several ways you can learn about the ingredients in medicine.

1. Speak to your pharmacist; if he does not readily have this information he should be able to obtain it for you.
2. Similarly, your doctor can check his *Physician's Desk Reference* (PDR), or ask the pharmaceutical company's representative to get the information.
3. Your local library should have a copy of the PDR, and they may also have the *Nurse's Desk Reference*.

The PDR can provide the name of the manufacturer of many medications, and a phone number to call. Most pharmaceutical companies will try to assist you.

Compounding Pharmacists

You may want to consider finding a compounding pharmacist; these professionals are likely to understand your need for medicines free of the most troublesome additives.

Most pharmacists purchase brand name and generic medicines and fill prescriptions by dispensing the number of pills, etc., requested. A compounding pharmacist has the ability to create medicines from the same components used by pharmaceutical companies. He will fill your prescription using ingredients you tolerate -- such as lactose-free, flavored with natural ingredients, made without dyes, etc. He could fill a capsule, create a tablet, or prepare the medicine to be delivered by a syrup, gel or spray.

Compounding pharmacists are also able to create fluoride preparations free of synthetic colors and flavors. You can obtain the name of a compounding pharmacist near you by calling the Professional Compounding Centers of America at 1 (800) 331-2498.

My child will require surgery and I'm concerned about the use of an anesthetic. Is there one that would be better tolerated by a Feingold child?

Pure Facts interviewed an anesthesiologist specially trained in pediatric anesthesiology. He and his wife were Feingold volunteers when their son was younger.

It is unlikely any of the anesthetics or medications the anesthesiologist will employ during surgery contain artificial colors, flavors or preservatives, nor would they be treated with BHA, BHT, or TBHQ as these are generally used to prevent rancidity in fats. (Similarly, nitrous oxide -- used in dental surgery -- should be acceptable for most Feingold members.)

Pain relievers are generally administered along with the anesthetic so the patient will awaken without undue discomfort. In the recovery room, oral medications like Tylenol can be given. (Feingold parents will need to be sure the Tylenol does not contain artificial colors or flavors. There are some versions of acetaminophen that are dye-free. Feingold adults who are salicylate-sensitive should be sure aspirin and medications with aspirin are not used. Also, request non-salicylate juices be available for the child or adult if these are given with medicine.)

Because a child is hyperactive or sensitive to synthetic food additives, you cannot necessarily assume he will be unusually sensitive to anesthetics. There is a very wide range of difference within the population; some people require very little anesthetic to achieve the desired effect, while others may need a great deal.

In addition, because a person has had a negative reaction to one medication, this doesn't mean he will be sensitive to all of them. Various classes of medicine are handled differently by the body. Our doctor noted that he has not observed any difference in the reaction hyperactive and non-hyperactive children have to anesthetics.

Any patient -- whether they are chemically sensitive or not -- needs to give the anesthesiologist detailed and accurate information prior to surgery. A person who uses alcohol, tranquilizers or certain drugs will require a larger dose of the anesthetic since their liver has "learned" how to metabolize certain drugs and get rid of them quickly. Dilantin, used for the control of seizures, also falls into this category.

Editor's Note: Some Feingold parents report their youngster has experienced adverse reactions to medication given during surgery, and some appear to require a much smaller amount than is typical for their age group, but they may simply fall at the far end of the spectrum of normal variations. Be sure to discuss all of your concerns with the doctors prior to surgery, and bring in printed information on the Feingold Program to give to the people who will be caring for your child. The Feingold Association can provide this material.

Inactive ingredients and active children

The couple carefully examined the package of children's vitamins, but could find no indication that it contained synthetic dyes.

They arrived home, opened the package, and poured out brightly colored pills. Then they called the Feingold Association.

The vitamin manufacturer is not obligated to indicate the presence of synthetic dyes since they are considered to be "inactive" ingredients. "Inactive," "non-toxic," and "harmless" are adjectives that frequently precede the words dye, or food coloring. But Feingold parents know only too well the damaging effects of these petroleum derivatives.

The role of "inactive" ingredients was investigated by the American Academy of Pediatrics Committee on Drugs, and in October, 1985, the results were published in the academy's journal, *Pediatrics*. The committee investigated a variety of additives, including synthetic dyes. They found that the dyes triggered a variety of physical problems, primarily affecting the skin and respiratory system.

The seriously ill child

When the problem is very serious, diet management is seldom considered.

Charlene has studied about illness and medical procedures for nearly four years. She is not a medical student, but a mother whose little boy has been beset with an unending series of problems for which there was no explanation. Johnny ran a constant low grade fever, had abnormal sleep patterns, chronic ear infections, followed by viral infections, and despite a high caloric intake, he did not grow or gain weight normally -- a condition generally called "failure to thrive."

He had symptoms of childhood arthritis, jaundice, allergies, and several episodes of hallucinating. Johnny was obviously bright, and spoke well and at an early age. But he simply could not slow down enough to sit and watch TV or listen to a story. His fine motor skills were poor, and his behavior became even worse after he left the "terrible twos."

Charlene describes herself as having been a hyperactive child, so Johnny's high level of activity was not surprising, but she hoped the defiance she saw in her 3 year old son was just a "stage" he would outgrow. But underneath the aggressive behavior, Charlene knew there was a sweet, loving little boy, and she was able to remain patient with him because she knew, somewhere, there was an explanation for all the problems he had.

Specialists from many medical disciplines tried to find the reason. In addition to numerous pediatricians, Johnny was seen by the following specialists: endocrinologist, gastroenterologist, rheumatologist, allergist, neurologist, and pediatric ENT specialist. He had CAT scans, body scans, EEGs, several bone age tests, food protocol, and was tested for cystic fibrosis, rheumatoid arthritis, liver disease, and hormonal disorders. Prestigious medical schools and children's hospitals repeatedly were unable to come up with any answers to this very little boy's problems.

Most of the professionals treating Johnny were compassionate with both their little patient and his parents. But Charlene bristles when she recounts the female gastroenterologist who blamed Charlene "for not feeding him enough" and the male pediatrician who told her, "Let me take him home with me for a week; I'll straighten him out." (She switched pediatricians.)

By this time Johnny was 3-1/2. He still had endless problems, and John and Charlene still had no answers. "As soon as he recovered from one crisis, another would follow. It kept us on the edge all the time. "John's mother learned of the Feingold Program from a colleague at work, who suggested it might help. The parents felt it was "worth a try," and joined their local association.

In the first couple of days, Charlene reports, there was a noticeable improvement in Johnny's behavior. He calmed down a lot, was less distracted, and could sit quietly to watch Sesame Street or listen to a story. Charlene doesn't know how many of her son's problems will be found to be related to his diet. But in the two months he has been on the Program, Johnny has grown more than he did in the previous year. The change is most noticeable to friends and family members who don't see him every day. His cheeks are filling out and his color is better. He's still an active preschooler, but he doesn't destroy his toys, as he previously did. Johnny now shows and receives affection, likes to cuddle, and seems genuinely sorry when he does something wrong.

The pediatrician is delighted with the improvement in her young patient, and will be closely monitoring his growth and progress. The ironic part is that the pediatric group where Charlene takes Johnny is very supportive of the Feingold Program. They just never thought something so simple could help a child with such serious problems.

First Aid Help to Have on Hand:

- Vitamin E capsules are great for scratches, scrapes and minor burns. Aloe vera is also excellent for minor burns; it is available in health food stores, or from your own aloe plant.
- Ammonia will relieve the itch of an insect bite.
- Rhus tox is a homeopathic remedy that many Feingold members use to both prevent and treat the rash caused by poison ivy. One of the nice things about homeopathic remedies is that they do not contain synthetic dyes and flavorings.
- Herbs and other natural remedies are now being taken seriously by traditional medicine. Two that are used by some physicians and their families are Echinacea for the common cold, and Lysine to prevent fever blisters.

Visit the Dentist -- But Avoid the Additives

Regular dental care is an important facet of maintaining a healthy body, but a trip to the dentist can be laden with artificial colors and flavors unless you take steps to avoid the chemicals.

The following is a letter received by the Hyperactivity Association of South Australia:

"Despite my instructions to the school dental clinic...they applied pink disclosing liquid to my son's teeth. He had one of the worst reactions since he started the Feingold diet. He went completely wild and punched up half the children in his class before being sent to the principal. Of course, instead of going there he ran home, arrived a crying wreck, collapsed exhausted and slept for the rest of the day.

"In addition to the behavioral and learning problems that may occur, a sensitive person may develop oral canker sores as a result of the artificially flavored and colored dental products. These mouth sores frequently recur and often fail to respond to usual therapy, according to the late Dr. Ben Feingold."

What can you do?

Most dentists will cooperate and help you avoid the colors and flavors that are present in so many clinical preparations if you discuss your sensitivities with them. Check your *Foodlist* for an acceptable brand of toothpaste; several are available at health food stores and at some drug stores. Avoid synthetically colored or flavored mouthwash and fluoride treatments. And refer to the *Feingold Handbook* for additional tips.

Fluoride

The Feingold Association acknowledges that some children appear to react adversely to fluoride in any form -- whether it is in their dental product, food, or drinking water. Beyond acknowledging this sensitivity, the Association does not take a stand either for or against the use of fluoride. But many others do.

Those infamous disclosure tablets

"The use of dyed materials for visualizing dental caries can precipitate acute episodes of hyperactivity. If the dentist has an alternate procedure, it is advisable to use it; otherwise the element of risk compared with benefit must be evaluated. If of sufficient importance the limited application of the dye may be applied with the knowledge that a period of disturbed behavior may be precipitated.

"The matter of carbohydrates must be considered. It is generally accepted that simple sugars predispose to dental caries. In addition, some children have a low threshold for simple sugars and develop hyperactivity. The matter of dentifrices should be discussed. Practically all toothpastes contain a variety of additives which should be avoided." (Contact FAUS for acceptable brands.)

Ben F. Feingold, M.D

SEASONS AND HOLIDAYS

Valentine's Day

The first holiday of the year where your child is likely to encounter synthetic additives is one that celebrates love, but doesn't do much to promote it. One of our talented volunteers put it so well in her article, titled:

"Love is not a lollypop"

I do not deprive my child. I do not limit or restrict her. Food additives can do that more certainly than a parent ever could. She would be too uncoordinated to swim, play soccer or ice skate. She wouldn't be able to sit still for a film, a meal or a car ride to Grandma's. How could she enjoy a field trip with her class if she couldn't stop touching things and couldn't stop fighting? How could she stay over with a friend? How could she go camping with the family?

Of course it is sometimes awkward, even embarrassing. And I do get tired of explaining, and reading labels, and making refreshments. But my efforts can give her back to herself. When she is free of chemical stress she is free to realize her true potential. Isn't that what we all want for our children? Love is not a lollypop.

Make a Valentine cake

The cake can be simply constructed by fitting together an 8" or 9" square cake and matching round cake:

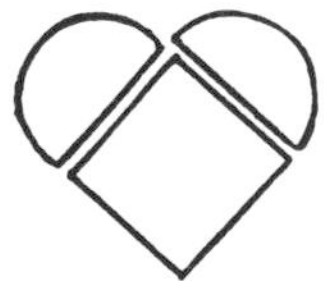

Decorate the cake with non-edible plastic hearts and/or flowers. Or use beet juice to color the frosting pink. There are many red juices for those who are on Stage Two.

Check your Foodlist for natural colorings that can be ordered.

Role reversal at the class party

If red cookies look nice on a white plate, then white cookies will look good on a red plate. Keep this in mind not only for a Valentine celebration, but next month when St. Patrick's day comes around. Green plates and plastic or paper cups will add lots of color for your white goodies and clear soda.

Enjoy a Feingold Easter

The Feingold Easter Bunny will need your help, plus some advanced planning to make this holiday a pleasant one for all.

Take the emphasis off candy by providing gifts. Small toys, costume jewelry, hair accessories, action figures, books, cassette tape or a new box of crayons will be welcomed.

A coupon from the Easter Bunny, good for an outing at a theater or amusement park, can be tucked in among the cellophane grass. Or how about a coupon book to play video games at the nearest shopping mall?

Use hollow plastic Easter eggs to hide coins or trinkets, or use them to hide treasure hunt clues (with each clue leading to another hidden egg, until the prize is located.) Don't forget nature's own candies such as dried pineapple, papaya, figs, dates, nuts. Just be sure to buy enough for the grown-ups!

Information on dying eggs with natural food colorings can be found in the *Feingold Handbook*. Or try the colorful plastic "sleeves" which need only be slipped over the egg and dipped in hot water.

Homemade cookies, miniature muffins, and dried fruits are more nourishing choices than candy. Limit the amount of candy in the basket and encourage your child to wait until he/she has eaten a nourishing meal before getting into it. Don't spoil the joy of the day by starting it with a lot of sugar on an empty stomach. If you want to include candy in the basket, refer to your Feingold information for acceptable brands.

*IMPORTANT: Carefully check the labels on the chocolate candy to be sure they do not contain "vanillin" (synthetic vanilla). Sweets on an empty stomach are a recipe for disaster, but for that special dessert after a nutritious meal, here's an idea for a bunny cake your children can help you decorate.

Bunny Cake

You'll need: 2 9" round layers from your favorite Feingold recipe

Frosting (see recipe)

1 1/2 cups coconut

cut up fruits, such as dates, papaya
black pipe cleaners or yarn
beet juice or natural colorings

Cut one layer as shown, and leave the other whole.
Tint a cup of the coconut pink by tossing it with natural coloring or beet juice.
Arrange the cake as shown, and frost it.
Sprinkle with coconut and decorate, using the pink coconut for the inside of the ears.

Creamy Frosting

6 Tbsp. butter
1 16 oz package confectioner's sugar
4 Tbsp. milk
1 tsp. pure vanilla extract

Cream the butter; gradually add in the sugar alternately with the milk. Add vanilla extract and beat well.

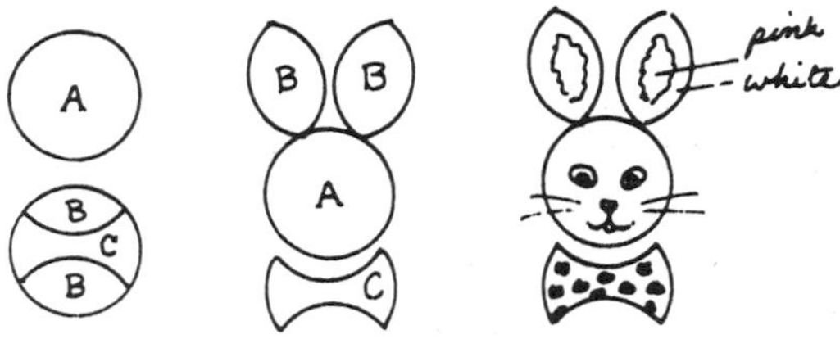

Suddenly it's summertime!

Here we go again - summer is just around the corner. Whether you're heading for the mountains, the beach, the park, or just the backyard, you can take the Feingold Program with you.

Are you sending your child off to spend a week with relatives? Plan ahead! Send a list (with brand names) of foods your child can tolerate. Feingold members can order additional Foodlist for any area of the U.S. Better yet, include a bag of groceries -- especially snacks. Kids generally snack more during vacation time.

On the road

Are you planning to travel by car? Some members bring their own natural feast; others take only some hard-to-find things. How much food to take along depends on many factors, particularly your degree of sensitivity and the length of time you've been on the Program.

If you're new to the diet or very sensitive, it's a good idea to pack more food, especially those things you may have trouble finding away from home. "Veterans," on the other hand, can often eat just about anywhere by choosing carefully.

Buy products like mayonnaise and salad dressing in small sizes; so you won't need to refrigerate them until they are opened, and you'll probably use them up before you get back home. Even though they are more expensive than the larger sizes, you will save a lot of money over restaurant foods.

For meals on the first day or two, load the ice chest with yogurt, hard boiled eggs, juices, soda, cold chicken, lunch meats, etc. You can always replenish at a supermarket.

Combine a rest stop and picnic on your travels. This gives the kids a chance to run off the excess energy while you are preparing lunch.

You can keep a box in the car with supplies such as drinking straws, plastic utensils, paper plates and napkins. A sealed plastic bag containing a damp washcloth is handy too. Pack in a few toys that can be used at rest stops.

Eat right; sleep tight

If you are staying at a motel/hotel, take along a box of cereal. You can always find a convenience store with milk. Consider making some muffins ahead of time; fresh fruit will complete the meal.

"Take along enough unbreakable bowls and disposable spoons for everyone in your family," suggests one volunteer, "for a breakfast of cold cereal in your room. If you'll be traveling to Canada or Mexico where you won't see many familiar brands, pack enough cereal for your Feingolder. Add fruit (canned or fresh) to complete the meal.

"If you feel it's necessary to warm things up, take along an old electric popcorn popper or electric skillet. You can manage without a kitchenette. But having one -- at least part of the time -- is wonderful; if it saves restaurant bills, it's worth the extra cost."

Check your Foodlist for shelf-stable meals that can be either boiled or microwaved. These will probably have to be mail ordered in advance, but are a wonderful convenience.

The extremely sensitive person may want to consider bringing along their own small microwave oven; the new compact versions will travel easily.

Traveling with a Feingolder does present challenges to your family and especially to Mom, who usually makes the food preparations. But the extra effort and planning make the trip more enjoyable for everyone. If you have ever traveled with an uncontrolled hyperactive child, then you understand.

Hotel room meals: the French student special

"A tried and true method of controlling your diet (and aiding your pocketbook) when away from home," notes one volunteer, "is to enjoy a little bread and cheese in your room, as students in Paris have done for centuries.

"Just as you keep a toiletry bag in your suitcase, also keep a mini-kitchen: a knife, small cutting board/plate, can opener, small salt & pepper, and utensils. When you arrive at your destination, instead of looking for restaurants, find a small grocery or deli and pick up items you know to be acceptable for your diet.

"With a little finesse, you can even turn your simple meal into a social gathering by inviting others to join you for bread, cheese, fruit and beverage in your room or in that inviting park across the way."

The summer dilemma -- away from home and hungry!

Close to home or far away, pick up your picnic at the supermarket.

We tend to think of the supermarket as just a place to do our grocery shopping, but modern supermarkets offer a wealth of possibilities at lunchtime. Even the less glitzy markets can provide the makings for an impromptu picnic.

Check out the salad bar. Are the bananas ripe? And do they offer melon halves ready to eat? Yogurt, cottage cheese and chilled fruit juice or milk are obvious choices. How about cheese with crackers or specialty breads?

At the deli section consider the sliced turkey or roast beef; they may even prepare sandwiches for you. Adult tastes suggest the croissants, and for the kids there's always a jar of peanut butter.

If you're not near a park, an elementary school playground might be just as much fun. Keep an old blanket in the car for picnicking. A wash cloth will stay wet for a long time if it's sealed inside a sealable plastic bag; it will take care of dirty hands and sticky fingers.

The convenience store

You're thirty minutes from home, the kids are hot, tired and hungry, and you spot a 7-Eleven down the road. Do you dare stop? There's a lot more to a 7-Eleven than Slurpees. If it's been a while since you browsed through a convenience store you may be in for a pleasant surprise. Hidden among the salty-sugary-chemical concoctions you can find real food: chilled fruit juices, yogurt, peanuts or milk.

For those times when a dessert is in order, look for natural juice popsicles or packaged snacks such as natural granola bars, pretzels, potato chips and corn chips.

Some more ideas on summer drink strategies

Before the thirsty season is upon you take some time to consider the many choices you have.

A jug of ice water in the back of the car is so obvious, many people overlook it. The kids might not be impressed, but they will drink it readily when they're away from home and thirsty. Spills aren't much of a problem. Take it to soccer practice and it can cool your athlete on the outside as well as the inside.

A cooler in the car will keep homemade lemonade or boxed juice drinks cool. Then use it to tote the ice cream home from the supermarket.

Fast food restaurants always have something to drink. Virtually any restaurant can provide ice water, a slice of lemon, and sugar. In other words, homemade lemonade. If all else fails, keep some small cans or boxes of acceptable drinks in the car. Any place that serves food should be able to supply a cup of ice (even if you have to pay them for it!) Pour in the drink and it will chill quickly.

Supermarkets compete with restaurants by offering snacks and drinks to go. You'll find small cartons of chilled juice, lemonade, etc. in the refrigerated section. If necessary, buy some paper cups or a box of straws and then keep them in the car.

Before you pile the kids into the car, mentally line up some possible watering holes so you can head for one while the thirsty howl is still a whimper.

Watermelon popsicles

This is a real treat for the kids and a good way to use up that melon that has been in the refrigerator a day too long and is getting "tired."

Cut up the melon and remove seeds; discard rind (or save it for watermelon pickles). Whirl the melon pieces in a blender and pour the juice into popsicle molds or small paper cups. Freeze them and enjoy!

Watermelon Gell-Oh

Prepare the watermelon juice as you would for popsicles. Follow the recipe on a package of unflavored gelatin, or use a recipe in the Feingold Association's recipe book.

Summertime notes

Some sensitive members react to insect sprays, lawn chemicals and various lotions rubbed on the skin (insect repellant, suntan lotion, etc.). Avoid these chemicals when possible.

PABA Ointment may be used for safe tanning and for burns of all kinds. Aloe vera and vitamin E oil are also natural remedies for burns. (Individuals who are very sensitive to benzoates may need to avoid PABA, which stands for para amino benzoic acid.)

Happy Halloween!

How can you make a major splash at the class Halloween party without artificial orange cookies? [Check Stage Two of your Foodlist for natural orange coloring.]

Try a Scary Night sheet cake. Use chocolate frosting to cover the cake, then add ghosts, gravestones, haunted houses or skeletons in white frosting. Coloring books are a good source of art ideas for decorated cakes. If pumpkins are a part of the scene, look for small plastic ones at a store that sells craft or cake decorating items. (Plan to get a lot of pumpkins to avoid fights over who gets to take them home.)

For cupcakes with a dramatic flair, try topping vanilla frosting with a black plastic spider or bat ring. (Oooh gross!) Or look for a colorful assortment of pumpkins and other seasonal plastic novelties; use them to decorate frosted cupcakes or cookies for treats that disappear quickly.

Ideas to help you enjoy the bewitching day -- and the days that follow

Ask a teacher what is the worst day of the year and you will probably hear "the day after Halloween!" A few school districts conveniently arrange to have a teachers' inservice day on the next school day. (I wonder why.) Here are a few ideas to get everyone through this holiday intact.

- If you have the time and interest, consider organizing a Halloween party, along with appropriate video movies. Or try a special evening at the skating rink, bowling alley or movies, followed by homemade treats.

- Arrange to buy back the treats your child collects, or have a bag of acceptable treats to swap with him.
- Send the kids out with full tummies, to minimize the risk of snacking. Or take along some "safe" treats when you accompany your child on the rounds.
- Deliver permitted treats to the homes of some of your neighbors beforehand and ask them to give these to your child when she comes by.

How moms have handled Halloween

A fair exchange - One mom described how she and her daughter went shopping together for a special new doll. She explained to her child that the doll would be Mom's for the short time until Halloween, and then the collected candies could be swapped for the new toy. Her child had the fun of collecting the Halloween candy, brought it back home, and gladly exchanged it for the new doll.

For the older children, nothing seems to beat the attraction of cold cash. Set a price for each piece of no-no candy, and you'll find them looking forward to the holiday as a favorite fund-raiser.

Carnival - A Texas member organized a party for Feingold kids at her church. The next year the church decided to hold a carnival. Her friends were very supportive, and made it a "safe" carnival with no forbidden treats or face painting. Prizes were stickers, puzzles, balls, patches, hats, pencils, novelty jewelry, posters, plastic toys, stuffed animals, etc. The teen-agers put together a spook house.

"Good dreams" holiday - An Iowa member writes, "I visited several neighbors earlier in the day and dropped off candies which were on the Foodlist. "When her dad took Amy out trick-or-treating he made sure they went to those houses, among others. When she returned home, Amy sorted her treats into two piles. (It was her idea.) She called them 'good stuff' and 'bad dream stuff,' which she gave away.

"The Feingold Association has been a great help to our family -- what a relief to begin sleeping most nights after three years of very little sleep!"

And what you will be giving out-

Balloons - These are great alternatives for Feingold families to give on Halloween night. (Look for a pump to help you supplement lungpower and to avoid ingesting the powder found inside them.) But be aware that uninflated balloons can be a hazard for children who put them in their mouth. The Consumer Product Safety Commission reports that inhaling an uninflated balloon or piece of a balloon is the leading cause of suffocation death in children.

Funny faces
When it comes time to transform your young trick-or-treater into his or her chosen role, take a look at the possibilities available with acceptable cosmetics. Traditional face paint can trigger a reaction.

Red: This has generally been the hardest color to create, but now that natural lipsticks are available in incredibly bright reds your little clown can sport a big red smile or rosy cheeks. Your older child can use it for vampire blood. Pinks and oranges are also available.
Check your Foodlist under non-foods for some natural lipsticks and other cosmetics.
Blue, Green, Purple, Brown, Black: Makeup designed to be used near the eyes is not permitted to be colored with synthetic dyes, so eye shadow and eye liner should be acceptable for Feingolders. (Check the labels for the BHA, BHT and TBHQ.)
White: You can create your own grease paint. Using a spatula, blend the following on a plate: 2 teaspoons white shortening, 5 teaspoons cornstarch, 1 teaspoon white flour. Add 3 or 4 drops of glycerin to form a creamy consistency. Glycerin is available at some drug stores.

Makeup will be much easier to remove if you first put a layer of cold cream on your child's face and allow it to dry, then apply the makeup.

Pumpkins!
Instead of carving your pumpkin this year, how about using paint, marker or crayon to provide its face? This is a great project for younger children. What's more, the pumpkin does not grow "peach fuzz" on the inside.

Feingold Assoc. of Southern California

One family writes, "We discovered a trick last Halloween that made our jack-o-lantern a little bit different, and made lighting it a lot safer.

"Instead of making the first cut around the stem on top, cut your opening around the bottom. No more reaching down inside to light the candle. Simply lift the pumpkin by its stem, leaving the bottom and the candle exposed, ready to light."

Caramel Corn

You will need a candy thermometer for this recipe. It takes a bit of watching, but the results are worth it.

1 batch of popped popcorn made from about 2/3 cup kernels
(don't add salt or butter)
unsalted peanuts or other nuts
unsalted sunflower & sesame seeds (optional)
1/2 cup honey (Honey is easy to measure if you first coat the
inside of the measuring cup with oil.)
1/4 cup water

Place the popcorn, nuts and seeds in your largest bowl or pot.
Combine the honey and water in a small, heavy saucepan.
Boil the honey/water until it reaches the soft ball stage, about 235 degrees.
If you don't have a candy thermometer you can test the syrup by dropping about 1/4 teaspoon of it into very cold -- but not ice -- water. Let it stay a moment and then pick it up. It should stay in one piece, but will not hold its shape.
Immediately pour the syrup over the popcorn mixture, stirring well to coat.

Thanksgiving!

If you're new to the Feingold Program, this year will probably provide much to be thankful for. You will be able to avoid unnecessary chemicals in your holiday feast by following some basic guidelines.

Turkey talk

At one time preparing a turkey for market was a pretty straightforward process, but today the bird is considered by many to be simply the raw material for another processed product. Colleen Smethers, president of the Feingold Association of Southern California, describes some of the tricks of the trade.

Sodium phosphate may be injected into turkeys to enhance water retention. This additive isn't likely to be a problem for the Feingold member, but it does mean we pay turkey prices for water.

The yellowish color of some poultry was once a result of the expensive corn and alfalfa feed used years ago. Today the Food and Drug Administration allows farmers to use feed additives referred to as "pigmentors."

Turkeys with the word "butter" in their name may not contain any butter at all, but are likely to be injected with a combination that can include: coconut oil, fat, water, salt, sugar, emulsifiers, antioxidants and artificial flavors and colors. All of these are unnecessary for the self-respecting turkey.

The newest wrinkle in turkeys is the addition of hydrolyzed vegetable protein (which contains **MSG**), and this may be found in fresh and plain frozen turkeys.

In most cases, the plain, unadorned supermarket brand fresh or frozen turkey is your best and most additive-free choice. If your family is too small to use up a bird before you grow tired of it, ask the butcher to cut it into two equal halves. (He can easily saw a fresh or frozen turkey.) Cook one half now, and freeze the other for a special meal in a few weeks. You will need to prepare the stuffing in a separate dish; turkey halves don't lend themselves to stuffing, but they're lighter and easier to handle.

Stuffing - Use your favorite bread. Add onion, celery, and other fresh foods; moisten with water or turkey broth, but not bouillon cubes.

Gravy - This can be a hassle if you're used to bouillon cubes, and now need to do without them. If you are roasting a turkey there will probably be enough drippings to make a rich and tasty gravy.

Feingolders can use other ingredients as well. Browned, sautéed onions provide both color and flavor. Soy sauce (stage one) and A-1* or Mrs. Dash's Steak Sauce* (both stage two) are good additions.

If you have the time and inclination, you can make your own beef broth by roasting beef bones and then making broth. Most commercial beef broths contain a hefty dose MSG. Check out health food varieties, but watch for salicylate flavorings in them.

The same is true with most canned chicken broth. But it's easy to make your own chicken or turkey broth and freeze it in portions for future use.

[* At the time of publication, these products are acceptable for use; however, brand name products are subject to frequent change. Please refer to a current Foodlist.]

Cranberries and Blueberries - New members are encouraged to skip the cranberry sauce until they are ready to go on Stage Two of the diet. Although cranberries are not always listed as one of the salicylate foods, Dr. Feingold found they affected some individuals, particularly those with eye-muscle disorder.

FAUS consulted the U.S. Department of Agriculture concerning the salicylate content of cranberries and blueberries. USDA informed us that cranberries and blueberries are members of the Vaccinium family of plants and thus contain benzoic acid, but should not contain salicylate. But we have seen that some members have trouble with these foods, so they should be treated the same as natural salicylates.

Vegetables - Most fresh, frozen and canned vegetables are acceptable. (Tomatoes, peppers and cucumbers are salicylates.) Vegetables packed in a sauce are likely to contain prohibited additives. A basic white sauce will turn fresh or frozen pearl onions into a holiday dish.

Sweet potatoes don't need to have marshmallows melted on them to be delicious. (However, there is a natural mini marshmallow available at press time.)

Mash cooked, peeled sweet potatoes with crushed pineapple plus its natural juice. Place the mixture in a greased baking dish and into the oven until it is heated through. The dish is so naturally sweet, your family will think you must have added sugar.

Relish tray - Carrots and celery are fine for people on Stage One, as are vegetables such as cauliflower and broccoli. There are several brands of olives on most Foodlists. Most brands of pickles (Stage Two) sold in supermarkets have added tartrazine, the name for Yellow dye No. 5. Dye-free versions can be found in health food stores.

Pumpkin pie - Most Feingold members use Libby's* canned solid pack pumpkin. This is just plain pumpkin, not the prepared pumpkin pie mix. Follow the recipe on the label, but leave out the cloves, which are natural salicylates.

Whipped cream - Take a look at the ingredient labels of whipped toppings in your supermarket. You may be surprised to find that some of them don't contain any cream at all! Pure heavy cream is an old fashioned treat if you can find it. To make your own whipped cream, whip 1 cup of cream with 1/4 cup confectioner's sugar and 1 teaspoon pure vanilla extract (or according to taste).

[*At press time Libby's canned pumpkin is on the Foodlist.]

Ice cream - Real vanilla ice cream is readily available. Look for the "vanillamark," or words like "natural flavoring" or just "vanilla." Steer clear of ingredient labels that list "vanillin" - a name for artificial vanilla. (Some vanilla ice creams contain yellow dye to give the appearance of added egg yolks.) There are also many acceptable ice creams in other flavors.

Nuts - Almonds are salicylates, and red pistachios are dyed. Check your Foodlist for brands of nuts, even those in shells, to avoid BHA, BHT, and TBHQ.

Cakes, cookies - Here again, the biggest problem for the cook who will be preparing her own homemade cakes and cookies is artificial vanilla. When you shop, look for pure vanilla extract. Then ask yourself: "if a manufacturer can afford to sell imitation vanilla at such a low price, what in the world is it made of?" Unfortunately, they are not required to tell us.

Refer to your membership materials for information on finding natural cake or cookie mixes.

To help Grandma cook with love, not additives, you may want to photocopy the above food information and pass it on.

Over the river and through the woods...

Whether you travel over the river and through the woods or take the elevator up to their condo, this is the season to get together with Grandma and Grandpa.

Holiday trips to Grandma's house are a warm and rewarding experience for some Feingold families; for others they are a potential disaster.

In some cases, Grandma and Grandpa have been so impressed by the change in their grandchild, they join the Association and improve their own eating habits. They feel better than they have in years, and food is not an issue.

But some grandparents have difficulty accepting the idea that foods and food additives can affect behavior. Rather than see their grandchild as a normal person, who simply can't eat petrochemicals, they see him/her as being singled out as "different."

One member described her holiday experience:

The holidays have arrived! Is it the same for you as it is for me? I have mixed feelings. I can just hear Grandma's usual refrain, "The poor dear, I feel so sorry for him. There really isn't very much he can have, is there?" Of course, she has to stand right next to him when she says it -- never remembering the many times I have showed her my 81 page list of approved foods, or made specific suggestions about where to buy what products.

What can you do? Be firm. Make it clear that yes, just one day of cheating will hurt. I find that telling people about my son's experience can be quite effective. Denny had started school in a new class where they didn't know about his diet. Under peer pressure he traded foods at lunch.

Some additives can cause vision and/or hearing deficits. Well, Denny walked out in front of an oncoming car and was hit. I have had to issue an ultimatum to the grandparents: "Because I love my son, either you will purchase or allow me to bring approved foods. You will not degrade his diet, or he will not visit you."

And do stick to your guns. Which would you prefer -- an offended Grandma or an injured child?

Work at gaining cooperation from the relatives

The Feingold Association of the Bay Area advises: Prepare Grandmother and other well-meaning relatives ahead of time. Take 15 minutes to call and ask what will be served at the holiday dinner. Then take another 15 minutes to drop them a note and list the acceptable brand names. Volunteer to bring some of the food; it's worth the effort to be sure you'll all have an enjoyable celebration.

Feingold members can purchase an extra Foodlist for any region of the United States to pass on to the relatives. Contact FAUS; we can send the Foodlist to you or directly to the relatives so it will be there when you arrive. Or, send your copy, perhaps with the familiar brands highlighted. Then order a new one from us. Some members prefer to take the relative shopping once they've arrived at their location, and buy all the needed food then.

Regardless of how your family likes to handle these visits, it is essential that you stick to your guns and not give in to the "just one little piece won't hurt" routine. Chemical sensitivity is not the same as a food allergy, where a little bit of cheating may be tolerated. The member who has been on the Feingold Program for less than a year, is likely to be extremely sensitive to even a tiny amount of the prohibited chemicals, and perhaps to salicylates.

Teaching your family about our program

Have you sent Grandma her copy of the School Year Calendar? Did you loan her your *Handbook*, or request an extra one from FAUS? Have you passed along an information brochure and some of your issues of *Pure Facts*? (You can obtain extra copies of these too.) Loan this book to her.

The Association can provide many aids in explaining the program to your relatives, but none is as good as our videotape. This 21 minute promotional VHS tape makes the Feingold Program and the scientific basis for it easy to understand. For a minimal cost you can order your copy from: FAUS Video, P.O. Box 6550, Alexandria, VA 22306.

If you find you need to bring out the big guns, check the section of this book on Coping Skills. But for many relatives, you will need only to provide information on the diet your family is using. The following letter to Grandma and others is something you may want to photocopy and pass out.

But first – a note to the experienced Feingold member:

Most of us who now use the Feingold Program started out not understanding it, and many of us thought it sounded pretty crazy to say that our kid's behavior had anything to do with our shopping list. Keep this in mind when you deal with skepticism.

Do you remember all the questions and doubts you had when you first learned of the Feingold Program? You may have wondered why a child who isn't overweight would have to go on a special diet; or you may have worried that being on this program could mean there's something wrong with your youngster. You may have imagined all sorts of unfamiliar foods you would have to eat -- possibly tofu and alfalfa sprouts three times a day!

You now know that the Feingold Program means normal food for normal people. You've had the advantage of observing the change in your child or in yourself. You KNOW how food additives/salicylates can affect a person's behavior because you've lived it.

We'd like to help you to explain the Feingold Program to your friends and relatives, particularly those who have a special place in their heart for your child. We hope this summary will make the Feingold Program more understandable to them, and that they will see how small a change is required to go from "synthetic" to "Feingold." Please feel free to photocopy it and spread it around.

***Dear Grandma and Grandpa,** doting aunts and uncles, teachers, and friends...There's a special child in your life who needs your loving support. The purpose of this letter is to tell you about a program that could make a big difference in the life of that child, and to show you how you can be a part of its success.*

Back in the 1960s a remarkable doctor began to experiment with certain types of allergic reactions, and this eventually led to an understanding of how various chemicals can influence behavior, as well as one's ability to reason and learn.

After a long and distinguished career as both an allergist and pediatrician, Ben F. Feingold, M.D., had reached the age where most men ease into retirement. But instead, he accepted the challenge to create the department of allergy for the Kaiser Permanente Medical Center in San Francisco, and to serve as its Chief.

One of his patients was an adult who did not respond to the traditional therapy. Suspecting that this woman may be sensitive to aspirin, Dr. Feingold researched the scientific journals and uncovered some surprising relationships.

He found that not only is aspirin a problem for some people, but other substances, commonly found in our food supply, have a chemical similarity to aspirin. This includes certain food additives as well as some fruits and a few vegetables. (The chemical name for aspirin is acetyl salicylic acid, and from this comes the term "salicylate," which we use to refer to those fruits and vegetables.)

Using the time-honored technique of an elimination diet, he asked patients to remove the additives and salicylates, and to observe if there was an improvement. The aspirin-sensitive patient was the first of many to follow Dr. Feingold's suggestion, and the results surprised and intrigued him.

Not only did some health problems diminish on this diet, but he kept hearing that patients became calmer and better able to concentrate when the additives and salicylates were removed. Children who were being treated primarily for allergies -- but who also had behavior or learning problems -- were suddenly functioning well, both at home and in school.

After helping hundreds of children and adults in his clinical practice, Dr. Feingold published the results of his work in professional journals, and in 1973 presented his findings to the American Medical Association. At the request of a major publisher, he wrote of his findings in the book, Why Your Child is Hyperactive.

Today this effort is being carried out by a network of volunteers -- parents, teachers, doctors, nurses, counselors, dietitians -- who have seen the program work for themselves, or their families, or for others they care about. Support groups have been established in the United States, Canada, Australia, New Zealand, Israel, Norway, Holland, Sweden, and throughout Great Britain. The literature has been translated into French, Dutch, Japanese, Norwegian, Hebrew and Spanish.

Children who follow the Feingold Program need to restrict their intake of the natural salicylates (apples, oranges, etc.) for a few weeks, and then may add them back one at a time. Only those that are not tolerated are removed. Beyond that, children on this program can eat virtually any kind of food; the change in their diet is that they eat the brands and flavors which have been researched and found to be free of certain synthetic additives.

Synthetic dyes are the most infamous of the additives we remove. You may have bought a box of little bottles of red, yellow, green and blue food color. They are powerful substances that are synthesized from petroleum, and are suspected of causing serious health problems, including cancer.

Most of the dyes originally used in foods have been banned, and those that remain have been found to trigger behavior and learning problems in sensitive children. Some studies suggest that these chemicals can "short circuit" the electrical impulses in the brain, interfering with the ability to think.

Like most additives, they were used in foods for decades before our government considered conducting any safety testing on them. But even today, there is no requirement that a food dye, or any other additive, be tested for its effect on behavior and learning.

The other problem additives are the artificial flavorings and three preservatives: BHA, BHT and TBHQ (which are also made from petroleum).

Because we are all unique, a compound that appears to be tolerated by one person may be a real problem for the next. Other factors include the age and weight of an individual, as well as the amount of the chemical they consume.

Synthetic food colorings, originally made from coal tar oil, have been around for more than a hundred years. You probably ate them as a child when you had an occasional lollypop, candy cane, or jelly beans at Easter. But the key is "occasional." Your day did not begin with red, white and blue toothpaste, followed by fluorescent cereal filled with colored marshmallow bits, imitation orange juice, and topped off with a synthetically colored and flavored chewable vitamin. Wasn't your toothpaste white, your cereal beige, and if your mother made you take vitamins didn't they taste awful? When you got sick, the medicine was probably dark and unpleasant tasting, a far cry from today's shocking pink, red, or purple artificially colored and flavored potions.

Well, the problem seems to be that our food supply has changed drastically in the space of a few decades (even Jell-O was natural when it was first introduced!), but little bodies haven't changed. The child who consumes petroleum derivatives may be getting an overload, taking in more toxic chemicals than his small body can handle.

Grown-ups can have a tough time coping with these powerful chemical additives as well. Here again some of us are more sensitive than others, and we have different thresholds of what we can tolerate. Dr. Feingold noted that, except for terminology, there is no difference between a chemical we call a food additive, and one we call a drug.

If all this sounds like a farewell to candy, ice cream, soda, and miscellaneous junk food, that really isn't the case. The secret is in knowing which candy bar, which brand of ice cream, etc. is free of the harmful additives. Of course, we ask you to hold off bringing out these foods until after a child has eaten a good meal.

The Feingold member can provide you with the names of acceptable products available in your supermarket. Whether you're looking for a pancake mix, salad dressing, vegetable oil, chocolate chips, or any other food, you should be able to find a suitable brand in our Foodlist. Chances are, you are already using many of these products.

You will probably be able to use your favorite recipes, but simply substitute one or two ingredients. For example, desserts would be made with pure vanilla, not artificial vanilla or "vanillin." Gelatin is made with real fruit juice and unflavored gelatin. Read the label on a box of the well-known mixes and see if you can find anything in that chemical concoction (besides sugar) that sounds even remotely like food!

Feingold cooking is basic old-fashioned real food, and you can find it whether you cook from scratch, prefer mixes, or use prepared products. You can even locate real food at the fast food restaurants; the secret is in knowing what to look for and what to avoid. That's where we can help.

Getting there

When your holiday travels involve several hours or more be sure you have some food with you.

If you're driving, it's easy to keep an emergency kit in the trunk of the car. Snacks like crackers, nuts, dried fruit, pretzels and individual boxes, cans or bottles of juice will keep for a long time.

Sandwiches made of nut bread, spread with cream cheese, are filling and easy to take in the car or on a plane. Cartons of yogurt are also portable, and require only a plastic spoon.

A volunteer's time to say thanks

...to all who have "cast their vote" each time they chose real food and passed up the make-believe. Thanks to the store managers and businessmen who knew us first as customers, and then as friends, as they became caught up in the exciting business of helping children.

We all owe thanks to those parents throughout the countries of the world who spent their lunch hour typing, or who took vacation days to help a fledgling support group become incorporated.

Thanks to the moms who fixed dinner for their families, phone cradled on their shoulder, while helping another family over the rough spots at the beginning; to the dads who didn't get dinner until 8:00; to the kids who watched Mom go out to another Feingold meeting (her third this week). To all who have collated and labeled, stuffed, stamped and stapled...thinking back to those first papers you received, and the difference they have made in your life.

And especially

Our affection and gratitude go to Dr. Feingold, the man who called himself the "oldest jet setter," traveling all over the world for children. (Who said doctors don't make house calls anymore?) But of all the thank you's, the biggest goes to our kids...the 3 year olds who turn down candy, the 9 year olds who pass up "bug juice" at soccer practice, the teens who display a wisdom beyond their years...we're so proud of you.

And thanks to a Delaware volunteer for this lovely thought:

If you want to touch the past
touch a stone
If you want to touch the present
touch a rose
If you want to touch the future
touch a child

Teacher's gifts

It isn't too early to be thinking about a holiday gift for your child's teacher. She may welcome something that can be used in the classroom, such as stickers. Mail order companies (Spencer, Lillian Vernon, etc.) and stores which carry teachers' supplies offer boxes of unusual stickers -- including dinosaurs and insects -- that would be a welcomed change from stationary and cologne. Please be sure the stickers are UNSCENTED.

Another useful gift is an introduction to the Feingold Program. FAUS will provide your child's teacher with a year's subscription to *Pure Facts* at a special rate. Contact the office for details. (800) 321-3287.

A really happy holiday

It's tempting to let your hair down as you get caught up in the hustle of the holidays. But this is a bad idea. There's nothing like a three or four day out-of-control reaction to ruin all of your hard work and happy anticipation.

You're going to want your child to be at his best, whether he is at a class party, a family celebration, or going shopping with you. Try to get goodies lined up early, whether they are homemade, mail ordered, or available at local stores. You may want to freeze some of them so there will always be a "safe" alternative to the unnatural temptations.

Eat before you leave the house, and then have a little stash in the trunk of the car, just in case you stay away longer than you had expected. Even foods your kids might not like very much will have a way of being appealing when they're hungry. This is something you may want to use to your advantage.

One mom was planning a railroad trip with her preschool son. It was to be his first experience with rail travel and he was very excited. She deliberately chose new foods her finicky little one would normally not want to try called them "railroad food" and packed them along with the other carry-ons. The same technique often works with bored kids on long car trips.

Seasonal notes

The **glues** on stamps and envelopes are often artificially flavored. Give your holiday helper a damp sponge to use instead of his tongue.

Most children like to eat **snow**, but if a child is very sensitive, the pollutants that accumulate in snow could cause a reaction.

Mothballs that contain naphthalene (such as camphor balls) can be fatal to children if they are swallowed. Infant deaths have been reported after the babies were simply exposed to blankets and clothing which had been stored with mothballs. Products containing paradichlorobenzene should also be avoided as they are suspected carcinogens.

Pollution Inside

Indoor pollution is a greater concern during cold winter months when windows and doors are kept closed. These chemicals are harmful for everyone, but are likely to be a particular problem for the chemically sensitive person. Among the worst offenders are: gas appliances, including gas and oil furnaces which may leak fumes; kerosene heaters; fires in fireplaces or woodstoves (never burn building scraps, as they may have been treated with toxic chemicals); filters on heating systems and humidifiers (they can collect dust, bacteria, mold); formaldehyde, which can be found in pressed wood furniture and paneling, carpeting, upholstery fabrics, insulation in walls and around pipes, particularly in mobile homes; cleaning products, especially those using chlorine bleach. Some of these problems can be diminished by venting fumes to the outdoors, and others by airing the house out occasionally.

Projects which use **paints, solvents**, etc. are best for the times when the weather permits wide open windows.

Stay calm while you stay warm this winter.

YOUR CHILD IN SCHOOL

Starting the new school year

"To tell or not to tell" is the issue faced by many Feingold families as their child enters a new school year.

Is it better to let the new teacher know in advance that your youngster is on the Feingold Program, or would that prejudice him/her and label your child as hyperactive, ADD, etc.? This all depends upon the people you will be dealing with. If you believe that it's best to provide your child's teacher with information and assistance prior to the start of school contact the FAUS office to obtain printed information that is designed for the educator. Bring this with you when you have your first meeting.

Your primary grade child's teacher is vitally important to his success at school, and can have an influence -- for better or worse -- that lasts long after the year is over. So this is a relationship that merits your best diplomatic efforts. In his book, *Helping Your Hyperactive/ADD Child*, Dr. John Taylor writes, "In maintaining the delicate balance between your firmness on behalf of your child and your understanding of the teacher's frustrations, show an awareness of the rights of other students in the class."

Once you have this rapport, it's important to work at keeping it. The child who goes off his diet, becomes a royal pain at home, and tries his parent's patience to the limits, is not going to be any more loveable in a classroom. In other words, don't conduct any brave food experiments when there's school the next day.

Feingold moms who are successful in helping their children tend to be more visible than the average. If you can possibly manage it, volunteer to be room mother -- or at least be in charge of buying the foods/goodies they eat. Even if you end up preparing treats, you'll probably find that baking a batch of cupcakes for the class is still much easier than coping with a three-day reaction after your child eats candy corn at the Halloween party. A good relationship with your doctor will go a long way toward winning cooperation in the school. Next time you are in the office, ask for a note, written on his/her prescription pad, which says something to the effect of: "Jennifer is on the Feingold Program and all food should be cleared with the parents beforehand."

Even if you are successful in gaining the school's cooperation in following the Feingold Program, you may need to work at obtaining special help if your child has a learning disability. Just as adults often think a hyperactive child could control his behavior if he really wanted to, they often think a child could do his schoolwork if he really tried.

Taylor notes, "When an ADHD child in the primary grades responds well to one-on-one attention from the teacher, a common mistake is to conclude the child is simply poorly motivated or trying to get attention. The labels applied most frequently by well-meaning school personnel to ADHD children are 'unmotivated,' 'immature,' 'under-achieving,' 'bright but not working to potential,' and 'won't settle down.'"

Girls are more likely to be overlooked since their learning difficulties are apt to be manifest as distractible or flighty behavior (airheads), rather than the more typically disruptive, overactive behavior of the hyperactive, ADD boy. But quiet, confused little girls need help too.

Once your child is identified and enrolled in a special program, you're still not out of the woods. Find out if synthetic candies are given as a reward in the resource room. What about smelly stickers, scented markers, stamps used on hands, or (Heaven forbid) face painting? When it's time to prepare the IEP, which is required for every learning disabled child, be sure to have the Feingold Program written into it. Once again, contact the Association and request Feingold literature; the special ed teacher also needs to understand our program.

Nursery school

I have just returned from parent's night at nursery school for our four-year-old. I must write to you about this experience.

The director of the school had to bring her husband (who had substituted one day for our son's teacher) over to us so that he could meet the boy's parents. The physical education teacher and his classroom teacher both told us that he has a terrific positive self-concept for a four-year-old. They said he is self-confident about himself, but realistically so. They think he is a neat little guy. His teacher says if he ever turns up missing we'll find him at her house. They said he has a great sense of humor. The physical education teacher wanted to know what we had done to raise him to promote such a positive self-image.

What music to the ears of these two parents! Can this be the same child who cried constantly from seven days old until he was 2 1/2? The same child who had a burr under his blanket constantly till age 2 1/2? The same child who could not tolerate any frustration at all?

As a toddler when he faced frustration he would run backwards, sit down, and slam the back of his head to the floor. If his head hit something soft, he would get up and do it again until he hurt himself. When something irritated him, he would physically attack the person he determined was frustrating him. Mommy said "no." Hit Mommy and scream at her. Then dissolve into tears and clutch Mommy, crying "Hold me. Hold me!"

So what happened at age 2 1/2 to change our little fellow's direction? We had been talking regularly with the pediatrician about how to deal with this behavior and had tried various approaches, but nothing seemed to make a significant difference. He was our second child, born four years after his brother, and we had not had any of these problems raising our older son.

This is our family's valentine letter to the Feingold Association for providing us with a Foodlist, a sympathetic ear, positive encouragement, and directions for following the diet for our 2-1/2 year-old. We've come a long, long way in these two years. Thanks to you, Feingold Association, for providing the key for enabling our boy to be himself.

Preschool problems

One mother wrote:

My three year old, Timmy, is enrolled in a preschool which he attends two days a week. He is already reading, and advanced in some ways, but I wanted him to have a chance to interact with other children and develop his social skills. The problem is that his teacher dislikes him and doesn't try to disguise her feelings. I've tried to speak with her, but she generally avoids me, and when we do talk she is very resentful. The other day she said that Eric "choked" Timmy, but that it was understandable since Timmy "is always in Eric's face." It was as though choking was excusable since Timmy irritated Eric. Afterward, Eric's mother and I spoke; she felt bad about the incident, and suggested we try to get the boys together so we could help them to get along.

Timmy does get too close to other children, and he touches them too much, but he's really a sweet little boy, and most other people don't have a problem with him.

Lately, he's begun to have nightmares and worries when he goes to bed that he will have more bad dreams. He talks cheerfully about the children and the teacher's aide, but refuses to speak about the teacher, or to even say her name.

I find myself scolding him more at home, as I feel I need to back up his teacher and try to help him to behave when he is at school. It all feels very wrong to me, but my friends all say to give him more time since he's only been in school for a few weeks. They think he will adjust and get along fine. What do you suggest?

A Preschool director responds:

No child should ever have to experience nightmares as a result of attendance at preschool! You have a right to expect the teacher to communicate with you and to discuss any concern you may have, no matter how trivial she may consider it to be. If the teacher is unwilling to work with you, speak with the director.

Be sure the diet is working for your child at home. This will make it easier to track down the causes of any behavior problems. Even a child successfully on the Program may take time to adjust to the new setting/distractions of the classroom. As the newness wears off he should adjust.

Both the teacher and director should be given information on your child's diet. Stress the importance of following it carefully and explain how your child's behavior will change when he is having a reaction.

Consider having your child's vision checked. If he sits too close to the TV, or tilts his head too close to an activity such as reading or coloring, this could be a clue to why he gets too close to other children. You can have the child look at a picture from several feet away -- a picture he has not previously seen -- and see if he can describe some of the details.

If the above check out O.K., Timmy's teacher should use 'time out' to demonstrate to the child that certain behaviors are not acceptable in the classroom. She should take him by the hand as soon as the unwanted behavior occurs, explain to him what he did wrong, and have him stay separated from the class for no more than 2 minutes. He needs to know that each time he repeats that behavior the time out will immediately follow. Children don't like to be separated from the class, and the behavior should go away.

Parents can reinforce the school's effort. When he is relaxing, watching TV or playing casually ask how school's going and about his friends there. Ask him if he knows what "time out" means, and if not, explain it to him. If he touches other children too much, explain that bodily contact such as roughhousing with Dad or hugs with Mom are O.K. at home, but not at school.

What it all boils down to is that when you entrust your child to the care of a preschool you are paying for them to interact and enhance the development of your child.

A Feingold mom responds:

I suggest you have him switched to a different classroom, and if that is not possible, take Timmy out of that school as fast as you can. Listen to your instincts, which tell you your child is very unhappy -- and you are paying the school for this "privilege." The nightmares and refusal to speak his teacher's name are red flags and a cry for help. (Be equally suspicious when a child seems to be abnormally eager to please a teacher.)

Not all teachers are good teachers; don't be intimidated by her title. One of the most important jobs the preschool teacher has is to help her little students learn social skills. But this woman is not only failing in her job, she is punishing your son because of what he doesn't know.

Don't be afraid to tell Timmy that you're changing the school/teacher, or taking him out because his teacher wasn't nice to him, and he is a good little boy who deserves to be treated nicely.

If you seek a new preschool, interview the teacher or director and ask them how they would handle the traits that Timmy is showing.

Also, consider some techniques that you can teach him at home. You could begin by showing Timmy "arm's length." Have him hold out his arm, and (getting down on his level) place yourself that distance away. Explain that this is how Eric wants to play and let him practice by pretending that you are Eric. Then switch roles and pretend you are Timmy. Let him tell you how far/close you should be to him. Remind him that "children play an arm away," and see if the sing-song rhyme of the phrase may be easier for him to remember.

If you and Eric's mom do get the boys together, Timmy will have had some practice. You may want to talk about "an arm away" with Eric and his mom, and ask Eric to remind Timmy if he forgets.

When Timmy was a baby, you knew his cries meant something and you did not ignore them. A three-year-old simply has a different way of crying for help.

Finding real food in your school's cafeteria

It will take some time and effort on your part, but you may find there are foods your Feingold child can eat after all.

Food service directors have a tough job. They are expected to provide a hot, nutritious lunch (and often breakfast), to please countless young tastebuds, charge very low prices, and stay within an incredibly tight budget.

Five times a week they are expected to have just the right foods ready at just the right time and in just the right quantity. To make matters worse, some school districts consider food such a low priority, they have combined the job of food service director with other duties. Dietitians may now find themselves ordering pencils and construction paper along with the hamburger buns.

It's no wonder the old-fashioned school cafeteria where food is actually prepared is becoming extinct. Pre-cut, pre-cooked, pre-packaged lunches generally save school systems money. The ladies with the white uniforms and hairnets may still be working on school lunches, but you're likely to find them standing beside a conveyer belt in an automated food manufacturing plant.

What can you do?

As discouraging as this sounds, it's not impossible for the average Feingold parent to track down *something* in the school cafeteria for her child to buy. If your Feingolder is only moderately sensitive or if you are certain of his/her sensitivities, this should work. However, if you are just beginning the Program or have a very sensitive child, you may need to simply make the best you can of the brown bag routine.

1. Contact FAUS and request information suitable for you to give to the food service director.

2. Don't contact the food service person yet since there's a good chance you will meet resistance. Instead, speak with the principal or write to the superintendent of schools. Explain that your child has some limitations and you would like assistance in finding suitable foods.

3. Most likely, your request will be passed on to the food service director, who will be told to deal with it. This way your concerns are not so likely to be ignored.

4. Try to arrange a conference with the director, and bring in your Feingold literature to help acquaint him/her with our program.

5. The food service office should have a detailed list of all of the ingredients for all of the foods they purchase. Being a veteran label-reader, you will probably be able to spot the no-nos and the potential problem areas. Of course, look for the obvious synthetic colors, flavors and anti-oxidants. But also be on the lookout for such tip-offs as: lard (almost always has BHA or BHT), "antioxidants," "color added," "certified color," "flavorings." And if your child is sensitive to MSG, watch for "hydrolyzed vegetable protein" and the many other places where this troublesome additive may be hidden: autolyzed yeast, sodium caseinate, calcium caseinate, flavoring, natural flavors, malt flavoring, high flavored yeast, soybean extract, seasoning, textured soy protein, yeast extract.

6. Ask for a tour of the pantry in your child's school. Here you can read the labels for yourself.

7. Have you found a few promising items? Maybe they're using natural (packaged) chocolate chip cookies, or it could be a good brand of yogurt. How about natural juice or lemonade? If the school has a salad bar this is a likely possibility. Does the fresh or canned fruit look O.K., or do they serve carrot salad? Even if you come away with nothing more than a carton of whole milk and an ice cream cup, it means your youngster can stand in line too, and buy something!

8. The length of time you have been on the program, as well as your child's age and sensitivity, will be important factors in deciding how much the foods could be eaten and how often. If you follow the program "by the book" (the *Feingold Handbook*) you should generally be able to detect a reaction. Test new foods cautiously, one at a time.

9. When you find a brand name product the school is using which your child seems to tolerate, please let the Feingold Association know about it. We can do the necessary research and gather information that will be helpful to other families.

Packing the lunch box

- Include a holiday napkin or a note.

- Pack some homemade candy with extra to share.

- Occasionally put some chocolate syrup in a small container so your child can add it to the milk bought from school.

- Vary lunch from day to day (unless your child likes having the same food day after day). When you bake or buy treats like cupcakes, cookies, etc., freeze half so she does not get the same treat each day.

- Special breads like banana, pumpkin, lemon or date-nut freeze very well and are easy to pack if you freeze them in individual slices.

- Small bags of popcorn, chips, seeds or nuts are a nice change.

- Dried fruits are sweet and nourishing.

- Look for alphabet pasta to add to your homemade soup.

- For the younger child, cut the sandwich out with cookie cutters or into different shapes for variety.
- Ask for permission to keep an emergency lunch in the school's freezer. An extra cupcake in case of unplanned parties is good insurance too.

Teenage or pre-teen lunch?

One mom won over her reluctant teen by hiring him to prepare his lunch each evening for the next day at school. She liked having the job delegated, he liked the income, and stopped complaining about brown bagging.

Too Much Candy!

It used to be just the bank and the barbershop where every child left with a lollypop in hand.

Doctor's offices climbed on board, as did scouts and Sunday school. Candy sales helped to fund school clubs and athletics. Candy machines joined the soft drinks in nearly every place visited by children. Shopping malls sport enormous gum ball dispensers. It's hard to find a place where children are not met with synthetically dyed and flavored confections. Now many are learning their "A, B...C is for candy" and being given it on a regular basis by their teachers.

Our society equates candy with love; just think of all the terms of endearment that use the words "sugar," "sweet," or "honey." Most parents are likely to see no harm in teachers rewarding the child for finishing a math assignment or writing all of the spelling words correctly.

But what about those parents who don't want their child to be given candy? The parent could be a dentist, a diabetic, an adult battling a food addiction, a Feingold parent, or a person who simply wants to be responsible for what her child eats. Whether the teacher gives candy to every child but one, or gives an alternative treat to that child, he is singled out and feels what most children don't want to feel -- different.

That is not the only reason to question this practice. What effect might this practice have on the school's goal of teaching that learning has its own reward? And why does the candy payoff bring to mind the morsel a trainer gives the animal that has performed a stunt?

While it may not be possible to talk adults out of giving rewards, you might be able to convince some of them to switch to the inexpensive trinkets available through mail order companies.

The End-of-School Fiasco

We received an interesting letter from the other perspective, written by a teacher who had recently learned of our work.

It was the last week of school a number of years ago. Teachers, parents, students and some pre-schoolers were all waiting for a bus to take us to a neighboring park for the school picnic. A downpour of rain forced a change in plans. There was no way we could go to the park for the picnic, so the buses were sent back and we made plans for the "picnic" in the school building. Since our school is small we decided to let the students sort of "do as you please" for most of the morning. We could hardly believe how well behaved the children were in spite of the fact that they had to stay on the grounds -- and inside the building. They were free to roam around or play games in any of the rooms, listen to music, whatever they wished. We had absolutely NO problems and the fact was remarked on by all of us who were in charge. Even the parents were surprised.

The truck that was to have brought the soda for the picnic arrived late. The driver had been lost so the children had nothing to drink except orange juice for lunch. Since it was getting late in the afternoon we decided to let the children drink all the soda they wanted (since it was already paid for). Drink they did!

Within ten minutes our well-behaved children turned into speed demons! They would not -- or could not -- sit still to play games or do anything they had done all morning. Parents and teachers alike (and even some of the children) could not believe what they were seeing. Needless to say, we were all happy when the busses came to take the children home.

There seemed to be only one answer to the problem - it had to be all the soda they drank. All of the teachers and some of the parents had attended a talk about a month before concerning the conduct of children and food additives; at the time of the talk most of them did not agree with what was said. Many times I have wished that I had a tape recorder so that I could have taped the comments of the parents on the hyperactivity of the children after they had consumed all that soda.

After forty-six years of teaching and administering elementary schools I am no longer an active teacher. I wish there would be some way to get parents to really listen when experts talk on WHY some children really do behave as they do.

Sister Paula L., St. Louis, MO

Strategies for dealing with the end-of-the-school-year party

You made it through Halloween. Thanksgiving wasn't hard, and you handled Christmas very well. Easter was a credit to your imagination. The baskets overflowed with Feingold-safe delights, and nobody seemed to miss the jellybeans.

Just when you think you're out of the woods and there are no more junk food holidays to contend with, along comes the last-day-of-school party. You're the mother of three kids (one Feingold, two Regular) holding down a full-time job away from home -- not to mention the full-time job *at* home. Baking cupcakes for half of the elementary school population is not your idea of fun. But you can't let your Feingolder "blow it," and your other two will feel slighted if they don't have goodies to take in to their class too.

You don't have to do everything in triplicate. Bake one batch of cupcakes, and give each child one third to take in and share with his friends. Add a container of approved brand lemonade and a bag of chips for each child's class. This will give you maximum benefit for a minimum effort.

As you wash the beaters, be comforted by the realization that nobody, thus far, has succeeded in connecting junk food with the 4th of July, and you'll have till the end of October to take it easy.

Tips on finger-painting

Dye can be absorbed through the skin, just as medicine is when placed on a patch.

If a child is not terribly sensitive, he might be able to finger paint, and then just wash his hands well after he has finished. For the sensitive child, it is not as simple. Some parents have purchased disposable gloves for the child to wear, but it is difficult to find these in a size small enough for the child to use them with ease.

Conney Safety Products is a mail order company in Wisconsin that offers a wide range of first aid supplies, including **disposable gloves**. They offer latex, vinyl and powder-free vinyl. The gloves are very small, but extremely stretchy, and look like they would be suitable for virtually all hand sizes.

If you suspect your child may be reacting to the materials in the glove, it would be worthwhile to try washing them first. Some sensitive people report this helps. The gloves are available from FAUS's mail order catalog.

The Sick School Syndrome

A former teacher who became ill as a result of working in a polluted environment has become a crusader for healthy school environments for both children and teachers.

While she taught Spanish in a newly built New Jersey high school, Irene Wilkenfeld would not have considered the word "polluted" to be an appropriate description of the building. But years later, she would make the connection between her deteriorated health and the toxic chemicals she had encountered there. Irene spent fifteen frustrating years searching before she found the medical help she needed to overcome the effects of the school chemicals. Today she is a free-lance medical writer who conducts workshops on how schools can recognize and clean up sick buildings.

Referring to the frequently cited decline in the performance of American students, Irene gives the educational bureaucracy a failing report card. She writes: "It's ironic to note that the institution mandated to nurture our students may often be an unwitting culprit in their toxic poisoning and in their learning disabilities. Educators must realize that all chemicals used in construction, furnishing, housekeeping, maintenance, renovation, pest control, food service and classroom activities can and do affect indoor air quality and subsequently the health of the building's occupants. The health of the human body is a barometer of the health of the environment. The health of a student and the health of his/her school environment are intimately interconnected!"

Feingold parents know the profound effect chemicals can have on a child's ability to behave, to learn, and function. If you find that after you have changed your child's diet you are still seeing reactions, consider the following possibilities.

Typical culprits in the schools

Even before your child arrives at school, a potential culprit is the school bus. Just as cars give off a "new car smell," new buses also contain many synthetic materials that release fumes from chemicals that are used in their creation and manufacturing process. A sniff test is a simple way to identify a possible problem; eventually, the smell will fade as the chemicals "gas off." If a cheerful youngster step into that shiny orange vehicle, and a grouch gets off at the school, step into the bus yourself and see if you detect an obvious smell; you may even notice that you have a physical reaction of some type. Speak with the bus driver. Has he/she noticed any effects after driving a new vehicle, compared to an older one?

What can be done? A school administration interested in minimizing off gassing can do a variety of things. Ideally, they would consult with experts in this field and insist the manufacturer use materials with low toxicity.

When traditional materials are used, allowing them to be exposed to the air for out-gassing would help. Permitting the finished buses to air out before they are delivered would lessen the problem.

The Dasun Company provides a product called NonScents, which actually absorbs gases and odors, and can be reused many times. For more information contact the Dasun Company at P.O. Box 668, Escondido, CA 92033, (800) 433-8929.

The inside of the school bus is not the only source of problems. A potent chemical, benzene, is given off in the exhaust fumes of gasoline and diesel fuel.

What can be done? Drivers can minimize children's exposure to these fumes by simply keeping the engine turned off while parked at the school.

Maintenance crews can check the engine exhaust system carefully for any leaks that could enter the bus.

Where is the air intake for the school's ventilation system? It should be located as far as possible from the exhaust fumes of cars and buses.

Inside the school

Everyone likes to come back to a freshly painted school -- provided the painting was done during the summer and the fumes have had a chance to gas out.

New carpeting looks great, but it can take a long time before the formaldehyde and other chemicals in synthetic carpeting have outgassed. Unlike hard flooring, carpets are prone to harbor mold, mites and any pesticides used in the building.

Leaky roof? The best time to spread tar on the school roof is when the building is empty. Asphalt and tar are powerful toxins. (Steer your teenager away from summer construction jobs that will expose him to these.)

Cleaning supplies, waxes, polishes and deodorizers can contain powerful chemicals that leave enough of a residue to cause noticeable problems for sensitive people. Alternatives are available. Safer forms of pest control are receiving well-deserved attention in some school districts. Integrated pest management (IPM) refers to techniques for controlling pests with the least toxic chemicals possible. There are several organizations devoted to promoting this. The art room, shop, chemistry lab, auto repair facility, cosmetology room etc., can all have potentially harmful chemicals.

What can be done? Cleaning up a school environment does not have to be an impossible (or impossibly expensive) job. Some substances can be replaced with safer products; a bit of extra precaution in handling others will help. And a major improvement will come by planning for the necessary ventilation.

Fresher air

Schools have contained strong chemicals for many years. It's true there are many more chemicals today, but the compounds themselves are not the only problem. Toxic fumes become a serious problem when they are kept sealed in tightly built, energy efficient buildings. These problems are just as prevalent in office buildings. Many new schools and offices have windows that don't open to let in fresh outside air -- which is nearly always far purer than indoor air.

Note: Portable classrooms can be comfortable places to work and learn (especially if they're just drafty enough to let in fresh air). But airtight mobile home style units can be filled with materials that emit formaldehyde.

Centrally controlled ventilating systems are supposed to keep the air reasonably pure, but they are often a major problem. Systems can malfunction. Filters can be dusty, dirty or moldy. Chemicals from one part of the school can be circulated throughout the building.

Since few school boards would be willing to cut holes in the walls and install windows, the next best choice would be to take a close look at how well the ventilation system works, and make any needed changes.

In your child's classroom

Of the many potential problems found in schools, the most obvious and (hopefully) easiest to change are probably found right in your child's classroom.

A major offender Feingold volunteers hear about is perfume. Perfume manufacturers have given their products an image that is not deserved. Far from being romantic, exciting, fresh, and lovely, perfume is a collection of harsh chemicals, many of which are derived from petroleum. (According to the California consumer group, Citizens for Toxic-free Marin, some of the chemicals used in perfumes are designated as hazardous waste disposal chemicals.)

As a rule, the younger your child, the less likelihood of being exposed to perfume from the other children. The chemically sensitive high school student may have to contend with fragrances from many sources, but for the typical first grader, the source is likely to be his teacher. Scented stickers, markers and other pens are also frequent offenders. Potpourri and room deodorizers can be a problem. Some dolls, doll clothes and other toys are now being treated with fragrance.

Of course, the most obvious source of trouble for the Feingold child is the food served in thc school cafeteria and sometimes given out in the classroom. He can refrain from eating the food, but cannot refrain from breathing perfumed air.

What can be done? If your child's health, behavior or learning is being affected, you'll have to speak up. I have no formula for convincing a teacher to stop using perfume, scented classroom products or giving out additive-laden food. But we can provide printed information and materials to support your effort. Don't expect others to take your word for it; you need to be ready to document what you are saying, whether you are speaking with a teacher, doctor, relative, friend, or neighbor.

Has your youngster's teacher seen the "before" and "after" child? Someone who has never witnessed a reaction has a right to be skeptical. If your child is unfortunate enough to have a reaction and there is some way his teacher can observe the effects without embarrassing him, she may be more understanding in the future. Seeing is believing.

One child had a very bad reaction as a result of a leak in the school's oil furnace. In such a case the child should stay at home until the problem is corrected, with the school providing a tutor.

A private school may be more receptive to making the changes your student needs. A modification that helps your very sensitive child will also help his not-so-sensitive classmates.

One Feingold mom got fed up with her son spending his days out in the hall, being disciplined because he was reacting to his teacher's perfume. The principal had to weigh an ultimatum to the teacher with the loss of a tuition check.

Another mom was astonished at her youngest son's angry, abusive behavior when she picked him up after school. He had eaten lunch in the newly painted basement lunchroom -- a room with no windows.

Additional information on safer schools is available from Irene Wilkenfeld. Contact Irene to learn how you can become a Safe School

Ambassador, alerting your community to the hidden hazards lurking in your schools. Ask her about her workshop, on detoxifying contaminated classrooms, and arrange one for your area. (Irene Wilkenfeld, Safe Schools, 205 Paddington Drive, Lafayette, LA 70508, phone (318) 269-1735.)

(You may want to photocopy the next section in this book, to pass on to a teacher.)

Especially for Teachers: That Kid Who Drives You Crazy!

You could run through an alphabet of symptoms: Aggressive, Belligerent, Clumsy, Distractible, Emotional, Forgetful, Gauche, Hyperactive, Impulsive...

There is evidence to indicate that many children like this are reacting to everyday substances; fortunately a great deal can be done to help them.

Do you wake up some days and wonder why you ever chose to be a teacher? Of all the challenges you face, let's isolate one, and take a closer look at it - and in this case "it" refers to a child we'll call Jeremy. He's bright. The tests show that, but you wouldn't know it from looking at his work. He understands a concept one day, and is bewildered by it the next.

He does foolish/destructive things even though he knows better. When you ask him why, and he responds, "I don't know," his answer seems genuine. His hands, legs and mouth appear to possess a life of their own. He says the wrong things, too loud, and at the wrong time. Most of the other children avoid him, although a few find him an easy target and convenient scapegoat.

As you speak with Jeremy's mother, you listen carefully for clues that would explain where she went wrong. But she's as exasperated as you are, and her other children are fine. "Poor parenting" just doesn't fit.

Is there "something wrong" with this little boy - something in his brain that doesn't work properly? Is there a defect he was born with? This is not a comfortable fit either, as his behavior is inconsistent. On some days he functions quite well, and on others he's impossible. Similarly, his mother notes there are wide variations at home. She also mentions that Jeremy was a contented baby during the time she was breastfeeding, but he had difficulty sleeping after she introduced table food. Both of you notice he's worse after holidays and parties, but conclude that he is just overstimulated.

Although various tests show Jeremy's brain is perfectly normal, your suspicion is correct that something is wrong with his "internal environment." A relatively new branch of science deals with this. It's called behavioral toxicology, and looks at the way a sensitive individual's behavior can be affected by external substances.

While the formal study of behavioral toxicology is new, the examples are as old as recorded history. Take an external substance called "wine." If a person consumed a large quantity of wine, and then behaved abnormally or couldn't remember how to solve a math problem, we wouldn't be mystified by the cause.

If we were to conduct an experiment with many individuals, we would see wide variations in the ability to tolerate this substance (wine). The reactions to it would depend upon the amount consumed and each person's degree of sensitivity to it - in other words, their individual chemical make-up would be an important factor.

There are many substances besides wine that can affect a person's behavior and ability to focus and learn. Some are believed to be transient and some are known to be permanent. Examples include: heavy metals such as lead, mercury and cadmium; alcohol of all types; nicotine; caffeine; drugs -- both legal and illegal; solvents and glues, such as airplane glue; petroleum.

Petroleum!? Who thinks about this, except when we fill our gas tank? Few people are aware that thirty seven percent of the crude oil used in the United States goes into the manufacturing of other products with which we come in contact every day. Derivatives of petroleum and crude oil are in our clothing, cosmetics, shampoos, detergents, perfumes, paints, plastics, pesticides, and - most significant of all, our food. We eat, breathe, and surround ourselves with the by-products of crude oil every day, and some of us are having a hard time coping with these powerful substances.

Let's take a look at the typical morning in Jeremy's life as he gets ready for school. (Every substance which is likely to be an irritant for a chemically-sensitive person is noted with an *.)

He wakes up between sheets that have been exposed to scented fabric softening strips*. He walks down the hall on new carpeting*, which still retains the smell of the chemicals used in its manufacture. An air freshener* adorns the bathroom, and competes with scented soap* and scented tissue*. The tub has been cleaned with a miracle spray*, and the scent of chlorine* clings to the tile floor. His toothpaste is green*. Breakfast is a bowl of sugar frosted grains and synthetically colored marshmallow bits*, all treated with the preservative BHA*. They float in a sea of low-fat milk which has BHT* hidden in the added vitamin A. What looks like juice is a blend of water, sugar, and synthetic dyes*, plus artificial orange flavoring*. An artificially colored and flavored vitamin* tops off the meal. If Jeremy is having one of his frequent ear infections, his mother adds a spoonful of bright pink, bubble gum flavored medicine*. He runs past the fragrant potpourri*, out the door, across the lush green lawn -- treated with powerful pesticides* -- across the newly paved asphalt* street. He has forgotten his homework and his lunch money (for the third time this week) and Jeremy's mother wonders why her son simply can't get his act together.

Reaction

A sixth-grade Feingold child was displaying behavior that was unusual for him since he started the diet. It turned out that he was reacting to the markers provided by the school. They are "fragranced" with scents such as mango, grape, orange, blueberry, lemon, cherry, licorice, etc. There are some children who are very sensitive to inhaled fragrances. (By the way, the label states that the markers are safe for children.)

Unexplained reactions?

A Feingold mom reports that her son was finding it hard to stay out of trouble at school. He kept having his name written on the chalkboard. After considering all the possible factors in Stephen's diet and environment she noticed they seemed to be eating out much more frequently - usually several times each weekend. She went back to home cooking and the behavior problems disappeared.

Experienced members can generally eat out, but if your child's behavior seems to have slipped, you may be overdoing it. Back up to your earlier Feingold days and see if this helps. Then enjoy the restaurant meals, but just not as often.

How I Saved Fairfax County $62,296.00

Money is scarce. Politicians are worried, and school boards are nervous.

Have you ever thought about how much money you have saved your state and local government by placing your child on the Feingold Program?

In Fairfax County, Virginia, it costs $5,336.00 (1990 figures) to pay for the education of one child for one year in an elementary school classroom. If that youngster receives help for a learning disability from a resource teacher, add $2,871.00 per year. And if the child's problems require him or her to be placed in a self-contained classroom for learning disabled children, the total annual bill is $12,671.00. That's ONE child, ONE year.

I added up the 13 years my daughter was in the public school system -- thirteen years she did not need to be in a LD class because she was on the Feingold Program. Then I figured the difference between the cost of a regular classroom and a special ed class. If you calculate that the costs have increased at the annual rate of about 4% for the thirteen years she was in school, the saving is $62,296.00.

For the child who has problems so severe they cannot dealt with in the public school, the county pays for "contract services" (spell that $ervice$!) which make my $62 thousand look like loose change. To learn how much money the Feingold Program has saved your school system, call the office of your school superintendent. They can refer you to the person in charge of the budget. Or ask the reference librarian at your local library; this is considered public information. Next time you ask for cooperation from your child's school, you may want to bring some figures along.

What's wrong with our schools?

Education is receiving a lot of attention these days. There is little dispute that something needs to be done. The "somethings" proposed are typically: give parents a choice, improve the caliber of teachers, lengthen the school year, and -- predictably -- spend more money. The following is taken from an article that appeared in *Business Week* magazine.

"In recent years a cruel paradox has been bedeviling observers of the US education system: On the one hand, statistics indicate that the US spends more on education on both a per-student basis and as a share of national income than virtually all of its major industrial rivals. On the other hand, numerous international comparisons of students' skills reveal that Americans are badly deficient in most areas of learning at a time when education and training are becoming an increasingly critical factor in determining national competitiveness."

Business Week 1/29/90

In all the well-meaning solutions suggested, the one vital element forgotten is the child -- the child who cannot concentrate, cannot behave appropriately and cannot learn. Paying higher salaries, lengthening the school year or giving parents a choice won't work if a child cannot read or spell. Spending more money won't help the youngster who can't keep his body in his chair or who forgets what she knew yesterday.

The concerned businessmen should go into the schools. They should observe the children, and speak with the teachers the day after Halloween, or even after lunch, and see what they have to say about food and behavior. Good food is not likely to be a panacea for the problems of our schools, but there's ample evidence that it can make a tremendous difference.

Better nutrition brings up test scores

In the spring of 1979, New York City's public schools ranked in the 39th percentile on standardized California Achievement Test scores. The following fall the New York City Board of Education began to change the foods served in the school breakfast and lunch programs. Gradually, synthetic colors, flavors and the antioxidant preservatives were removed and sugar was reduced.

Four years later, in the spring of 1983 the students scored in the 55th percentile! The only change that was made in the 803 participating schools was an improvement in diet, and the result was a whopping academic percentile increase of 15.7%.

The study was conducted by Stephen J. Schoenthaler, Ph.D., Walter E. Doraz, Ph.D., and James A. Wakefield, Jr., Ph.D., of California State University. It was published in the *International Journal of Biosocial Research*, Vol. 8, No. 2, 1986.

Edward and the K.I.S.S. Plan

Feingold mom, Diana M. is a crusader on behalf of children whose needs are not being met by the school system. She shared some of her experiences with members attending the 15th annual Feingold Conference.

Dr. Feingold had addressed the problem of a child who has had unhappy experiences in school, and continues to feel the effects even after his behavior and learning ability have improved on the program. He recommended one-on-one instruction for these children, and encouraged parents to remove their child from a school that failed to work with them for the student's benefit.

Like many of these youngsters, Diana's 9-year-old son, Edward, still has negative school experiences to overcome. After a year in a rigid, punitive atmosphere, they found an excellent private school with an approach that has worked very well.

Many schools use the terms "structure" and "discipline," Diana noted, and as a teacher, she was aware of the theories. She defines structure as: knowing where you're going and how to get there. Discipline, she continues, is just a matter of accomplishing the task. But too often what is called structure and discipline end up being rigidity and punishment.

Fortunately, the next school was able to help her son overcome the mistakes of the first.

Stressing the positive

The technique St. Mary's school successfully used with Edward is based on chips. Diana bought ordinary poker chips, and designated a color for each class. On the white chips she used a marker to note additional classes, such as P.E., or to give to the bus driver.

Each of the teachers had a supply of chips, and Edward had the opportunity each day to earn chips by behaving well, completing his work, etc. Every day he had the chance to proudly show Mom how much he had accomplished by the number of chips he earned. If one or two chips were missing, they could talk about what went wrong that time, and how he might try a different approach tomorrow.

The best part of this system, Diana noted, was that if he "blew it" at 9:30 in the morning it didn't mean the whole day was a loss. He still had the chance to earn a chip in the next class or the next hour. The entire emphasis for Edward was on success. It allowed the school, the parents and the child to focus on what he is doing right, and on what is wrong with the behavior, not with the child.

Everyone understood the clearly defined rules. They are listed by levels of consequences, beginning with number one, which is the least serious, going all the way to five, when it's time to pull out the big guns. The beauty of the system was that things seldom had to go very far, and never to level 5.

1. Verbal warning by the teacher. This might be for a minor thing like daydreaming. Edward would know that he wasn't going to get a chip then, but if he could get it together, there could be another chip on its way in the next hour.

2. Lost privilege, such as having to sit by himself at lunchtime.

3. In-class time out. There is a study carrel (not a cardboard box!) in the class. A child would be asked to remove himself from the rest or the class and take his work into the carrel so he could calm down and pull himself back together. When he felt he was ready to rejoin the class, he could come back to his seat.

4. In-school time out. There was also a carrel in the school office. In each instance, the teacher's words were gentle (but firm). "Edward, you seem to be having trouble settling down, so I'm going to ask a monitor to help you take your books to the office so you'll be able to put yourself back in control. As soon as you feel that you're ready to rejoin the class you may come back here."

5. The final step would be a conference with the parents. Each step is seen not as punishment, but as a chance for the child to modify his behavior. The assumption was that he was able to do so, and also that he would succeed. Every chip earned was a reinforcement to him that he was indeed capable of success in school.

Talking it over

Diana reinforced this approach when she spoke with her son. "What do you think went wrong? I'll bet you can remember to ____________ tomorrow and bring home a chip."

At the beginning when he may have been able to bring home only one chip for the entire day, it was still a success for Edward. In some cases, the school had to work hard at finding something worth rewarding, but they always found a way to let him know he had the ability to do well.

The payoff for the child is at the end of the week when he trades in his chips for a reward. Parents are told the payoff has to be non-monetary and non-material. They discuss it with their child and find activities both can agree to as rewards. For Edward's family, it's a trip to the beach, a picnic, a special movie, going skating, fishing or spending extra time at Grandma's. One of the benefits of such rewards is that they generally involve the parents and child spending time together.

Eyes on the prize

In the early weeks, Diana made sure the number of chips Edward would need to earn was a small, easily attainable number. "Attainable" is really the heart of this technique; each success builds upon the previous ones, until the child becomes accustomed to succeeding. For most children, the crucial thing is to break the pattern of failure by being given many opportunities to be successful.

He may need to earn an average of only 2 chips a day, in order to get the prize. Diana gradually raised the stakes, but he never failed to reach it. When she suggested Edward could bring home 15 chips the coming week, he seemed ready to accept the new challenge. "He began to have a different mind set," Diana notes, "he began to feel that if he really buckled down he could succeed. Before that he saw himself as a 9-year-old failure."

In addition to using chips, there were certain "target behaviors" for Edward to work on, and ordinary index cards were the tool used here.

Changing behaviors -- one at a time

One behavior is isolated and they may work on it for weeks. An example is "refrain from making noises in class." Each day, Diana sent in an index card divided into two sections: morning and afternoon. When Edward would forget and make noises, he would be reminded "That's what we're working on." A noiseless morning would earn him a smile sticker, and a mistake in the afternoon would mean a frown. This worked out to be so much more effective than punishment, and each day was a clean slate.

The school uses what Diana describes as the "KISS system." This stands for "Keep It Simple, Stupid." (Not very easy on the adult ego, but hard to forget!) Giving a child a token, a pat on the head, or initialing an index card doesn't take very long, and can be implemented even in a large class. The key to the effectiveness of these techniques, Diana believes, is the quality of the administration. "If you want to know how good a school is," she advises parents, "check out the administration."

The KISS technique, along with patience and positive encouragement, have clearly paid off for Edward. This year he made the honor roll and his national test scores rose from the 60th percentile to the 90th. He doesn't exactly love school, but he certainly no longer hates it!

Social Skills

Feingold parents understand what an important part diet plays in behavior. But there are many other factors that contribute to the difficulties children experience when they interact with others.

The youngster who begins the Feingold Program prior to age 5 or 6 might escape the destructive effects of being "the kid who doesn't fit in," and may not have trouble socializing. When the Feingold Program isn't started until later, a child may have a hard time catching up with his peers, and may always lag behind in social skills.

For some children, social difficulty can be the result of highly stressful experiences (see the story of Jenny, later in this section), and others, even after their behavior improves, just seem to remain out of sync with the rest of the world. One of the saddest things about social skills deficits is that the child generally has no idea why he or she doesn't get along with other children; even when the child grows to adulthood, the characteristics can still be present.

Stephen Nowicki and Marshall Duke are clinical psychologists at Emory University who have studied the problem of social rejection and have developed some practical "how to" strategies which parents and professionals can use to teach the skills a child lacks.

Helping the Child Who Doesn't Fit In, Duke, (Peachtree Press, Atlanta, GA) is based on many years of work with these children. The authors have coined a new word to describe the problem: dyssemia. "Dys" means difficulty, and "semes" stands for sign or signal. Together it describes difficulty in using and understanding nonverbal signs and signals. *Helping the Child Who Doesn't Fit In* describes characteristics of dyssemia and offers techniques for teaching a child to overcome them.

Planning a response. When John attempted to hold a conversation with another child his mind was so busy planning what he was going to say that he didn't pay attention to what the other boy was telling him. He needs to let go of programming himself, and focus on what he hears, then respond with a brief reaction to let his partner know John listened and understood. Children are not likely to be shunned simply because they don't speak a great deal; and everyone appreciates a good listener.

The "Uh-huh" factor. Recent research indicates that the way men and women speak is very different, and can lead to friction. Briefly described, the differences are:

When a group of men speak among themselves, one man is likely to be "in control" of the conversation. Then another gains control and speaks his mind. It's seen as a type of contest over who holds center stage.

Conversations among women, in contrast, are likely to be more like a tennis game, of back and forth dialogue. When two women speak and inject phrases like "really?" "Uh-huh," "Oh my gosh," this is taken as a sign the other woman hears and empathizes.

When a man speaks to a woman and she injects these phrases, he considers it an annoying interruption. When a woman speaks and a man is stony silent, she assumes it means he is not interested or isn't listening.

The dyssemic child may not understand that others feel uncomfortable when their comments to her are met with dead silence. "It's like talking to the wind; she makes me feel like I'm invisible."

Another characteristic is the child who avoids eye contact. This may be seen as disinterest or dishonesty. Avoiding eye contact is appropriate in some cultures, but considered rude in our society. The dyssemic child may do the opposite, and stare intently at the speaker, with equally bad results.

Creating Social Skills Problems

She had been an outgoing toddler, and approached anyone approximately her size with a smile and welcoming gesture. Jenny was stubborn, however, no doubt about that! In pre-school and later in kindergarten she would select a toy and hang on to it no matter what. "Time to put the toys away" meant nothing to her, and eventually her insistence triumphed over even the most determined adult.

She wandered away from her class, and would turn up in unlikely places in the school building. She was the child who could take any harmless toy and turn it into a disaster; it wasn't that she was mean or spiteful. She just did things her own way.

But all of these quirks didn't seem to create problems for Jenny's peers. When her family began using the Feingold Program the behavior extremes disappeared, so she became an easier child to be around, both at home and school. Things were looking very good -- until she moved from first to second grade. Jenny's first grade teacher seemed to have unlimited patience, and seldom spoke above a whisper. The children were comfortable with her and she was an effective teacher.

Second grade was the opposite. Jenny's new teacher ran on caffeine and seldom spoke below a shout. The little girl who had been confident and interacted easily among the other children began to change. Jenny retreated into a world of her own, as though she had crawled into bed and pulled the covers over her head. Like many chemically sensitive children, she was especially vulnerable to loud noises and constant stress -- the atmosphere she was in for about six hours a day.

When she shut the world out, she stopped interacting with other children, and stayed in her lonely isolation for years to come. Her social skills remained at the seven-year-old level. By the time Jenny eventually wanted to venture back out into the world, she had missed the years and experiences that would put her at her appropriate age level. Her inability to interact successfully further isolated her and made it difficult for her to practice the social skills that were so in need of work. Jenny's way of protecting herself from the daily assault was to emotionally withdraw, but when the stress was over, when she moved on to the next grade, she remained in her own world.

The hard lesson her parents learned is that chemically sensitive children are very vulnerable to stress of many kinds: loud noises, bright lights, sometimes even to touch. They are generally unable to cope in situations where there is constant tension, especially when it is accompanied by shouting. The younger the child, the greater the potential for harm.

Asperger's syndrome

The Feingold Program has been a help – a huge help, especially with your child's behavior, but there are still problems, especially with his peers. Here is one possibility to consider.

Asperger's syndrome was first identified by a Viennese pediatrician more than 50 years ago but it is only recently that this collection of characteristics has begun to gain recognition. One reason may be the dramatic increase in children with autism, which shares many traits. (There is disagreement over whether Asperger's is a form of autism or a separate syndrome.) Another reason we have not heard much about it is that the characteristics can be so close to what we perceive as normal behavior, with the difference being only one of degree. For example, many children become fascinated with a particular subject (dinosaurs, astronomy, etc.) but for the child with Asperger's the interest is too intense and too limiting.

How many of us have known a colleague, playmate, relative or professor who has narrow interests in one subject, to the exclusion of others? He is intelligent, but seems to lack common sense, especially when it comes to social interactions. We consider his behavior to often be rude, or at least inconsiderate, but if we suggest this he is truly baffled. A hallmark of Asperger's is the individual's inability to see how his words and actions affect us, his lack of empathy. If his senses are overloaded, if they are unusually affected by loud noises, bright lights, etc., he is likely to react in ways that seem irrational to us, and this further removes him from the mainstream.

"The patterns [of Asperger's] include a lack of empathy, little ability to form friendships, one-sided conversations, intense absorption in a special interest and clumsy movements."

Asperger's Syndrome, A guide for Parents and Professionals, by Tony Atwood. Jessica Kingsley Publishers, London, 1998.

"But the salient feature of the disorder is the child's preoccupation with a favorite subject...and will talk about it, often in a monotone or in strangely affected speech patterns, at great length and at inappropriate times. Nor will the child detect, understand or heed attempts by others to stop. He or she will often avoid making eye contact with others..."

"How to tell Asperger's from autism" by Edward Susman. *The Brown University Child and Adolescent Behavior Letter*, Jan 1996.

Children with Asperger's are likely to have a normal or high IQ, and this leads others to expect them to function as other children do, both in academic and social situations. One mother of a child with Asperger's writes, "When he cannot do this, he is accused of deliberately being disruptive. Because the child's inner world is one of chaos, he feels a desperate need to organize his surroundings; as a result others see him as too controlling.

"Few adults understand that the child with Asperger's is behaving in a way that seems appropriate to him, and even fewer children understand this. These are the children who are teased unmercifully by the other kids. This is one of thc saddest parts of the syndrome. The child is so close to 'normal' that he is expected to act like others. He is bright, and understands that he doesn't fit in, but he does not know what to do to change this.

"Such a child might be helped by a variety of interventions, including: sensory integration therapy, diet management, removal of gluten and casein, the rote teaching of social skills, and structured support in the classroom. The good news is that, if they are provided with the help they need, these children can learn to fit in better with their peers. They can be taught the appropriate behaviors that come so naturally to others."

WHAT IS "ADD" AND HOW CAN IT BE TREATED?

Understanding ADD -- How does a brain work?

Our brain is made up of cells, and the ones that enable us to think are the nerve cells, or "neurons." The body of each neuron has one long cable extending from it; this cable is called an "axon," and is a tube, filled with chemicals. Like the twigs of a tree, the axon branches out into little offshoots, ending in knob-like structures called "axon terminals." Each of these terminals can make a connection with other nerve cells, but it does not physically touch the other cell. The space between the axon terminal and the next nerve is incredibly tiny -- only about one millionth of an inch. This space separating the two parts is called the "synapse."

Thoughts are formed when electrical discharges move from the bodies of nerve cells, down their axons. When the electrical impulse reaches the end of the axon (the axon terminal), chemicals are released. These chemicals are called neurotransmitters. The neurotransmitter molecules travel the tiny distance across the synapse, and fit into receptors, located on the adjacent nerve cell. A brain contains billions of neurons, and each has many terminals, so the number of connections which can be made are virtually countless.

How foods and additives affect the brain

Robert Sinaiko, M.D., described possible mechanisms by which foods and food additives relate to attention deficit disorder (ADD).

Dr. Sinaiko, an immunologist practicing in San Francisco, was privileged to work with Dr. Feingold for several years. He later began a private practice and to date has treated approximately 1300 ADD children.

He is an enthusiastic supporter of the Feingold Association, and feels that Dr. Feingold's work has not only been validated by parents using the Program, but also by the scientific literature. He specifically mentioned studies by J. Egger et al published in *The Lancet* in 1992, and by C.M. Carter et al published in the November 1993 issue of the *Archives of Diseases in Childhood.* Dr. Sinaiko noted that Carter's group undertook the study to *disprove* previous studies linking diet and ADD, but their own results convinced them of the benefits of dietary treatment. The Carter study also showed the reliability of parental reports of children's behavior.

The workshop focused on "What's happening biochemically inside the body to cause behavior changes when certain foods/food additives are consumed?" There are two major pathways involved.

The pharmacological pathway

Dr. Feingold called the first pathway the pharmacological or toxic pathway. Small molecules such as artificial food colors or naturally occurring salicylates can be carried from the intestine to the brain through the bloodstream. In the brain, these molecules interfere with the chemical and electrical functioning of our brain cells. The effects can be produced by drugs, cosmetics, food additives and preservatives, and it takes very little of the offending chemical to produce the toxic effect.

Immunologically mediated pathway

The second major pathway Dr. Feingold considered is the immunologically mediated pathway. This occurs when we eat a food to which we are allergic, such as wheat. Our body identifies the wheat as a foreign substance and responds as it would to an invading infectious microbe. This allergic response has been shown to reduce the levels of neurotransmitters (small messenger molecules) in our brains. When neurotransmitters are in short supply in the brain, behavior can be affected.

Neurotransmission

This is the method by which our brain and nerve cells communicate and send messages to our body, shown in the simplified drawing.

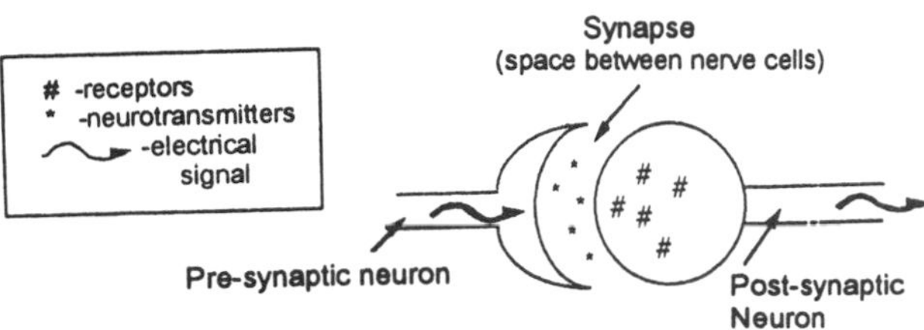

In neurotransmission, an electrical signal travels down a nerve cell (pre-synaptic neuron). When it reaches the synapse (space between two nerve cells), the electrical signal changes to a chemical one. The pre-synaptic neuron (nerve cell which is sending the message) releases chemicals called neurotransmitters into the space between the two cells. The nerve cell receiving the message (the post-synaptic neuron) has receptors on its surface to "catch" the neurotransmitter molecules being released. When enough neurotransmitters are "captured" by the receptor molecules, the post-synaptic neuron begins a new electrical signal to be transmitted down the second neuron. The process is repeated along many neurons as they transmit nerve impulses around the brain and to the rest of the body.

After nerve signals have been transmitted, the excess neurotransmitter molecules in the synapse are almost immediately destroyed by special enzymes. This ensures that the neuron does not continue to send signals when it shouldn't. At any point in this process, interference with the delicate balance can disrupt the workings of the system.

Phenols

Many of the additives which trigger problems in children with ADD have a chemical structure based on phenol (see below). Norepinephrine, one of the neurotransmitters, is also based on phenol. Phenolic compounds can dissolve in both water and in fat. This is important because cell membranes are composed of both water and fat. This means that phenol molecules can easily cross membrane barriers and can get into the brain.

One of the reasons children with "ADD" are unable to tolerate additives such as vanillin (artificial vanilla) and BHT, Dr. Sinaiko suggests, could be because these molecules can act as "counterfeit" neurotransmitters. Note how similar the chemical structures of the additives and salicylates are to the chemical structure of the neurotransmitter norepinephrine.

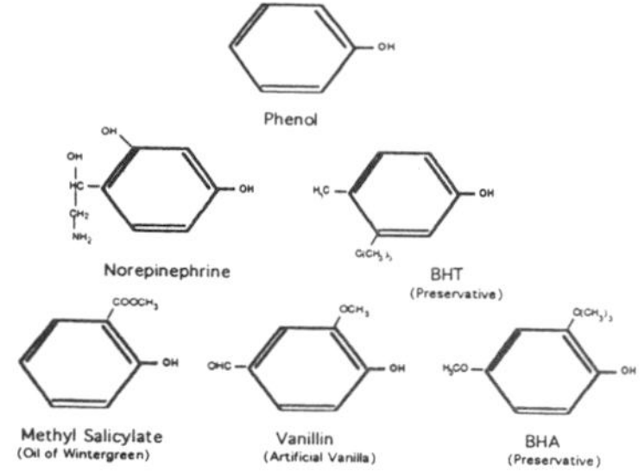

Petroleum-based additives such as dyes, BHA, etc. can act as "neurotoxins," binding themselves to the receptors. In other words, instead of a real neurotransmitter connecting with a receptor on the next nerve cell, the BHA molecule takes its place. The nerve cell (post-synaptic neuron) thinks that it has received a real neurotransmitter, and fires a false electrical signal. The neuron was "excitable" and transmitted a signal when it shouldn't have. The result of this is like having static, or unwanted noise in the brain.

A word about phenols: Although some of the chemicals with a phenolic structure cause problems for Feingold members, there are others that do not. Not all phenolic compounds act as neurotoxins. In fact, some naturally occurring compounds, such as the amino acid tyrosine, contain phenolic structures. In addition, there are some chemicals that affect ADD children that do not have phenolic structures; an example is Yellow No. 5. So this concept is not simple, nor is it well understood at this time.

Enzyme deficiency

Another potential problem is a deficiency in certain enzymes. Enzymes are needed to break down the leftover neurotransmitters in the synapse. You might say the enzymes clean up those neurotransmitters that are no longer needed, and dispose of them. If the extra neurotransmitters are not disposed of, the nerve may continue to fire randomly, producing "noise."

Enzymes have another job to do; they get rid of excess phenolic compounds such as those found in the high salicylate foods. Since phenolic compounds can easily get into the brain and cause problems, the body normally produces an enzyme called "phenol sulfotransferase" to detoxify them and allow them to be eliminated from the body. This means that naturally occurring phenols (found in apple juice, oil of wintergreen, and many foods) are prevented from interfering in the transmission of nerve impulses.

It is estimated that about half of the children identified as autistic are deficient in the enzyme phenol sulfotransferase. Researchers in England have developed a test to measure the amount of this enzyme in the bloodstream, and many autistic children have almost none of the enzyme at all! It is possible that this inability to detoxify phenolic compounds in the body may disrupt the ability of the brain to send messages, resulting in autistic symptoms.

Receptors

The third area of possible interference in neurotransmission is a change in the number of receptors on the post-synaptic neuron. The number of receptors on the surface of a nerve cell can vary.

We referred to the fact that ongoing allergic reactions can reduce the availability of neurotransmitters in the brain. If we are exposed to an allergen (something to which we are allergic, such as milk or dust) over a long period of time, our brains compensate for the loss of the neurotransmitter, norepinephrine. Our brain creates more receptors so that even though there are fewer neurotransmitter molecules coming across the synapse, there is a better chance of many being "captured" -- of connecting with a receptor. In other words, someone who was drunk would find it easier to unlock a door if there were twelve keyholes instead of just one.

Although the increase in the number of receptors means that more of the neurotransmitters are caught, there is a down side. With the extra number of receptors, the nerve cells are now more excitable and have a harder time distinguishing between a real message and background "noise." For example, imagine that you are trying to listen to a distant radio station with a weak signal; you need to turn the volume way up in order to hear the speaker's voice, but this produces so much extremely loud static that you can barely make out what is being said.

Neurotransmitters have many roles

When a child's brain is affected in any of the ways described above, there can be many symptoms. Neurotransmitters are involved in a number of essential areas where ADD children have difficulties. They are involved in waking up, in experiencing pleasure and in focusing.

Neurotransmitters are essential for the "orienting response" which is so important for athletes such as tennis players. When you play tennis, your brain functions in two very different ways -- it must constantly switch back and forth between an "organized" and "disorganized" state. The organized state is needed for hitting the ball; you are performing a task that has been practiced over and over. But as you wait for your partner to hit the ball back to you, your brain needs to be in a highly disorganized state. You have no way to predict where the ball will come and how you will need to react. In a disorganized state, your brain is ready for whatever action must be taken.

ADD children seem to be able to focus, but they focus on their own dreams and ideas. They have trouble making the shift between the disorganized open mind ready to respond to sensory input and the highly organized mode in which well-rehearsed behaviors are performed. This shift requires that neurotransmitters be available in sufficient amounts. The use of stimulant drugs such as Ritalin locks the brain into the organized state. The reason some children do not seem to learn well on medicine is because they are not able to switch to the receptive (disorganized) state.

Antifungal drugs

Fungi normally live in relatively small numbers within the intestine, but after repeated courses of antibiotics, fungal populations flourish. Like foods, abundant fungal overgrowth in the intestine can cause an ongoing allergic response, an immunological activation that depletes the available supply of the neurotransmitter norepinephrine, reducing chemical signal amplitude in the brain. In addition to allergens, fungi produce a wide variety of phenolic compounds, which in the absence of adequate phenol sulfotransferase will accumulate in brain tissue, further degrading brain function by adding to chemical "background noise."

Future research will tell us if the benefit of antifungal treatment (about half the autistic children treated with antifungal drugs were shown to improve) is a combined effect of reducing both allergen and toxin exposures, with improved nerve transmission due to higher signal amplitude *and* reduced chemical background noise levels. Based on what we now know, this seems likely.

Summary

Dr. Sinaiko discussed many different mechanisms, and it is likely that all of them play a part in the connection between diet and behavior/

learning disabilities. Allergies weaken the nerve transmission signal, while toxic effects raise the background noise level of false signals. Both effects disrupt the critical chemical balance at the synapse.

Recent work has not only validated Dr. Feingold's clinical observations, Dr. Sinaiko stressed, but has gone on to implicate the biochemical mechanisms which may be responsible for the effects of food additives and common allergy-inducing foods on behavior and learning disabilities in children. Although many pieces of the puzzle are still missing, research is progressing rapidly in this area and is leading us to a much clearer understanding of behavioral reactions to foods. It is very important to recognize that more than one mechanism is involved here. While diet modifications can help most children significantly, this is too complex a problem for one single answer.

References:

Carter, C.M. et al. 1993 *Arch. Dis Child* 69:564-568.
Egger, J. et al. 1992 *The Lancet* 339:1150-53.
Levitan, H. 1977 *Proc Natl Acad Sci USA* 74:2914.

Editorial note:

Dr. Gerald Klerman of the New York Hospital-Cornell Medical Center noted: "I'm pretty convinced that something rather profound happened in our society from about 1950 to 1980 and that it had its greatest impact on young people." Dr. Klerman concluded, "It could be some virus or some toxin in our food or water..."

Dr. Feingold traced the increase in behavior and learning problems to the years following World War II, when foods began to change from minimally-processed to additive-laden. Each year, more synthetic chemicals are consumed by more children, exhibiting more disturbed behavior.

EEG Confirms Food-Induced Abnormalities in ADHD Children

A specialized form of EEG enabling researchers to map the brain's electrical activity has provided objective proof that some children diagnosed with an attention *disorder* do not have any disorder at all. They are simply reacting to a food or food additive.

Uhlig and colleagues write, "during consumption of provoking foods there was a significant increase in betal activity in the frontotemporal areas of the brain. This investigation is the first one to show an association between electrical activity and intake of provoking foods in children with food-induced attention deficit hyperactivity disorder." That means that "certain foods may not only influence clinical symptoms but may also alter brain electrical activity."

The children were selected because it was shown prior to the testing that they were sensitive to these foods and additives and experienced a change in behavior when they were exposed to them.

Uhlig, T.; Merkenschlager, A.; et al. "Topographic Mapping of Brain Electrical Activity with Food-Induced Attention Deficit Hyperkinetic Disorder." *European Journal of Pediatrics* 156(7):557-561 (1997).

ADD Abroad

During the summer of 1994 *Time* magazine carried a feature article on ADD in children and adults (July 18, 1994). The writer noted that European nations like France and England report one-tenth the U.S. rate of ADHD. In Japan the disorder has barely been studied. This comes as no surprise to Feingold members who are aware that Europe allows fewer synthetic food additives than the U.S., and the typical Japanese child has a vastly different diet.

While the numbers may be smaller, the problems are as agonizing for parents of children living in other countries as they are for us. Dr. Feingold's work led to the establishment of other parent support groups similar to ours. One of these organizations is the Hyperactive Children's Support Group in Great Britain. Sally Bunday, who has long directed the fine work of this group, writes that stimulant medication is now being heavily promoted in the United Kingdom. This is a sharp reversal of past policy where drugs were rarely used.

A massive promotion of stimulants for children is being carried out, apparently by pharmaceutical companies and by ADD support groups that advocate the use of medication. Previously, only psychiatrists and consultants were allowed to prescribe these drugs for children, but as a result of the current campaign family doctors will be able to prescribe as well. She adds that for children under age 16, all medication is paid for by taxes, further encouraging its use. Sally is particularly distressed at the practice of using strong drugs for babies. She writes, "21 month olds on Pemoline is, I feel, most unacceptable."

The Hyperactive Children's Support Group can be reached at: Mayfield House, Yapton Road, Barnham, West Sussex, England. For a listing of current international volunteers, contact FAUS at P.O. Box 6550, Alexandria, VA 22306.

Mark

We called our son "Scooter" when he was a baby because he rocked so hard in his crib that he would scoot it all the way across the room. Mark had problems from the beginning. First it was colic, then speech problems, and later it was an inability to read or spell.

He was not at all like the typical "hyperactive" child I had learned about in nursing school. Mark was a quiet little boy who enjoyed listening to stories; in fact, he could sit for hours, drawing tiny little pictures.

It was clear our son was bright, so why couldn't he learn? The school thought perhaps the problem was that my husband's job caused us to move so frequently. I didn't agree, but couldn't come up with an answer either. Our daughter, who was three years younger, didn't have these problems. Virtually every professional we encountered told us the same thing, which was, in effect: "Michelle is fine -- what are you doing wrong with Mark?"

When he was 9, we were told that Mark would be placed in a "LD class." I asked for a copy of the results of their tests and was told he had not been tested. There was no way I was going to agree to any such placement without some solid information. Testing then showed Mark to be close to the 98th percentile in all subjects.

He had been moved along from grade to grade even though he wasn't able to keep up. In the earlier years it was less crucial, but now, since he couldn't read he couldn't learn, and this began to damage his usually sunny disposition. He wasn't happy with himself, and the other children began to exclude him.

By the time Mark reached fifth grade, things were getting desperate. "If Mark would progress any slower," I was told, "he'd be going backwards."

The fifth grade teacher suggested Mark may be hyperactive. This prompted me to go to the library and do some research on the problem. I recalled seeing Dr. Feingold on the Donahue show, and then found his book, *Why Your Child is Hyperactive*. After reading it I began to recognize that other symptoms -- what is now called attention deficit disorder -- seemed to fit Mark. With my newfound information, I attacked the cupboards with a vengeance.

After we began the program he no longer had problems which we hadn't even identified as problems! He could come to the dinner table and sit down without spilling everything, could go to sleep without rocking, and stopped talking out in his sleep. He stopped incessantly teasing his sister, being argumentative, and could now turn off the TV without a confrontation.

Mark had become so unhappy with his life by the time he was ten years old, he welcomed a chance to change things. I soon received a letter from his teacher, which says, "Mark is a pleasure to have in class." After ten years of worry and searching, I can't describe the feelings this brought. Needless to say, I still have that letter.

We began the diet in November, and by the end of the school year Mark had brought his skills up to almost grade level! He had no problems with reading or spelling after that, and sixth grade was a real success story.

It's been 12 years since we first learned about the Feingold Program, and I've been an active advocate, both as a diet assistant, and in my work as a nurse. Moms who learn of the program when their children are toddlers are so fortunate; there's so much we had to go through. If this sounds like I feel sorry for myself, nothing could be further from the truth. The day our ten-year-old told us, "I really like me the way I am now," I knew no amount of effort would have been too much.

Summer School for Keri and Me

My granddaughter was diagnosed as an ADD child in first grade, and now she was showing poor prospects of passing from third to fourth grade.

Her math ability was above average but there just seemed to be a mental block where reading was concerned. She skipped words, or reversed them, and labored over every word until she lost the meaning. As a result, all subjects suffered progressively to the point of total frustration for her bright little mind.

I am a schoolteacher, but teaching reading is not in my field. However, the urge to try to help became too great to ignore and I made plans with my family to spend the summer tutoring Keri. Shortly before I was to leave, I learned about the Feingold Association and received their literature.

We began our reading sessions on Monday and the Feingold diet on the following Wednesday. One day during that first week Keri became so frustrated she burst into tears and cried, "My mind just won't let me do it right!" The sixth day on the diet, Keri read a chapter in her reader without stumbling. From that time her progress has been steady, and today she is doing well in school.

Parents Under Pressure

The school has let you know -- subtly or otherwise -- that your child should be on medication to control his behavior. What can you do?

First, take a good look at how you feel about yourself as a parent.

Most parents of a difficult child will say "terrible." But the problems you encounter do not start in September of the first grade. You've already had six ego-bruising years, and if the child is your first-born, your confidence may be in shreds.

"As first-time parents we really believed that if we did 'all the right things' we would be rewarded with an adorable, intelligent little baby," reports one member. "When 'all the right things' didn't work, we were devastated." If your six-year-old is less than the ideal child, you are accustomed to others implying/declaring your inadequacy.

The fallacy of this is that your child's personality and behavior may have very little to do with you, your ability as a parent, or your methods of raising children. (This concept is beginning to find its way into the professional literature, but your mother-in-law isn't likely to have read about it.)

Most couples don't really appreciate the vast difference in children's temperaments until they have a second child. "As Matthew's mother, teachers are courteous to me, but they are tense and speak carefully," a mother told *Pure Facts.* "As Danny's mother, the smiles come readily; the talk flows easily with facial muscles relaxed. I'm still the same me, but my adequacy as a parent and a person depends upon which classroom I happen to be in." If Matthew suffered from an obvious physical disability his mother would not be held responsible. But because his handicap is invisible -- a sensitivity to synthetic chemicals which affect his behavior -- Mom gets all the blame.

When parents accept psychological factors as the only cause of behavior problems they get locked into a no-win situation. They must either: 1) admit their inadequacy as parents and follow whatever direction is given, or 2) deny the child has a problem. Most parents are caught up in a nebulous middle ground somewhere between these two options. Neither choice is likely to solve the problem.

It is important for you to realize that your child's behavior really is a problem.

Chances are he/she is driving other people nuts! Once you accept that a problem exists, you have taken the first step toward identifying the cause/causes and exploring solutions. Let your child's teacher know you understand that your child's behavior is making it difficult for him/her to teach. Explain that you are actively researching and exploring the choices that are available to you. Don't allow the situation to drag on in hopes that it will get better. Generally it gets worse.

Try to imagine how it feels to be your child. How would you feel if you lived inside a body that talks endlessly/touches everything compulsively/always says the wrong thing? And no matter how hard you try, you're always on a collision course with the world? It's easy to forget that a child's behavior may cause as much distress for himself as for those around him.

Dr. Feingold stated, "Most of the children don't want to be bad. They don't want to be on drugs. They don't want to be in learning disability classes. They are not sub-intelligent. In my opinion they are chemically abused. These children are normal. Their environment is abnormal."

Consider your choices

Parenting skills counseling: Who wouldn't benefit from that? But if your child is chemically sensitive, this will not address the problem, and is likely to be of limited help until after the offending chemicals have been removed.

Behavior modification: If you don't object to carefully weighing every word you say, every action you take, and if you are willing to spend most of your time watching your child, this may make a difference. But it, too, doesn't address the cause of a chemically sensitive child's problem, so results are likely to be disappointing.

Counseling for your child: Just as it is unreasonable to try to counsel an alcoholic while he is drunk, it is difficult to change the behavior of a child who does not have control over his own actions. Once the offending chemicals have been taken away from the chemically sensitive child, counseling can be very helpful in teaching new ways to behave and in restoring a damaged self esteem.

Remedial help for learning disabilities: A child who cannot pay attention cannot learn. Removing offending foods and/or additives will not teach your child math, but it may enable him to focus on the task; then he can learn. Fortunately, most 'Feingold kids' are bright and with appropriate help they can catch up with their peers.

Medication: This option is very popular with many professionals. No doubt a major factor is that they have seen so little improvement from techniques such as those mentioned above. With medication, one is very likely to see results quickly.

Since hyperactivity is not due to a Ritalin deficiency, however, the use of this or similar drugs will not address the cause of the problem. Not only are the side effects potentially serious, but the drug may mask other problems.

Dietary management: As a technique which incurs no risk, very little expense, and generally yields fast results, dietary management should be the first to be tried.

With a Foodlist and other detailed information provided by a Feingold Association, parents will know in several days to a few weeks if chemical sensitivity is a factor in their child's problems. It is not unusual for a young child to respond to the Feingold Program in a few days. For the individual on medication, it might be more difficult to see the clear improvement in behavior. Thus families should try dietary management before considering drugs.

How about diet + medication?

Dr. Feingold found that in many cases the use of behavior-modifying drugs interfered with the effectiveness of the diet. But we do hear from parents who report they can combine the Program with a small dose of medication. Some report that prior to using diet, their child quickly built up a tolerance to the prescribed drug, but by using diet plus an uncolored version of the drug, they were able to see a sustained improvement without having to increase the dose or switch medicines.

We also are aware of parents using stimulant medicine, who find that food additives interfere with the effectiveness of the drug.

If you are considering using the diet in combination with medication, ask your doctor or pharmacist for assistance. They may be able to help you obtain the drug in an uncolored form, and can adjust the dosage to your child's need. Even a little yellow pill can sabotage a sensitive child's successful response to the Feingold Program.

What should a parent know about stimulant medicine?

The following information is based upon an interview with the Deputy Chief of the Drug Control Section, United States Drug Enforcement Administration.

Drug Schedules -- a means for classifying abuse potential

Dexedrine and Ritalin are listed as Schedule II drugs by the Drug Enforcement Administration, although there is pressure to place them in less restricted categories.

There are five categories under which a drug may be classified:

Schedule I - an illegal drug with no legitimate medical use.

Schedule II - has accepted medical use but has the highest potential for abuse, and may lead to a severe psychological or physical dependence.

Schedule III-similar to II, but the danger of abuse is less than a Schedule II drug.

Schedule IV - less danger of abuse than II or III. Cylert, a central nervous system stimulant sometimes used on hyperactive children, is in this category.

Schedule V - as with all drugs these have potential problems, but they offer the least danger of abuse.

Ritalin production increases

The production of Schedule II drugs in the United States is controlled by the Drug Enforcement Administration (DEA). This agency sets quotas that reflect the valid medical, scientific, and research use for each drug. When the demand for a drug increases, manufacturers petition DEA to raise the quotas in order to meet that demand. For the past four to five years DEA has granted increases in the quota of methylphenidate (Ritalin), based upon documented increased sales. Prior to 1982 the use of this drug was gradually declining. "The evidence suggests over-prescribing," the Deputy Chief said in 1995, "The United States is using five times as much as the entire rest of the planet combined."

"What does this increase mean?" he posed the question, "Is the drug being more widely advertised or is it being more vigorously promoted? Most of all, does this sharp increase constitute good medical practice?"

Behavior modifying medication - Some comments from professionals

"Various side effects have been reported with methylphenidate (Ritalin) treatment including insomnia, abdominal pain, adverse behavior changes, and an increased incidence of seizures. There is evidence of exacerbation of Gilles de la Tourette syndrome in certain children while receiving the drug.... Probably the most well known complications are the suppressive effects of methylphenidate on appetite and subsequent growth retardation as reviewed in 1979 by Roche and colleagues."

Linsey K. Grossman, M.D., and Nell J. Grossman, M.D. *The Journal of Family Practice* Vol. 20, No. 3:302-304, 1985

"Stimulant medications, including methylphenidate, dextroamphetamine, and pemoline, may cause a variety of motor disturbances.... Stimulants have been reported to aggravate tics in Tourette's syndrome and to worsen motor dysfunction in tardive dyskinesia."
Charles D. Casat, M.D. and David C. Wilson 111, M.D. *Journal of Clinical Psychiatry* 47:44-45, 1986

"It is not known how frequently CNS (central nervous system) stimulants may unmask latent Gilles de la Tourette syndrome (GTS) or worsen preexisting tics. GTS is a disorder of presumed neurological original characterized by the childhood onset of multiple involuntary motor and vocal tics. More than 50% of affected children also manifest the behavioral symptoms of attention deficit disorder (ADD), with or without hyperactivity."
Gerald Erenbert, M.D.: Robert P. Cruse, D.O.: and David Rothner, M.D. *Neurology*, 35:1346-1348, 1985

Letters to the Feingold Association

"My 5-year-old daughter was put on Ritalin at age 3. Called 'very hyperactive' she was on 45 mg each day until I started her on the diet two weeks ago and began to cut down the drug. Day 4 of the diet was beautiful and she only needed 17 mgs Ritalin for the whole day. By Day 8 I got the Ritalin down to 15 mg and the doctor was delighted.

"For the first time in her life she's able to wear a braid and a bow in her hair without tearing it out. Two mothers of hyperactive children led me to the Feingold diet. Yellow No. 5 was the first time I noticed a relation of behavior to additives. Donna had already taken 30 mg of Ritalin when I fed her packaged macaroni & cheese for lunch, and the yellow dye counteracted all this Ritalin... as if she had none and worse. That day I vowed she would never see food coloring again and I started the diet as best I could without much information.

"I noticed the smaller doses of Ritalin 'lasted' longer and were more calming than the larger doses without diet management, so I hope to eliminate Ritalin altogether one day by completely following the Feingold diet."

*****

"Just recently my son was taken off his medication at my request. (The doctors agreed.) He has not grown in height at all in two years, nor has he gained much weight (5 pounds in two years). He was on his medication for three years. Anyway, since he has been taken off his medication, I don't want another doctor to put him on anything else, which is what the school wants. The school is preparing to put my son in a severely emotionally handicapped class. He is already in the emotionally handicapped class now.

"The diet has been controlling my son's behavior as well as Ritalin did, and without the side effects. He has started eating better and putting on weight.

"Just a note of interest, my baby (not yet 2) had bronchial asthma and although he is not on the Feingold diet I have eliminated yellow dye and sulfites and he has improved at least 50%! He no longer needs his nebulizer treatments."

Better Ways to Help ADHD Children

One of the speakers at our 15th Annual Conference was Paul Lavin, Ph.D. Dr. Lavin is a licensed psychologist practicing in Maryland. He is the author of many publications, journal articles and books, including *Parenting the Overactive Child: Alternatives to Drug Therapy*. His undergraduate work was in elementary education and he holds a master's and doctorate in both guidance and counseling. In addition to his private practice, Dr. Lavin is currently a therapist at The Children's Home in Catonsville Maryland, Associate Staff Psychologist at Taylor Manor Hospital in Ellicott City, Assistant Professor of Psychology at Towson University, and a consultant with the Division of Vocational, Rehabilitation and Disabilities Determination Services.

Medication is a court of last resort. I think it's a tragedy in this country that at this time we have an estimated one million kids on Ritalin. (Editor's note: That number has greatly increased.)

It makes sense to me that the diet should be the first line of offense -- not defense, but offense -- in the treatment of ADD. If we look at the current research evidence (Kaplan, Egger) they had excellent results. Professionals may say the diet doesn't work, but there is sufficient evidence now to indicate that the diet does work, and it works with a significant number of youngsters. Although the diet takes time, effort and commitment, it has no negative side effects. Try that with medication.

There were magical beliefs attached to medication: what it could do and not do; and despite the fact that there was evidence that it doesn't do half the things people claim that it does, these kids were plied with medication, and that was the only thing they received. This is contrary to the PDR (*Physician's Desk Reference*), which recommends medication be used only with other methods.

I'm not going to say there aren't some cases where it may be warranted...we can always find cases where medication is effective. However, I want to stress the fact that Ritalin is a potent drug, classified as a Schedule II drug by the Drug Enforcement Administration. The DEA describes Schedule II drugs as having "a high potential for abuse and may lead to severe psychological and physical dependence" so let's make no mistake about it, Ritalin is a powerful medication and needs to be carefully prescribed and carefully monitored.

The PDR clearly specifies a number of negative side effects associated with the use of these drugs. Yes, we can alter or change the medication so the negative effects will disappear, but the point is when you take a youngster who is still developing, who's still young, why take the chance when you've got other methods which can be more viable?

Another factor to consider -- this is a quote from the PDR: "Sufficient data on the safety and efficacy of long term use of Ritalin in children are not yet available." So over the long run we don't know what it does. Further, it states that Ritalin should not be used with children under 6 "since safety and efficacy in this age group have not been established." And yet there are many children I have seen under the age of 6 that have received stimulant medication. Even the evidence supports that it's not that efficacious with younger children, so it doesn't make sense to prescribe that as the first line of offense.

The American Academy of Pediatrics, 1987, states that "medication for children with Attention Deficit Disorder should never be used as an isolated treatment."

There's a book I recommend, called *When Children Don't Learn*, by Diane McGuinness. She does an excellent job of pulling together much of the research on ADD. She clearly indicates that the research overwhelmingly supports that Ritalin doesn't improve academic performance, self-esteem or social adjustment. McGuinness cites a number of studies where the long-term effect of nonmedical intervention (behavior modification) have had excellent results. So even though these methods are more time consuming and require greater effort, they're much more efficacious over the long haul. *[Note: This book may not be easy to locate. Dr. McGuinness wrote an article for parents, titled "Stimulants and Children" which is available through the Feingold Association, P.O. Box 6550, Alexandria, VA 22306. Please include a long, self-addressed, stamped envelope along with your request.]*

I will not deny that medication has some benefits; it does. It calms the child and makes him more compliant. However, that's it. It doesn't do any of the other things that people propose it does. The thing to consider is that the kids who only take medication are under-treated. They are not receiving the full regimen of treatment that they need in order to be successful.

In the long run these kids are at high risk for failure in school. They are also at high risk for failure in the community. These kids not only wind up as dropouts and do poorly academically, they also become antisocial, lots of them. That means as a society we pick up the tab at a later point in time.

The other thing that I want you to consider is that there is no drug that I know of that teaches responsibility. If that were the case, this country would be in great shape right now, wouldn't it. There is no drug that teaches skill. There is no drug that develops character. Those things come about by intervention -- intervention techniques that are well designed and well implemented. If you give a child medication, that becomes the excuse for success or failure; it's not the kid's own initiative, it's not the kid's drive that does it, it's other factors, and that's not something that I think we want to foster with kids. IT made me feel better; IT increased my self-esteem; IT improved my academic performance. If it's "IT," it's outside of us, and we want something inside that's responsible for successful achievement over the long run.

Developmental Psychology, by Liebert, contains excellent information on achievement motivation -- characteristics that lead to success. It also has a good synopsis of the research. Internal vs. external locus of control: People who are successful [have an internal locus of control] believe there is a direct connection between what they do and the benefits that follow -- and the failures. They take responsibility. It's not other things, it's them. Kids who achieve success believe that their behavior is responsible for what happens. The opposite of that is external locus of control -- luck, fate, or other people that are responsible for whatever happens. Have you ever worked with delinquents? Did you ever see a delinquent take responsibility for his own behavior?

If we want people to succeed in life then it's important that we foster the internal locus of control. How do drugs do that? They go quite contrary to that, in fact. We're saying "you take a pill, and it's responsible." I think that's a mistake. I think that what we need to say is "don't take a pill; start being accountable, responsible. We're going to help you with that, but you've got to make choices."

You have to start early. It's very difficult for a kid of twelve or thirteen who's been on medication for years, for you to say, "Now you're responsible for your behavior." As you well know, adolescence is of itself often a "disease," even without having ADHD. That's tough enough to deal with -- I know, I've got a couple of them now. But when you add the problem of ADHD, then the kid is also stubborn and oppositional, as you well know, and it doubles the misery that a parent is required to face.

We need to train kids to be independent and to make decisions, and to assume responsibility. That's something we can train if we use the proper techniques; you can do that with the diet every day, can't you? The kid has to make choices. The choice is "Am I going to eat the junk food and go wacky, or am I going to say 'no' and assert myself and make the choice to be in control?" We can train kids to make those choices, and a kid who can stand up in the face of that adversity is one who's going to have character and he's going to have self control and he's going to be a person who has the potential to make something of his life. A person who caves in to peer pressure, and has to eat the junk food in order to win peer approval because they want immediate gratification, is not going to be that successful. We train that. That doesn't come from any pill.

Finally, let me just pull together some of the combination of methods we need to consider in working with ADHD kids. I think the proper nutrition and diet should be the first line of offense. I think every kid should be given the opportunity to participate in that program.

Secondly, we need a highly structured environment using behavioral techniques and principles, and that is not very simple, at least in principle. The basic principle behind it is "if you eat the peas, you get the ice cream." Remember Grandma's law? That's it. So we have to train kids that when you behave appropriately, good things happen; when you behave negatively, negative things happen. This is a logical occurrence in life. Oftentimes we give too much, or feel guilty, or overindulge and feel sorry because the kid's got a problem. So we don't set up a high degree of accountability and structure and therefore the kid doesn't learn to be responsible. What they learn to do is whine and fuss and complain instead of taking responsibility for their behavior.

A good example of this is the kid who wants Crispy Crunchies in the morning, and then dawdles with them and they sit in the milk and become like cardboard. Then he whines and fusses because the Crispy Crunchies don't taste good and he doesn't want to eat them. Ten o'clock in the morning he comes back again and what happens? "I'm hungry," so Mom fixes him a pancake for breakfast. So what have we taught the kid? Not to be responsible, not to make good choices.

So what I'm suggesting is that we have to modify the environment so a kid learns early in life that there are consequences. If you don't eat the peas, you don't get the ice cream. That's the way life happens to be. And you have to set up in very clear behavioral language what those contingencies are going to be, and it doesn't mean the kid's going to approve of it. You have to stick to it firmly and consistently. If you want to modify behavior, that's what you have to do. Remember, consequences happen. That's life.

We have to arrange the environment to get the child's attention. This means you've got to remove competing stimuli -- sight and sounds. Open classrooms drive these kids crazy. We need to train the child to listen, to remember, and to carry out instructions. Have the child repeat the instructions to you, then carry them out. This needs to be done consistently over an extended period of time.

Here's a tough one -- getting close cooperation between the home and the school, and daily accountability via a checklist keeps you on top of your kid's academic performance. If that child needs tutoring, extra help, then you can get it done. But every 6 weeks, when a "death notice" comes home about all the things the kid doesn't do, it's too late. The kid's already behind the eight ball, with the negative feedback, and the long epistle pointing out all the things the child's done won't make a bit of difference. It's too late; the kid's partially down the drain at that point, so we need structure and accountability right in the schools. Yes, it's aggravating, and yes, it requires extra time and commitment, but the long term benefits of that far outweigh the short-term aggravation.

Another thing I've found to be helpful is that kids get proper sleep -- that's not easy, as you well know. But these kids fatigue easily and when they get tired they're miserable.

Self-control training First, the child has to recognize he has a problem, to understand that he has some behavioral deficits, and strengths too. All of us have strengths and weaknesses. We all have problems. If you have a problem it doesn't make you a bad person. That is the first step in making good decisions, in overcoming those adversities. Then we have to involve the child in helping himself. The child can learn to read labels, he can learn to be assertive, can learn to say "no."

Self-control training [also means] learning to generate positive and sensible statements, and ways to cope with life's adversity using cognitive mediation. We can teach kids "here's what you can say, here's what you can think, and this is what's likely to follow. Let's take a look and plan and anticipate."

"See if we can plan some strategies together as to how you're going to solve the problem of the cookie jar when you see all those goodies in there and somebody tempts you. How are you going to handle the field trip or the class party with cookies and K----A--?"

It's very important to keep ADD youngsters motivated. People say they don't achieve as well as normal control groups. However, the research belies that. Kids who are hyperactive, ADHD kids, can do just as well as normal kids if they're encouraged and reinforced -- even on boring repetitive tasks.

We need to focus on the kinds of people we want to produce. We don't want to just produce calm, compliant people. We want kids with positive social and personal characteristics who are viable contributors to society; and that does not come about easily or effortlessly.

I think medication is an oversold bill of goods. It doesn't do what a lot of proponents claim it does, but it's certainly got a lot of clout in this country at this time.

Paul Lavin, Ph.D.

"Once prescribed primarily as an adult stimulant medication to be taken for short periods of time, Ritalin is currently prescribed as a childhood behavior suppressant to be taken for several years. And it is prescribed with such regularity that critics have coined their own term for the substance: the teacher's and parents' relief drug."

Dianne McGuinness, Ph.D.

The Four R's: Reading, Ritin, Rithmetic and Ritalin

The Feingold Association receives reports from parents who are being told that their child has a chemical deficiency, and that the use of the powerful drug, Ritalin, is a "replacement therapy." In the past, some laypersons have (mistakenly) compared giving drugs to a hyperactive child with giving insulin to a diabetic. It is unsettling to learn that some parents are now hearing this from professionals.

Depressing news also comes from parents of very young children who are being urged by their physician to put the youngsters on drugs. The *Physician's Desk Reference* includes the statement from Ciba Geigy, the manufacturer of Ritalin, that "Ritalin should not be used in children under six years, since safety and efficacy in this age group have not been established."

In the same section, the manufacturer states, "There is neither specific evidence which clearly establishes the mechanism whereby Ritalin produces its mental and behavioral effects in children, nor conclusive evidence regarding how these effects relate to the condition of the central nervous system." (*Physician's Desk Reference*, 39th Edition, page 865).

Pampers, Pacifiers, and Prozac

By 1998 the trend of prescribing stimulants for very young children had accelerated.

Prozac, clonidine, dextroamphetamine and Ritalin are being given to children as young as one year who have been diagnosed with attention-deficit-hyperactivity disorder, says Marsha Rappley, an associate professor at Michigan State University. Various other drugs are also being used on this young population, Rappley learned. In studying 223 children under the age of 3 who exhibited developmental/behavioral problems she found that 127 of them have been treated with drugs. Twenty-two different drugs had been used, but the primary ones were Ritalin, clonidine and dextroamphetamine.

The development of a mint-flavored liquid Prozac for children brought a storm of criticism when it was introduced, but the overwhelming majority of children (90%) being treated with drugs for ADD/ADHD are on methylphenidate (Ritalin).

Inconsistencies, confusion in the treatment of ADHD; NIH panel finds diet "intriguing"

In November of 1998 the National Institutes of Health (NIH) held a consensus development conference titled "Diagnosis and Treatment of Attention Deficit Hyperactivity Disorder."

Scientists and practitioners from around the country gathered to answer key questions. Portions of the panel's report are provided, and comments are italicized:

1. What is the scientific evidence to support ADHD as a disorder?

"The diagnosis of ADHD can be made reliably using well-tested diagnostic interview methods. **However, we do not have an independent, valid test for ADHD, and there are no data to indicate that ADHD is due to a brain malfunction.** [emphasis added] Further research to establish the validity of the disorder continues to be a problem."

How can a reliable diagnosis of a disorder be made if professionals are uncertain that it exists?

"The reported rate in some other countries is much lower. This indicates a need for better study of ADHD in different populations and better definition of the disorder."

Children in most other countries eat far fewer synthetic additives than in the United States. The dramatic increase in additives such as food dyes has paralleled the increase in learning and behavior problems in the U.S.

2. What is the impact of ADHD on individuals, families, and society?

"Children with ADHD...experience peer rejection and engage in a broad array of disruptive behaviors.... These children have higher accident rates, and later in life, children with ADHD in combination with conduct disorders experience drug abuse, antisocial behavior, and accidents of all sorts."

"Families who have children with ADHD...experience increased levels of parental frustration, marital discord, .and divorce...the direct costs of medical care for children and youth with ADHD are substantial."

"...these individuals consume a disproportionate share of resources and attention from the health care system, criminal justice system, schools, and other social service agencies....additional national public school expenditures on behalf of students with ADHD may have exceeded $3 billion in 1995. Moreover, ADHD, often in conjunction with coexisting conduct disorders, contributes to societal problems such as violent crime and teenage pregnancy."

How much money is saved by families for whom non-drug approaches are successful? How much money could be saved and how many social problems could be reduced with the use of proven alternatives?

3. What are the effective treatments for ADHD?

"A wide variety of treatments have been used for ADHD including, but not limited to, various psychotropic medications, psychosocial treatment, dietary management, herbal and homeopathic treatments, biofeedback, medication, and perceptual stimulation/training. Of these treatment strategies, medications and psychosocial interventions have been the major focus of research."

"Until recently, most randomized clinical trials have been short term, up to approximately 3 months. Overall, these studies support the efficacy of stimulants and psychosocial treatments for ADHD. However, there are no long-term studies testing stimulants or psychosocial treatments lasting several years. There is no information on the long-term outcomes of medication-treated ADHD individuals in terms of educational and occupational achievements, involvement with the police, or other areas of social functioning."

The panel's statement is in conflict with the work of Swanson et. al., who reviewed studies evaluating the long term effects of drugs for these children. They found that there were no long-term benefits. Their review was published in Exceptional Children, *Vol. 60, No. 2, 1993.*

"These short-term trials have found beneficial effects on the defining symptoms of ADHD and associated aggressiveness as long as medication is taken. However, stimulant treatments do not 'normalize' the entire range of behavior problems, and children under treatment still manifest a higher level of some behavior problems than normal children. **Of concern are the consistent findings that despite the improvement in core symptoms, there is little improvement in academic achievement or social skills."** [emphasis added[

"There is a long history of a number of other interventions for ADHD. These include dietary replacement, herbal exclusion or supplementation, various vitamin or mineral regimens, biofeedback, perceptual stimulation, and a host of others. Although these interventions have generated considerable interest and there are some controlled and uncontrolled studies using various strategies, the state of the empirical evidence regarding these interventions is uneven, ranging form no data to well-controlled trials. **Some of the dietary elimination strategies showed intriguing results suggesting future research"** [emphasis added]

4. What are the risks of the use of stimulant medication and other treatments?

"Although little information exists concerning the long-term effects of psychostimulants, there is no conclusive evidence that careful therapeutic use is harmful."

"No conclusive evidence" of harm is not very reassuring. Shouldn't psychostimulants be required to be proven safe and effective before they can be approved for use, particularly when they are given to children and (more recently) to babies as young as one year old?

"Finally, after years of clinical research and experience with ADHD, our knowledge about the cause or causes of ADHD remains speculative. Consequently, we have no strategies for the prevention of ADHD."

ADD groups

Pressure can also come from parent support groups. There are numerous groups that have formed around the country to help parents of children diagnosed as having ADD or ADHD. Support groups can be of enormous help, especially for the parent who is having difficulty obtaining special services from their school. But take a good look at the group.

* Is it operated by parent volunteers or by a professional who may have a vested interest in promoting one form of treatment, or who receives clients/patients from their association with the group?

* Is information available on more than one approach to ADD, or is the literature obviously supplied by pharmaceutical companies?

* If you are using the Feingold Program, are the group leaders interested in hearing about your experiences with the Program?

* Are the group leaders aware of the many studies supporting the diet/behavior/learning connection?

* What is the source of funding for the group?

In defense of Ritalin

Dear Editor,

Our family has been using the Feingold diet with great success for more than 6 years now, and can't imagine how we would have managed without it.

However, I have been concerned about some of the 'bad press' Ritalin has been getting lately, both in Feingold publications and in other media. For the past 5 years our oldest son (who I will call Ray) has been on Ritalin, and I can't imagine how we would have gotten along without it either.

Ray went from an easily distracted infant to a toddler with behavior problems. I had asked my pediatrician on several visits if he thought Ray was hyperactive. Our doctor always said that if he could watch TV quietly for 15 minutes he was not. (Our pediatrician has since learned a lot more about what is now called ADD, and realized that was not a good criterion to use.)

By the time he reached second grade Ray's lack of self-control was a serious problem, and his self-esteem was headed downward. "I know I'm smart," he complained, "but no one else seems to know it."

After extensive testing by an educational psychologist, and consultation with our doctor, we chose the Feingold diet. Our doctor recommended Ritalin because he believed the diet probably wouldn't work and was very hard to follow. But I was determined and found neither prediction to be true.

The diet improved things for all of us. Ray was calmer as well as less restless and moody. He was able to stay dry at night, except for those times he went off the diet. He was better able to handle problems at school, but some nagging ones remained. After an extensive workup by a pediatric neurologist showed he still had problems focusing his attention, we decided that Ray needed more help. He began third grade on both the diet and Ritalin. Since then things have constantly gotten better.

I continue to do a lot of reading, attend ADD support groups and workshops, work closely with the school, and provide the structure Ray needs at home.

Today our oldest son is enrolled in advanced classes, is in the gifted and talented program, an honor roll student, an editor of the school newspaper, has many close friends, and -- most of all -- is happy with himself. When he goes off the diet he is moody, excitable, and often gets sick. When he forgets his Ritalin he is noisy and has trouble with self-control and paying attention. We tried testing him for allergies by eliminating certain foods, but the only things we saw reactions to were the artificial colors and flavors.

My experience, research, and participation in various groups leads me to believe that there are some children who may only need a change of diet to alleviate their problems, while others may be helped by Ritalin or other interventions. I do wish Ritalin could be made without artificial colors. We have used the 10 mg, even when we had to cut it in half; our son does not seem to react to the slight bit of blue dye in this form, but I would still like to see a dye-free Ritalin become available.

We found that Ray would lose his appetite if he took the Ritalin on an empty stomach; we were able to bend the rules so he could bring it in his lunchbox and take the pill then. This had another advantage. He was not teased as others were for having to go to the clinic to take "hyper" pills. He has always been on a much lower dose than other children his weight, and I often wonder if the diet is the reason for this.

Ray wasn't the only member of the family affected by food additives. After we went on the Feingold Program we realized that our youngest son frequently got sick when he ate away from home. But sticking to the diet, he no longer has diarrhea and ear infections, which had previously been frequent. He never exhibited the distractibility or impulsiveness of his older brother, but was moody and difficult when he ate the wrong foods.

Our success on the diet explained many things to me. When I was growing up we never had a lot of artificially colored foods, except at Christmas when we decorated cookies with brightly colored sugar. I always became terribly sick after Christmas. At college the (brand name) gelatin salads were a novelty and I ate them frequently; I was often sick in college as well. My husband and our 15-year-old daughter don't seem to be as affected by food additives, but since none of us are sensitive to salicylates it's easy to use the same diet for the entire family. We feel, however, that both the Feingold diet and Ritalin have been our solution to having happy healthy, well-adjusted children.

Editor's Response:
Are stimulant drugs good or bad?

Feingold members are not likely to pass judgement on other parents. We know only too well how that feels!

The mother who wrote the above letter exemplifies the Feingold Association's view on this emotionally charged issue. It's a view that is not likely to be found in the volumes of literature published on this subject.

To ask if a drug is "good" or "bad," "safe" or "dangerous" is missing the point. Aspirin, once thought to be harmless, is accused of triggering the often-fatal Reye syndrome in children. The same drug that can ease pain in some adults will bring about a severe reaction in the salicylate sensitive. The drug itself is neither good nor bad; only its use can be judged. If chicken soup were as effective as antibiotics, which would you select? If fiber works as well as laxatives, which is preferred? The current interest in the effect of nutrition on health mirrors our growing interest in the "gentler" approach.

Given the choice between diet therapy and drug therapy, one should ask: How do they compare in effectiveness, in difficulty to implement, in cost, and in side effects? No responsible person can feel comfortable about giving powerful drugs to children -- especially the young child -- unless there is no alternative. This is why the Feingold Association believes diet should be the first approach tried. If diet proves to be ineffective or of limited benefit, then parents and physicians need to compare the risks of other treatments with their benefits. For Ray it is clear that using a small dosage of Ritalin, along with the Feingold Program, has brought benefits, with no serious side effects being apparent.

The Feingold logo states "Nutrition is a better way," but it does not say that nutrition is the *only* way.

Moms who use Ritalin love their kids too

If the doctor had told me there was a pill that would make my child behave, I would have grabbed the prescription and run to the nearest drug store.

Back in 1975, before ADD had been invented, the diagnosis for a child who didn't behave appropriately was "poor parenting," which translated to: "What is Mom doing wrong?"

I was so sold on the idea that behavior is based solely on psychological factors that it was several years before I approached the pediatrician with the question that perhaps Laura had some sort of "chemical imbalance" which would explain her exasperating behavior.

The response to my question was a booklet on discipline. The response a mother receives today frequently depends upon the approach favored by her physician, and can vary from: referral to the Feingold Association, to a prescription, to a brush-off of "He's just an active boy."

The guilt glands

In the prenatal classes nobody ever mentioned that once I produced a child, there would be a mysterious physiological change. I would grow a set of guilt glands. No diagnostic test has ever been able to determine where these little critters are located, but every mom reading this knows they are there. Well, it seems to follow that moms of overactive kids have overactive guilt glands -- like insanity, we inherit it from our children.

By the time she is told the problem is not her fault, the typical mom of an ADD child has been badgered, blamed and bruised. Pressure from the school, reassurances from her doctor, understanding and support from other parents using it, plus the promise of relief are powerful incentives to go along with a trial of drug therapy. If there is an improvement a parent is understandably reluctant to give up any benefit, even when it is minimal. That's when the guilt glands go into high gear.

Feingold parents see the signs often. When you first begin talking about hyperactivity or ADD with the new teacher, she sympathetically tells you that her child has the same condition. But when you mention that you are using diet to address the symptoms, there's an awkward pause, and she changes the subject.

The congressman and the congressional assistant both have children who "used to be hyperactive." Their eyes take on a glazed look as you explain how a dietary approach could help families while saving taxpayers enormous amounts of money. These people don't hear you because they are undergoing their own personal inquisition. When you tell them the Program helped your child, they translate that into an accusation that they failed to use it and chose a different path.

A major ADD support group, which is drug-oriented, told Feingold volunteers they will not allow a speaker from the Association to address their group because we "would make their members feel guilty." There was never any dialogue as to what a Feingold speaker would say or what her philosophy is. The group leaders appeared convinced that either: a Feingold speaker would automatically sit in judgement, or that members need to be shielded from the guilt that could be generated by telling them of other options.

It can be exasperating to try to discuss the subject with a parent who has such overactive guilt glands, but it is also clear that these parents care deeply. If they didn't, their choice would not be so painful for them.

Some Feingold kids do well on Ritalin

One of the Association's board members recently came to the decision to try giving her son a small dose of Ritalin. The diet had helped enormously, but he had long been having trouble getting his act together when it came to schoolwork. At first she was appalled by the idea, but eventually decided she needed to at least see if the drug would help. In this child's case a small dose of Ritalin seemed to help, and there have not been any noticeable side effects. Other members occasionally report similar experiences, and find that because they stay on the Feingold Program they are able to obtain maximum benefits while using a small dose.

We don't understand why the same chemical that seems to interfere with the effectiveness of the Program at the beginning may be tolerated once a child is well established on the diet. (Naturally, members attempt to get the uncolored or least colored pills.) We do find that once a person's system has been free of the petroleum-based food additives, they tend to be able to tolerate many chemicals that previously would have caused problems.

What's the controversy?

The food, chemical and pharmaceutical lobbies are only too glad to supply parents, professionals, and ADD groups with their opinion of dietary management. To have their profits defended by parent volunteers has got to be a marketing executive's dream.

But parents should not and need not be adversaries. I don't use the Feingold Program because of any moral superiority, but because it worked so well, and by the time I learned of Ritalin, I was convinced that diet was much easier. We have long been able to eat a tremendous variety of delicious foods, including restaurant food, convenience food and junk food. In addition to feeling so much better, my family has been spared the expenses of medical treatment and the problems of dealing with a child whose medication has worn off.

No parent should be pressured into choosing a treatment they don't want to use, whether that treatment is drugs, behavior modification or diet. Each family has a unique circumstance that deserves to be acknowledged and respected -- by professionals and by other parents. Each has the right to be given the facts, without the contamination of personal philosophies or vested interests, and to choose the option that is the best fit for their family.

A Review of the Studies on the use of Stimulant Medication for Children with Attention Deficit Disorder

This article, published by the Council for Exceptional Children, is a comprehensive review of the studies on the long-term effects of stimulant medication for children with attention deficit disorder. The author was James Swanson et al., and it appeared in *Exceptional Children,* Vol. 60, No. 2, 1993.

Interpretation of the Swanson paper, by Syte Reitz, Ph.D.

The use of stimulant medicine for children with ADD offers short-term improvement for the majority of children, but with potential side effects and no long-term improvement in behavior, learning or social development.

The Swanson article uses a new "review of reviews" methodology to condense the existing findings in recent scientific literature on the use of stimulant medication for children with ADD. Nine review articles (traditional, meta-analytic and general audience categories) were included, as well as other references spanning 1975 to the present.

The methodology used in the article is complicated, and the reading is rough, because the existing literature is filled with conflicting aims, observations and conclusions concerning medication of hyperactive children. Swanson and colleagues attempt successfully to sift facts, effects and observations from aims, predisposition and opinions, and remarkably, they come up with some consensus from the existing literature.

The factual material where the various researchers are in agreement is summarized in one table and one figure.

Table 1 lists and compiles the findings of three individual review papers that are typical of information found in the literature. Despite differing interpretations and recommendations, the eye-opening conclusion all three reviews arrive at is that stimulant medication is seen to have **only short-term effects** on the behavior and attention of ADD children.

The "effect size" reported in Table 1 is not clearly defined in the article, but presumably it corresponds to % improvement seen in ADD children after treatment with drugs. Thus treatment with stimulant drugs produced an average (short-term) improvement rate of 0.83 or 83% in the areas of behavior and attention in ADD children. In the areas of IQ and achievement, short-term improvements averaged 35%. Considering the fact that Barkley (1977)* reported about a 30% placebo response rate, the above figures for stimulant medication translate to real numbers of about 50% short-term improvement in behavior and attention, and practically no improvement in IQ and achievement (short-term or long term).

No long-term effects of stimulants have been documented, according to Swanson et al., and most patients discontinue stimulant treatment within two years. The short-term improvement is also not specific to children with ADD, since these drugs exhibit the same effect of improved attention and concentration in normal children.

In the short-term, stimulant medicine can bring about a significant improvement in some very distressing symptoms.

The disagreement in the literature appears to rest in the interpretation of the above findings. Not all authors agree whether the short-term improvements are worthwhile improvements in themselves or whether they interfere with treatment by acting as a short-term crutch, preventing or postponing the use of more effective non-pharmaceutical approaches. Some authors point out that drugs may have greater relevance for stress-reduction in caregivers than intrinsic value to the child.

The paper summarizes what can and cannot be expected from the use of stimulant medication on ADD children.

Temporary management of the following symptoms will be expected to occur using drugs:

a) over activity
b) inattention
c) impulsivity

This will lead to temporary improvement in the following areas:

a) deportment (increased compliance and effort will be observed)
b) decreased aggression
c) social interactions (decreased negative behaviors)
d) academic productivity (increased amount and accuracy of work)

When using stimulant medications to treat ADD:

1) There will be **no** paradoxical response. This means that the stimulant medications produce the same effects on all children and all adults (improved attention and concentration), regardless of ADD diagnosis or "normal" label. Thus the stimulant drugs cannot be correcting a biochemical defect or physiological or neurological abnormality. They are simply helping teachers and parents to cope with the ADD child.
The researchers are essentially in agreement that stimulant medication does not provide any long-term benefits to the child.

2) There is no way to predict if stimulant drugs will help. Drugs do nothing for 25% to 40% of hyperactive children. The response of a particular child to drug treatment cannot be predicted in advance by any known neurological, physiological or biochemical test.
3) Absence of side effects cannot be expected. Frequent side effects of drug treatment include appearance or increase in tics, problems with eating and sleeping, and possible psychological effects on cognition and attribution (the ability to reason and to understand cause and effect relationships).
4) Major long-term improvement in skills or learning cannot be expected (no long-term improvement in reading, athletic or game skills, or positive social skills occurs).
5) Improvement in long-term adjustment cannot be expected. No improvement in academic achievement is seen, no reduction in antisocial behavior or arrest occurs.

Clearly, when editorializing and opinion are sifted out from the literature, a surprising consensus emerges about the expected benefits and the acknowledged limitations of stimulant medication in children with ADD.
Some researchers express concern that the use of medicine makes it more difficult to identify the cause(s) or the child's learning problems and to find solutions for them.

Drug treatment of ADD children has no long-term beneficial effects. Short-term effects are limited to temporary suppression of one subset of symptoms.

Some authors feel that stimulants may be overused in the United States. High doses of stimulants may produce cognitive toxicity (reduced ability to think and reason). Many children have adverse responses to stimulants. Most patients discontinue treatment within two years. Clearly the benefits of stimulant treatment of ADD children are limited.
*Barkley, R.A. (1977). A review of stimulant drug research with hyperactive children. *Journal of Child Psychology and Psychiatry,* 18, 137-165.

Dr. Reitz received her bachelor's degree in biochemistry from the University of NY at Stonybrook and her doctorate in biochemistry & molecular biology from Rutgers. She did her post-doctoral work at Princeton and was assistant professor of biochemistry and molecular biology at Oakland University in Rochester, MI.

ON THE PROGRAM AWAY FROM HOME

Steering Clear of Additives in Your Church or Synagogue

Feingold members represent many different faiths and philosophies, but all face a similar challenge when it comes to staying on the Program while they participate in religious activities.

Most religions observe at least one ritual that involves food. Wine, grape juice and bread are often used, and wine is the most likely to cause a problem. In addition to being a natural salicylate, wine may contain sulfiting agents (a problem for asthmatics), and other additives, including synthetic dyes. Since alcoholic beverages have little or no labeling it is very difficult to determine the ingredients. Grape juice is more likely to be free of additives, but it would still be a problem for the member who is very salicylate-sensitive.

Communion wafers and matzos are traditionally made of just wheat flour and water. If cubes of bread are used, your decision would be based on the individual's degree of sensitivity. In the case of an extreme sensitivity or allergy, it would be best to speak with your clergyman about refraining from participation.

Feingold mom, Nicki, says that the Mormon sacrament uses ordinary bread and water, and -- just to be on the safe side -- a Feingold member generally contributes the bread. Like some Mormon families, Nicki stores a year's supply of food in her home. She finds it isn't hard to avoid preservatives by sticking with basic grains (which are packed airtight) and with canned foods.

Barbara found the drinks served in the Methodist church vacation Bible school to be a problem. The easiest answer is simply to supply the drinks for her child's class during that week.

Drinks are something Trish always brings along when the family attends social events at their Catholic church. "When we were new to the diet and had to be more careful, I would sometimes feed my kids ahead of time, and then bring a dessert they could safely eat." Picnics are easy since there are always hamburgers and generally fresh fruit. Trish likes to bring a watermelon to share with the other families. Then when she bakes for a bazaar or bake sale, her cookies have a card stating they are made with all natural ingredients and are Feingold-safe.

Judy notes that the wife in a conservative or orthodox Jewish family expects to spend a considerable amount of time preparing food, particularly for the traditional Friday night meal. Since this generally means cooking from scratch, it isn't hard to be certain the ingredients are free of unwanted additives. All packaged food brought into the kosher home must have a designation certifying that it has been prepared in compliance with the religion's dietary guidelines.

The word "kosher" means "clean," but it does not necessarily mean the food is free of unwanted additives. Unfortunately, kosher hot dogs and lunchmeats usually contain nitrites. (Nitrites are not excluded from the Feingold Program, but many members prefer to avoid them.) It is not difficult to cook food at home that is both kosher and Feingold-acceptable. But preparing all of the food for your child's bar mitzvah, using the kitchen in the synagogue, is a different story. Brenda suggests you start making plans far in advance. By the time she reached her third bar mitzvah, Brenda says it got a lot easier.

Jackie finds that the Feingold Program fits in easily with their dietary preference for fresh, unprocessed foods. Like many Seventh Day Adventists, her family avoids meat. Their children are sensitive to grape juice, but can have cranberry-blueberry juice, which looks just like grape. Families that do not eat meat, and substitute soy-based products made to resemble meat, should be wary of the additives they often contain.

Gayle has come up with some innovative ideas for dealing with social events which include food. Since her mom lives nearby, and is also a member of the Church of God, they coordinate the dishes they bring to potluck suppers. If one brings an entree, the other will fill in with salad or vegetable, etc. so they all can enjoy a full meal. Gayle has introduced several other church families to the Feingold Program, so they often work together to provide foods all the children can enjoy.

These ideas may be helpful at any occasion where a meal will be served. Gayle told *Pure Facts* that the elementary school in their area has an annual Thanksgiving dinner for the children, and some of the foods served would not be OK for her boys. She plans for the dinner a few weeks in advance. When the family has roast chicken or baked chicken breast, Gayle saves some slices and freezes them. Another meal will include mashed potatoes, and two servings of that go into the freezer. When the family has green beans for dinner, she makes a little extra and puts aside some of them. With very little extra effort, Gayle prepares two "TV dinners" with foods that look like the upcoming Thanksgiving dinner. (The cranberry sauce the children make at school is natural.) The day of the big event, Gayle is one of the moms in the kitchen. She puts her boys' dinners into the school's microwave oven, heats them and slides them onto plates. Adam and Darin are served their food right away while their classmates must wait in line. "The other kids think that mine get royal treatment," said Gayle, noting that being on the Feingold Program has some unexpected pluses.

"Why I Don't Go to Church Anymore"

"The only time I really fit in at church is during a funeral service; then it's OK to cry."

This was the comment of an adult Feingold member who has been on our program for eleven years. She is extremely sensitive to perfume, and exposure to it will quickly bring on depression and uncontrollable crying. Another member realized that her daughter became ill when she was exposed to the new carpeting in their church. Sadly, her observations were greeted with ridicule.

Bobby reacted to church in a different way; as soon as the organ began to play, he covered his ears and screamed. Like many chemically sensitive children, his perception of noise was greatly exaggerated. What the other members of the congregation experienced as a loud, but pleasant sound, was painful to Bobby.

Children who are unable to be calm just don't fit in at most religious activities. Their disruptive behavior often means that families stay home rather than face embarrassment.

Sharon, a Feingold Mom, has conducted workshops on this subject for Sunday school teachers. She points out to the teachers that, "whenever we see pain, we have the opportunity to reach out and help." Her workshop, titled "How to minister to the child you wish were in another classroom" always draws a standing-room-only response.

Sharon notes that religions traditionally believe that children should be "seen, not heard." They are not set up to deal with the hyperactive child, nor are they equipped to provide help to their families. And yet, behind every difficult child there is a grieving family, including siblings who are hurting.

Members of your fellowship can be a wonderful help when they understand about chemical sensitivity. They can show their support by taking care in preparing foods -- perhaps even offering "Biblical foods" in place of the junk drinks and cookies. They can support you by skipping perfume and after shave lotion, or even just by opening the windows to let in fresh air. If you're less fortunate, the members of your congregation may tolerate your child being on a special diet only as long as you provide all of the allowed foods. Or you may have the misfortune to find that nobody wants to upset Mrs. Whoever -- the person in charge of the chemically laden snacks and church suppers.

A View from the Other Side of the Pulpit

It's difficult enough when you're a member of the congregation and your child is hyperactive. What do you do if you are the minister or rabbi, and the terror of the nursery is yours?

Pure Facts spoke with member families for some insight to share with you. First of all, assuming Dad is the clergyman, it's Mom who deals with the brunt of the problem. Once successfully on the Feingold Program, the child isn't likely to be treated differently than the other children in the congregation unless he/she is having a reaction.

The attitude of the clergyman tends to set the tone for the congregation. If he shows sympathy and understanding to people with special needs, a family's food choices are more likely to be respected. A pastor who has young children of his own is likely to be more understanding of others', and not so inclined to get upset when the children's choir gets restless. Of course there are times when a child needs to be removed from the ceremony, and parents should be able to do this without having to feel any embarrassment.

One pastor's wife found it was easier to find cooperation when they dealt with small groups, but the larger the numbers, the more complex it became. Speak to people in small group situations, she advised. Gently ask for their help, and don't become militant. Demanding a perfume-free section of the church won't work, but more modest requests may be honored as those around you gain understanding.

While she's a pastor's wife, she feels her role as a mother comes first, and puts her children's needs ahead of church obligations. Her husband's advice was similar. He feels a family must put the welfare of its members first. "It's OK to change churches if you don't have the support of the pastor and a segment of the population. If you are not happy in your present church, find one where you feel comfortable."

Going to Camp

Many Feingold children are able to go to summer camp, but it takes some effort -- both by the child and parents. If this is your child's first experience with summer camp, start out small with a one-week program. Many camps would not be willing or able to make the necessary dietary adaptations for a long stay. Thinking small is also a good idea when you are considering the size of the camp. There is likely to be much more flexibility on the part of the director and kitchen staff.

Most of the suggestions that follow are geared toward the overnight camp, but many would apply to day camps as well.

Camps generally fall into one of three categories. They are run by organizations such as the scouts, by religious institutions, or are private. Some private camps are geared to a particular interest: horsebacks riding, dance, computers, or weight loss. A nature-oriented program might be more likely to provide basic, wholesome food.

Finding the right camp

Check with the reference librarian in your public library for books on summer camps and summer schools.

Even if you believe your child will not be ready for camp until next year, it's a good idea to begin gathering information early. The Sunday newspaper may have advertisements for area camps and schools in the back of the magazine section.

Major cities hold camp fairs during the winter. This provides an opportunity to speak with representatives. (You may even be lucky enough to find a camp that serves natural food!) To learn about fairs to be held in your area, contact the American Camping Association at 5000 State Road, Route 67 North, Martinsville, IN 46151. Phone (317) 342-8456 or call (800) 966-CAMP.

The next step

Once you have a list of camps, send a form letter to the director of each, asking if they can accommodate your child's diet and any other special needs. Explain that you will be willing to supply any foods not available in their kitchens.

Even after you've found the ideal camp, some may not have any openings. On the other hand, as summer draws closer, the camp director who still has vacancies is likely to be more willing to accommodate a child's special requirements. Fortunately, people who are in the business of operating camps tend to believe that the most important consideration is for the child to have a great summer experience.

Be sure the camp director has a current set of Feingold literature. If you each have a set of the information you may be able to compromise over the phone. Contact the Association for extra copies of our material.

Your child's part

Not only is it important that your child is secure in saying "no" to unacceptable foods, but he or she should feel comfortable in questioning the ingredients used in a dish. You can discuss what should be done when nothing being served is acceptable. (If your youngster is content with a peanut butter sandwich, he'll always have something to eat!) Find out whom your child should consult about substituting foods, and arrange for them to meet before you leave the camp.

Some problem areas

Breakfast - Cold cereal is the mainstay of many camp breakfasts. Check your Foodlist for suitable brands, and don't forget the health food store as a source of acceptable cold cereals. In the past few years, there has been a big increase in the selection of natural cold cereals that look very similar to the supermarket brands. If eggs are served, be sure they are fresh, not imitation or powdered.

Lunch - If sandwiches are served and the camp is large, you're likely to run into a generous use of margarine. When the kitchen staff prepares large numbers of sandwiches, they will probably coat each slice of bread with margarine to prevent it from becoming soggy while the food is held until lunchtime. The bigger the camp, the more likely the food will be prepared in advance.

Drinks - Whether the campers are off on a hike, or eating in the dining hall, drinks will be an important consideration. Fortunately there are plenty of boxed drinks and juices, including "safe" lemonade and iced tea. Plan to supply a large quantity of stage I or II drinks.

Dinner - This will probably be the least problem for the Feingold camper. But watch out for foods that are deep-fried. A few commercial oils are made without BHA, BHT or TBHQ, but it's unlikely you'll be lucky enough to find them in use at the camp of your choice.

Desserts - The toughest part of dinner will come when dessert is served -- and this often means pudding made from a mix. But you will be able to supply a good selection of treats that will make your camper's buddies wish they were on the Feingold Program. Hopefully, the camp staff has already agreed to give you a corner of their freezer (or refrigerator) to stow a week's worth of goodies for your child.

If your family is new to the diet, stick with desserts found on your Foodlist. But if you're old timers and are able to experiment, you may already have found cookies and individually packaged desserts that are tolerated. (Test these out before camp begins!) You won't have trouble finding acceptable ice cream, and even if your child has food allergies, health food stores have some delicious frozen desserts based on soy and rice.

Non-food culprits

Try to get an idea of the activities and crafts that are planned. Will they be tie dying with synthetic colorings? A pair of plastic gloves would come in handy here. Will aerosol sprays be used inside the buildings? They often contain chemicals that will bother a sensitive child. Do the campers rub mosquito repellant on their skin? Does the nurse have suitable first aid creams or lotions? How about uncolored/unflavored acetaminophen? If you have been on the Program for awhile, you will know which things affect your child.

The do-it-yourself camp

It is possible to run your own Feingold Camp if you have enough youngsters who want to attend and some dedicated parents. This is what volunteers in Pennsylvania and Maryland accomplished a few years ago. Contact the camps in your area and ask if they will rent out their camp for a week during the summer. Facilities run by the scouts, churches, or a "Y" are a good prospect since they often are in need of additional income. You may want to seek out a camp designed for learning disabled children as some of them feature natural food.

It is important to find a camp that already has their counselors and a program director in place. You will also need to find a professional who has experience in food services and in purchasing food in quantity. You may be able to hire the camp's food director and cook, but it will be necessary to have a Feingold mom in the kitchen. It is also very desirable to have the nurse be a Feingold mom, and in these families where a parent works, the child gets to attend camp free. If these essential services can be supplied it will leave you and your colleagues free to handle the other tasks, especially registering children and dealing with finances. Girls and boys attending camp should be well established on the Program and not be ultra-sensitive.

As for the finances, develop a budget first, and then figure out how many children you must have attend in order to break even. Find out what the requirements are for insurance. Be sure to let the association know of your plans early so we can let other members know about the camp.

One more alternative

A nice compromise between selecting a camp and doing it yourself would be to interest a camp director in switching to foods free of toxic additives. As our program gains in recognition and acceptance, this may become easier to achieve. Contact the association for information suitable to send to a camp director.

Vacation Time -- with Restaurant Food

Food is an important part of a vacation; with some strategic planning, Feingolders can have as much fun as everyone else (and a lot more fun than families whose kids are acting wild)!

The amount of planning you need to do depends upon how sensitive your Feingold member is and/or how long you have been following the program. For most people, the longer they remain on the program, the less likely they are to have a serious reaction when there's a slip-up. (We don't recommend deliberately going off the diet.) Where are you going and how long will you be gone? A week at a beach cottage will take much different planning than three weeks in Europe.

Traveling

Airlines claim they can prepare food to your dietary needs, but don't bet the farm on it, cautions Feingold member/travel agent Susan, of San Jose, CA. If you're traveling on Canadian Air ask if you can order a "Feingold" meal. They were available at one time. As far as the other airlines are concerned, of the many special dietary meals they offer none will provide a meal of natural food. If it's a short trip, bring some snacks with you, and if it's a long trip, bring some more snacks -- just in case.

For car trips, a generous size cooler is a must. (Put it in the back seat to separate two kids.) You shouldn't have trouble getting ice to refill it at each lodging. Muffins, nut breads and large pretzels are satisfying, and if you can limit in-car drinks to water, spills won't be a major problem.

Be sure your car is stocked with a kit that includes: a can opener, bottle opener, plastic utensils, roll of paper towel, damp washcloth inside a Zip Loc bag, plus a blanket to spread out at a park when you want an impromptu picnic. If there's no park in sight, try the playground of an elementary school; it provides lots of equipment.

Supermarket lunch

You'll probably find it's easiest to eat breakfast in your room, then take a break and stop for lunch. If you're in unfamiliar territory, consider checking out a supermarket for lunch. Most markets have a huge assortment of Feingold-safe edibles that can be enjoyed without the benefit of a real kitchen. (You have a portable kitchen in your car, remember?)

Deli department: Sliced turkey and roast beef are generally fairly pure. If the meat is displayed in the glass case, you may be able to read the ingredient label. If it's too hard to see, ask the clerk to bring out an unopened package so you can read the ingredient label. If you explain "we have a lot of allergies," you won't be entirely accurate, but it should gain cooperation.

If your Feingolder is not extremely sensitive, you should be able to get away with most bread: white, whole wheat or rye. Avoid the dark breads that may contain raisin syrup and by all means, stay away from any bread, roll, or pastry that looks yellow. That color does not come from egg yolks! Although Feingold Foodlists note the presence of calcium propionate (the preservative generally found in baked goods) many members tolerate it.

Produce section: Salad bars and ready-to-eat fruits and vegetables may be inviting...at least for the adults. Salad bars are not likely to use sulfites anymore, but the dressings will probably contain one or more of the no-nos. If need be, you can select a bottle of one of the natural dressings. Look for Paul Newman's face, but watch for salicylates. Most plain cottage cheeses are straightforward, if you want to get some at the salad bar or dairy section. Don't even consider adding the "bacon" bits to your salad. If you don't believe me, take a look at the ingredient label.

If all else fails in your effort to satisfy young appetites, every store has a small jar of peanut butter and loaf of bread for finicky eaters.

The baby section should have pear juice. You may be able to tear off the label with the baby's picture and use the juice for your salicylate sensitive child (who would be humiliated at the idea of drinking something with the picture of a baby).

Health food stores

Even the little cubby at the mall will have natural drinks, probably both juice and natural sodas. If you're lucky, you'll find a health supermarket with a big selection of natural food; or you might locate a shop with an attached dining area. The meal may be heartier and the desserts heavier than your family is accustomed to, but if they're hungry enough you could be surprised at how fast the organic twelve-grain bread disappears. (One caution: Try to stay as close as possible to the familiar; this is not the time to test out tofu hot dogs.)

Fast food restaurants

If you travel for more than 30 minutes without seeing a burger sign, then you must be in Alaska driving on moose paths in your Land Rover. Hopefully, you'll have a copy of the Feingold Association's latest fast food information in your glove compartment (along with a few photocopies, just in case). It appears periodically in *Pure Facts,* and lists suitable foods available at McDonald's, Wendy's, Burger King, and others.

Don't overlook the fast food spot if you just want a drink. They always have soft drinks, and may be able to get you a container of real juice, even though it's way past breakfast time. Even if they only provide a cup of ice for you to add your own juice, it will be a refreshing stop.

Restaurants

Yes, Feingold families do eat at conventional restaurants. It isn't possible for us to provide any guarantees, but here are some suggestions.

Susan's family gets out the Yellow Pages when they arrive at their destination. They look for restaurants that are not part of a chain and phone those that look good. (Phone or visit restaurants during off hours when you have questions to ask.) They ask the chef if he can prepare a special meal for their Feingolder and describe what they need; then they make reservations for the following evening. Susan says they've had great results doing this. If you can visit the restaurant and speak with the chef in person, be sure to give him a copy of the Feingold brochure so he can have it as a reference. FAUS can provide literature.

One adult member called, worried about the plans she and her husband had made to eat dinner out with friends that evening. It was early in the afternoon, a good time to call the restaurant and ask to speak with the chef. Don't name all the things you cannot eat, and expect him to come up with a meal that fits your needs. Instead, have a brief list of some of the foods you enjoy and tolerate before you call, and ask him if he can prepare one of them for you that evening.

Perhaps you would like a fillet of fish, sautéed in olive oil and fresh garlic, with lemon. It could be accompanied by a baked potato with real sour cream or real butter. Green salad might have a lemon juice/olive oil dressing. The chef may be able to offer a grilled T-bone steak with no marinade and only salt, pepper and garlic to season it. Noodles tossed with butter could round out the meal. Sliced chicken breast, dipped in flour and sautéed is a dish easily prepared; corn on the cob and a green vegetable may be added.

Perhaps they have fresh fruit, fresh vegetables and boiled shrimp; these could turn a salad into a meal.

Quality restaurants probably have a good selection of basic ingredients on hand; look upon them the same way you do when you prepare food in your own kitchen. Maybe the fresh orange slices or pineapple chunks are designed to go in the mixed drinks, or the lemons are kept for use with iced tea. But that doesn't prevent you from enjoying fresh fruit with your meal or a glass of lemonade made to order.

Chances are, the chef entered the profession because of a love of good food, and may be just as interested in additive-free eating as you are. When I speak with chefs, I say that I would like them to fix me the sort of food they prepare for themselves when they are in their kitchen at home.

The most important thing to remember when you go to a restaurant is SKIP THE DESSERT. Look for a Haagan Dazs* ice cream shop, or pick up a pint of Ben & Jerry's* to take back to your home or hotel room, if you like; but don't trust what the restaurant has to offer. The chance the restaurant's dessert will be OK is slim. [*At press time, both brands had many acceptable varieties.]

Here are some suggestions on various types of restaurants:

Chinese: If you want to avoid MSG it's best ask if they can prepare food with "no MSG" before you sit down. Unless the restaurant is incredibly Chinese, they should be accustomed to this request. Don't order the egg rolls or soup since they already contain MSG.

Some other dishes to avoid are: sweet & sour dishes -- some chefs add dye to the sauce; lemon chicken may have yellow dye added; pork dishes (because red dye may be brushed on the outside of the meat). Your best bet is a dish they prepare to order. Things like chicken and mixed vegetables, shrimp and snow peas, etc., should be available without unnecessary additives. Be aware that some Chinese chefs use food dyes in unexpected ways to make a dish more colorful. And for the very sensitive child, avoid dishes with nuts, which may have preservatives added.

Remember to keep any doggie bags in a refrigerator or cooler that has plenty of ice.

Japanese: While MSG is not as likely to be used in Japanese food, anything's possible.

Italian: The atmospheric little spot run by Mama, Papa and the boys will probably have a lot to offer a hungry Feingolder. The pasta itself should not be any problem -- this is one food that has not yet been mutilated by chemistry. French and Italian breads are not likely to be a problem either, especially if they're the kind that would go stale by tomorrow if there were any left over. Make sure that the butter they serve with it really is butter.

Speaking of butter, your salicylate-sensitive child might enjoy pasta with butter and garlic, or perhaps a white clam sauce? Olive oil and garlic adds a type of "sauce" for those who must forgo the tomatoes. Mushrooms should be fine, both canned and fresh.

If you can eat the tomato sauce, then order what you like, but stay away from sausage, pepperoni, or anything more exotic than beef and chicken.

Seafood: Plain broiled fish fillet with lemon shouldn't be hard to get. It's the breading, sauces and seasonings that are likely to contain iffy additives. Ask if the scampi is prepared in real butter, and what other ingredients are used. If you splurge on lobster, boiled or steamed should be a very safe choice.

Steak houses: If the meat has not been marinated or otherwise treated, it should be acceptable. Since your children will probably want a hamburger anyway, that's fine; most Feingold members can get along very well with a hamburger from practically any restaurant. [The meat used on pizzas, however, is a different matter. Pizza meats are generally loaded with additives and may contain more filler than meat.] Contrary to what many people think, most hamburgers are made with plain old chopped beef, and adding coloring to hamburger is highly illegal. The reason chopped meat is brown in spots and bright red in others is due to oxidation, not dye, and should be a natural occurrence.

If you order roast beef, specify that you don't want anything other than, perhaps, salt and pepper. Request they not use seasoned salt, Accent, or pour "natural juice" over it.

Baked potatoes are widely served, and should be fairly safe. Ask the waitress if they use real butter (not margarine) and real sour cream (not make-believe).

As with the supermarket salad bar, the lettuce and vegetables are not likely to be treated with sulfites, but the garnishes and dressings are highly suspect. If you can be happy with a squeeze of lemon, that's easy; or consider bringing a purse big enough to hold a bottle of salad dressing.

Drinks: Any restaurant should have: water, ice, lemon and sugar. Presto! You have lemonade. If you order 7UP*, be sure that's what they serve. To many people, any lemon-lime drink can be called 7UP. (*At the time of this writing, Sprite contains sodium benzoate and 7UP in bottles and cans does not. 7UP served at a fountain may contain the preservative. Do not use the diet or flavored versions of 7UP.)

Real juice is generally easy to find, unless you need to avoid the salicylates. Consider a blend of juice and Perrier or other sparkling water. Many Feingold members can tolerate regular Coke and Pepsi (not diet). The reason they are not on our Foodlist is that the companies will not fill out our inquiry forms. Secrecy is big in the cola business.

If there's a natural chocolate milk or cocoa available in restaurants, we are not aware of it. Similarly, you're unlikely to find a natural chocolate or fudge sauce at ice cream shops.

The mall: Most shopping malls have some likely offerings. Soft pretzels are not apt to have many additives, and there is generally a place to buy your favorite variety of salted nuts. Import shops may have products that look fine, but one member family in Switzerland warns us that labels in other countries may be even less accurate than those here in the U.S.

If the mall has a food court, consider a hamburger, or a baked potato, or cup of fresh fruit, or tossed salad, or perhaps there's a place that will make up a tuna or egg salad sandwich. Skip the pickle, but the little bag of chips that accompany the sandwich might be OK. Examine the label.

Breakfast:

Suppose you decide to eat breakfast out. It doesn't get much purer than a hard cooked egg. (Some day they'll figure out how to add BHT to that too, but so far we're safe.) Add some toast and real butter, if they serve it. For a sweeter topping on your toast, try a sprinkle of sugar, or ask the waitress for cinnamon toast. Honey may be available too. Consider the little packets of jelly if you can tolerate the salicylate fruits and corn syrup. Jam or jelly can be a good stand-in for pancake syrup, or can add flavoring and sweetness to hot cereal.

Another way to get a fairly pure breakfast is to request an "egg roll" -- not the Chinese version, but a hard cooked egg, sliced, served on a buttered French roll; add lettuce if you wish. It's popular in France, and you'll see why when you taste it.

If you take a chance on pancakes or waffles (highly risky in most restaurants) spread them with jelly or honey as mentioned above, instead of the syrup -- which is bound to be loaded with unmentionables. "Blueberry" muffins or pancakes may contain gelatinous little dyed blue blobs in place of the more expensive real berries.

Prunes (salicylate) are not likely to have anything more than corn syrup in them. Grapefruit is fine if they can remember to keep the cherry off.

In the room:

When you make reservations consider asking if any rooms come with a microwave and refrigerator. Chains such as Embassy Suites provide a very workable little kitchenette.

If you're near a carryout restaurant, you could bring dinner or breakfast back to the room. And some hotels have a selection of menus from area restaurants.

You may want to ask if they have non-smoking rooms. If you have a family member who is sensitive to fragrances, ask if the hotel has any "green rooms." These accommodations are not sprayed with the many better-living-through-chemistry deodorizers, sprays and cleaning compounds that may be used in motel or hotel rooms. A "sniff test" when you arrive may be enough for the sensitive member to know if there will be a problem.

Amusement parks

If you are going to Disney World, call their Guest Relations office before you even leave your home; when you arrive, you will find it located at the entrance to the park. They should be able to provide information about special diets, such as vegetarian (which would probably contain fewer additives), but at this writing they cannot provide information about additive-free eating.

Chances are the staff will suggest you contact the restaurant you want to visit a day or so ahead of time, and speak with the chef during off-hours. If you specify what you would like them to prepare for your Feingolder you should be able to do quite well.

Here is some advice I gave to a family planning a vacation at Disney World. They were concerned about how to deal with their daughter's many food allergies. I encouraged the mom to type up a list of all the foods her child tolerates and enjoys -- no meals, just the foods alone. This might include, for example: brown rice, noodles, oats, macaroni, walnuts, pecans, cashews, cantaloupe, pears, lemon, pineapple watermelon, blueberries, banana, kiwi, green beans, sweet potatoes, onions, cabbage, peas, carrots, broccoli, squash (all types), lettuce, beef, chicken, lamb, flounder, salmon, tuna, eggs, cocoa, white sugar, honey.

She made multiple copies of this list and when the family arrived at the park, Mom visited the restaurants that looked promising (off-hours), taking copies of the list of foods. She asked each chef if he could devise several meals using those foods; then she gave the days and times the family would plan to eat at that restaurant.

Before the family set out for each day's activities, a call to the restaurant reminded the chef that they would be arriving for that day's lunch or dinner. We believe that most accomplished chefs will gladly accept the challenge (and may welcome the opportunity to use their creative talents).

Other places where you will be eating. A similar technique may be helpful whether you are arranging for special airline food or speaking with a neighbor who has invited your child to stay overnight. Make your suggestions clear and specific; for example, you might ask the airline representative if they could provide a peanut butter and honey sandwich, banana and whole milk for your child's meal. Your suggestions to your neighbor could be grilled hamburger, Fritos* and 7UP*, with Breyer's vanilla ice cream* (be sure it's the natural version) for dessert. For breakfast, Crispix* cereal with whole milk and pineapple juice is not a difficult request.

Note: *At press time, these brand name foods were acceptable for use on the Feingold Program, but ingredients can change at any time.

Back to Disney World Some of the lodging facilities located within Disney World have kitchens, and if you have a car it shouldn't be hard to find suitable foods in nearby supermarkets. There is a small grocery store in the park as well.

When you speak with the dietitian at any major amusement facility, you are welcome to give them the phone number where they can reach FAUS (1-800-321-3287). The association will be glad to speak with them and to provide printed materials. This is best done several weeks ahead of time. If a facility does not have one or more staff dietitians, it is unlikely you would get any satisfaction or assistance.

Whether your destination is a large or small amusement park, it's a good idea to call ahead and get an idea of what you'll be up against. Do they stamp everyone's hand with dye? Ask if there is a different method of showing the entry fee has been paid. Don't be surprised if they want to see a note from your doctor! If you can get this, it's a good idea to carry it with you.

Some amusement parks sell real lemonade, and others have watermelon slices. We know of just one that tries to avoid unsavory additives (Sesame Place in Langhorne, PA).

If you don't expect to find much in the real food department, you may need to bring in your own snacks. Here again, you could encounter static at the entrance. If there's a little one in your family, just stash the food in an extra diaper bag. As far as we know, no amusement park guard has ever insisted on looking inside a diaper bag!

The Feingold Traveler Abroad

Our advice to travelers is to stay as close as possible to the basics: meats without gravies, vegetables without sauces, pure fruit juices or acceptable sodas, water, or milk. If you want to avoid MSG don't order soups and be wary of Oriental food.

There are some foods that are more likely to be free of the prohibited additives. These include white cheese, peanut butter, fresh fruits and vegetables, most breads, plain rice, and pasta.

Foods that contain dyes are often obvious, but flavorings and hidden preservatives can be a problem in prepared foods. While food in other countries is likely to contain fewer additives, there are many pitfalls, particularly for those who are salicylate-sensitive.

Feingold mom, Gabriela Ehrlich, is a native of Switzerland. She has provided us with this outstanding summary.

Restaurant food

Higher priced restaurants (especially in France and Switzerland) rarely use coloring or flavoring as it goes against their honor. Homemade desserts will often be available, but ask for ingredients just to be sure. In other restaurants, stay away from desserts and ice cream.

When you eat out, look for plain food cooked in butter or flour with only salt and pepper added. Some restaurants have containers of seasoning mixes on the table, next to the salt and pepper shakers. These contain BHA. Soups and sauces are likely to be made with cubes and powders that contain BHA. Most sauces also contain some wine (salicylate), and cheese fondue is made with cherry alcohol.

Mustard and mayonnaise will probably be natural, but are made with grape or apple vinegar (salicylates). If you'll be doing your own cooking and need non-salicylate vinegar you can obtain rice vinegar in Japanese or Oriental shops. You can also substitute fresh lemon juice, but avoid the canned and bottled lemon juice.

Most restaurants use only natural butter; as in the U.S., avoid margarine.

Salicylate sensitive members can generally find honey to use in place of jams that contain apple pectin. You are not likely to find American style pancakes and syrup; if you do, the mixes could be a problem. On the other hand, fresh crepes served in France and Switzerland should be fine, but watch for salicylate fillings if you are sensitive to them.

A continental breakfast with rolls and butter should not present a problem; but avoid toasts, cereals and frozen croissants.

Steer clear of chocolate drinks. Chocolate products of all kinds can present a problem for the Feingold member in Europe. Gabriela writes, "All branded chocolates I know of (and trust me, I know them all) contain artificial vanilla -- vanillin." It came as a shock to learn that the famous Swiss chocolates contain this cheap additive. Other candies and chewing gum are also likely to be off limits.

Finding help in the health food stores

The Ehrlichs rely on health food stores for chocolate, other candies, and for ready-to-eat cereals. Here are the names for health food stores in various countries:

Germany - Reformhauser
Switzerland - Reformhauser, Biona, magasins dietetiques
Denmark - Helsebutik
Sweden - Halsobutik

Most people speak English, and should be able to help you find suitable foods, and to suggest restaurants and bakeries which offer additive-free foods.

Buying groceries

Supermarket shopping in Europe and the United Kingdom is not very much different than in the U.S. Processed food labels are not always accurate or complete, and additives already present in the oil, etc., may not be listed.

Good choices are: fresh fruits and vegetables; white cheeses; plain pastas; freshly baked breads; plain meats, fish and poultry.

Proprietors of small shops should be able to give detailed information about the ingredients in their foods.

"E" Additives to Avoid

In Europe each food additive is assigned a number, and most are preceded by the letter E. The following are ones Feingold members should exclude.

E102 Tartrazine (Yellow 5)
E104 Quinoline Yellow
107 Yellow 2G
E122 Carmoisine (red)
E123 Amaranth (Red No. 2)
E124 Ponceau 4R (red)
E127 Erythrosine (Red No. 3)
128 Red 2G
E132 Indigo Carmine (blue)
E133 Brilliant Blue FCF
E151 Black PN
154 Brown FK
155 Brown HT
E320 BHA
E321 BHT

Other additives to note:
E211 Sodium Benzoate
E250 Sodium Nitrite
E251 Sodium Nitrate
621 MSG

These additives should not pose a problem for most people:
E100 Curcuma or Tumeric
E101 Riboflavin (yellow color)
E140 Chlorophyll
E160 Carotene
E162 Red color from beets
E200 Sorbic acid
E260 Acetic acid (from vinegar)
E270 Lactic acid
E281 Sodium propionate
E282 Calcium propionate
E300 Ascorbic acid (vitamin C)
E334 Tartaric acid (E335 & E 336 are sodium and potassium tartrate)
E337 Potassium bitartrate (cream of tartar)
E406 Agar-agar (thickener derived from seaweed)
E410 Carob-bean flour (thickener)
E411 Tamarind-seed flour (thickener)
E420 Sorbitol
E440 Pectin

Traveling in France

by Mme. Margaret Serandour-Kerr

In a recent issue of *Pure Facts*, Gabriela Ehrlich published a complete guide to traveling in Europe with a Feingold child. It was so exhaustive that there is little to add except information concerning France. Here are a few thoughts that should be useful to those visiting Paris or the provinces.

Most high-priced restaurants can be trusted to use fresh food. But since even the profession of restaurateur has a few bad eggs (excuse the pun; it was irresistible) it would be a good idea to consult one of the good French restaurant guides. They generally mention if the chef does the shopping himself or uses fresh food. You can ask to speak with the chef and explain your needs.

To minimize costs, buy the fixings for the midday meal yourself. Bakers in France are not permitted to put additives in the baguettes, so you are safer if you buy bread from bakeries and avoid commercial sliced bread.

Many large supermarkets have a health food section, or "rayon de produits de regime," but check these labels as carefully as you would all others. You may find some health food products that you have used in the U.S.

Some of the chocolate in the health food section contains vanillin, particularly the dietary chocolate. On the other hand, the higher grade Lindt & Sprungli or Cote d'Or chocolate in the regular food section is made with real vanilla. [Information on brand name products is always subject to change.] Most large supermarkets sell a full range of qualities of chocolate, from the best to the very worst. Make sure the label says "arome naturelle de vanille" or "vanille en gousse" or "vanille naturelle." Some contain a blend of natural and synthetic vanilla.

If your child can tolerate salicylates, you can buy fruit juices in the supermarket. Government regulations oblige the manufacturers to state clearly on the label when the juice is not 100% fruit or when it contains additives. (Most additives are illegal in fruit juice.)

Breakfast in France

If you suspect your hotel is giving you croissants made with margarine at breakfast, just nip out to the local bakery (most of them open very early) and ask for croissants au beurre, which you can trust. Most jams and jellies in France are made with no additives, but they do contain apple pectin. Read the label carefully before you buy British and Dutch jams/jellies.

Butter in France should be fine, and the French are partial to sweet (unsalted) butter. Avoid margarine unless you get it in a health food store.

Avoid the cereals most hotels offer at breakfast, as they are just French versions of the American cereals we have all learned to avoid. You may occasionally find fresh-made oatmeal, which would be fine. Health food stores will have a variety of cereals that can generally be trusted, but many of the products are based on mueslis and many contain pieces of salicylate fruit. Lima, Cereal and Kentaur are brands that can generally be trusted.

Health food stores are a good resource

Health food stores can be found in moderate-sized towns. They are generally called "magasins de regime" or "magasins dietetiques," and one national chain is called "La Vie Claire." As Mrs. Ehrlich said, they can help you find a good restaurant or a bakery, and sometimes they may even be able to recommend a good local butcher who makes his own cold-cuts.

In two of the small towns where I have lived I found a butcher who made most of the delicatessen products he sold and would even smoke a ham on special order.

French bakeries

Buy your breads and desserts in bakeries, rather than supermarkets. France being France, a lousy baker will not last long unless he is the only one in town. On the whole, you can judge the quality of a baker by the line of people buying bread early in the morning or upon returning from work. In the Paris area there are a few really famous bakers whose products you can trust as well as one or two American bakeries (and here you can discuss the ingredients before making your purchase).

A taste of home

American grocery stores carry the best and the worst of American food, but you may stumble across products that are familiar. In any case, everyone speaks English and you can discuss ingredients. If you don't wish to venture out of the center of Paris, try Fauchon, the fancy grocery on the Place de la Madeleine. The grocery section carries many imported products, including American.

Cosmetics and toiletries

The best advice I can give is to bring what you need from home. Most products, except those sold in health food stores, do not specify all of their contents on the label. If you run out of toothpaste, however, try buying the homeopathic toothpaste called Homeodent, manufactured by Laboratories Boiron and sold in most pharmacies.

If you are traveling in Provence, you might want to drop by the factory store of L'Occitane (route de Forcalquier, Volx, in the department of Alpes de Haute-Provence). They make and sell all-natural toiletries and soaps as well as toilet water and flower essences. (Sensitive people may react to some of the natural salicylates or to natural fragrances.) You can also order these products through the chain of stores called Sephora.

Increase in additives used in Europe

The *Journal of the Hyperactive Children's Support Group* in Great Britain regretfully reports that it is becoming more difficult for consumers in Europe to avoid synthetic additives.

As the nations of Europe break down barriers to trade, some of the protection afforded by food regulations are being sacrificed. Many food additives used in European countries must contain an "E" designation, followed by an identifying number. The United Kingdom had allowed about 300 of these additives, while Germany and Greece permitted about half that amount. Now, with the harmonization of trade and food standards, the number of separately listed additives has grown to over 400. This does not include the enormous number of chemicals used as artificial flavorings -- approximately 3700 in the U.K. alone -- which do not have to be specifically identified.

Le supermarket

Don't be surprised if your visit to a European supermarket brings you face to face with familiar American cereals. The mammoth General Mills has teamed up with PepsiCo to export snack foods, and with Nestle to market their cereals abroad. Kellogg's has long been in the European market.

Australia

Families in Australia seeking to avoid harmful additives face as much difficulty as those in the United States. The Health Association of Australia reports, "One small ray of hope is that the Department of Health has acknowledged that chemical additives in foods result in severe and dangerous consequences for some people. They have issued a booklet of chemical additives so that families are able to identify potential hazards on food labels when they go shopping... At least one section of the bureaucracy now recognizes that additives can be a danger to health."

Contact the Feingold Association at P.O. Box 6550, Alexandria, VA 22306 for names of contacts abroad.

Thinking About College

When the Feingold member thinks about finding a college, it's tempting to wish for one that serves "Feingold food." Alas, we don't know of any to recommend.

"Look for the college first," advises high school guidance counselor, Ruth P. Narrow the choice down to a few, and then see what sort of arrangement you can work out with the administration at each college. It may require an adjustment as minor as assigning the student to a dorm that has a kitchen.

Pure Facts interviewed two college-age members who have been on the Feingold Program for many years. The good news is that they have been able to stay on their diet while living away from home. The relative ease with which they have combined college with their diet is the result of two important factors: motivation and reduced sensitivity. Both are on the diet because it is their own decision: they assumed responsibility for their food choices years ago. And both have been on the Program for a long enough time that their sensitivities are no longer as severe. They can be relaxed about an occasional infraction while eating out with friends, and are well acquainted with the subtle signs that tell them when it's time to get back to more careful eating.

Kathy

"At any college the food is fattening," noted U of Pennsylvania junior Kathy, "and to stay slim you pretty much have to stick to salads, fruit and potatoes." Kathy passes up the breaded and deep fried, sauced, or greasy entrees served in the dining room, and avoids both calories and additives.

Since the cafeteria has a fairly good selection, she can always find suitable foods. Having been on the diet for 8 years, Kathy has a good understanding of what to look for (less processed, fresh foods) and what to avoid (obviously brightly-colored foods, sauces, and highly processed dishes). Her friends like to bring their own bottle of salad dressing to the dining room, so Kathy's additive-free dressing isn't the least bit conspicuous.

There's always a good selection of sandwiches at lunchtime: tuna, egg, and chicken salads, as well as sliced turkey or cheese. They present no problem. Since the school Kathy attends is very large, there are many food options: vendors sell fresh fruit on the campus, there are Grocery stores and restaurants are nearby, including a Chinese carry out/restaurant where she can request foods with no MSG. Like most freshmen, Kathy had to live in a dorm, but hers had a kitchen where she could prepare her own food. Stir-fried chicken fillet, egg dishes, salad and soup are some of her favorites. As a junior, Kathy is now able to live off campus, so she is in total control of her diet.

Staying on the Feingold Program isn't very hard for the student who wants to stick with it. But as Kathy points out, "I have to want to do it."

Aaron

Aaron sent a questionnaire to the Food Service Directors of the colleges that interested him, and then telephoned those who responded positively. He received a wide variety of responses. Some directors were not interested in cooperating, while others were glad to open their kitchens and pantries to label-readers.

Having been on the Feingold Program for 12 years now, Aaron has a clear understanding of his sensitivities - which additives cause the most trouble, and how "relaxed" he can be before he will begin to experience reactions. He is particularly careful during the time when exams are given, so he can concentrate more effectively on his studies.

Once he was able to live off campus, life became much easier. As a graduate student, he preferred to cook on the weekend and freeze dishes for the coming week. He has since earned his master's degree and become an accomplished cook.

"Nobody worries about being different in college," both Kathy and Aaron noted, "because everyone's different!" The homogeneity of high school -- the concern about being singled out -- simply didn't exist once these Feingolders got to college. Just about everyone eats, dresses, thinks, or lives differently, they found. And even if classmates knew they were on the Feingold Program, "nobody cares." One of the few characteristics that college students share is a dislike for the food provided, and a strong desire to seek out alternatives.

Finding the right college

Deciding upon the right college or post-high school training for any teenager is a challenge. For the student with a learning disability or for one who has a hard time handling stress, the decision may be more difficult. There are numerous books available for the college-bound LD student. Your high school's guidance department may have several. Other sources are the school or public library and the Learning Disabilities Association (LDA) 4156 Library Rd., Pittsburgh, PA 15234.

BABIES AND ADULTS

Predisposing Baby to Hyperactivity

by Ben F. Feingold, M.D.

Hyperactivity is not new. It is as old as the human race; it is as old as mankind. It has always been with us and perhaps always will be with us.

If we go back into medical writings as far as 400 BC, we encounter descriptions of symptoms which are identical with the symptoms and deficits that we identify with hyperactivity today.

Now this is not remarkable when we recognize that women at the time of conception and gestation have always been subjected to potential mutagens and teratogens in our whole ecosystem. Mutagens (and teratogens) are substances that alter the genetic profile, alter the genes.

Mothers have always been exposed to the atmosphere, water, soil, and food that contain pollutants. They've always been exposed to forms of radiation that have a mutagenic potential They've always been subjected to infection, hemorrhage (bleeding), toxemia (blood poisoning) and jaundice (a blood disorder) during pregnancy. Each of these has the potential, the power, to produce alteration in the genetic profile.

But now, more recently, we must also consider medications, tobacco, and alcohol. And by alcohol I am not necessarily referring to fetal alcohol syndrome caused by heavy drinking. I'm referring to social drinking which has also been demonstrated to have the potential to change the biological profile. The mutations in the genetic profile can be activated by the appropriate compound in the environment, natural or synthetic.

Then we have the period during delivery. We have hemorrhage, infection, toxemia, and jaundice. And we have to take into account the contemporary obstetrical practices: with the mother lying recumbent with her thighs flexed on the abdomen, and the legs on the thighs. This position predisposes the baby, in some cases, as it passes through the birth canal, to a slight compression of the vascular system that may induce temporary and transitory anoxia and hypoxia (insufficient oxygen) affecting the brain.

And then in the baby itself we consider hemorrhage, asphyxia, prematurity, and immaturity.

I've labeled all these as predisposing agents, not causes. Why? Because they are not the direct cause. They provide the groundwork, they provide the alterations in the biological profile that makes it possible for them to react with anything in the environment, whether it's natural or synthetic. Anything may be a factor.

It must be borne in mind that these agents do not act singly or at a particular site. They occur in showers at random, hitting the entire biological profile. It is conceivable that these numerous mutagenic alterations in the genetic profile may lie dormant. We know from genetics that most of the mutations in the genetic profile are not active. But under certain conditions they can be activated and what activates them is the appropriate compound in the environment which may be anything, natural or synthetic. Depending on what the mutation is, what the chemical is, will determine the clinical pattern we observe and the reaction that occurs.

Hyperactivity and smoking

Mothers who smoke heavily during pregnancy almost double their child's risk of becoming hyperactive and impulsive by age 7, according to Dr. Paul L. Nichols.

Nichols is a research psychologist and behavior geneticist at the National Institute of Neurological and Communicative Disorders and Stroke, National Institutes of Health. He found that while only 7 percent of the children of non-smoking mothers were hyperactive, 10 percent and 13 percent of children of smoking mothers (who smoked two and three packs per day, respectively) became hyperactive by age 7.

The study, presented to the American Academy of Neurology, included 30,000 children who have been studied since birth.

Inter. Med. Tribune

The problem baby

"For some children, food dyes behave as a drug, with the youngest being the most vulnerable." *Bernard Weiss Ph.D., University of Rochester School of Medicine & Dentistry*

Most people now understand that hyperactivity is not limited to children, and can persist into adulthood, but babies are often overlooked. Perhaps the head banging, crib rocking, sleepless, screaming infant attracts less attention than the hyperactive child because he disrupts the lives of fewer people. Furthermore, it's easy to diagnose the cause as "nervous mother." A woman who has not had a restful night's sleep in several weeks would indeed be nervous. And calling it "colic" doesn't cure anything.

The practice of blaming parents for everything from colic to autism is finally losing favor. But this leaves the pediatrician with the unanswered question of why the infant behaves as he does. And if formula-switching doesn't help, the options are: 1) do nothing or 2) use medication. Even medication does not always work, and the bright red syrup that sedates some infants has an opposite effect on others.

Amphetamines were banned as diet aids for adults because of concern over their safety; but amphetamine-like drugs are now being administered to very young children. Many of the medications being given to very young children are close to the "street drugs" causing havoc among our adolescents. Teen-age baby sitters must wonder why the drug they are told to refuse is given to the three-year-old in their care.

Dr. Feingold had something better for babies than drugs. Not only is the Program easy to use with babies, it has an extremely high success rate, often producing a dramatic change in 36 hours. Our babies deserve the best we can offer -- a nutrition program that offers no risk and no harm.

The Best for Your Baby

by Barbara Hoffstein, R.D.

Preparing for Your Baby

The best way to prepare for your baby is to be healthy and well nourished *before* conception. Nutrients from your tissue nourish the embryo before you even know you're pregnant. Eat from the basic food groups and concentrate on foods with high nutrient density. (For example, a baked potato has more nutrients per calorie than French fries.)

During pregnancy, a good diet and healthy lifestyle will continue to be vitally important to your developing baby. We join your doctor in encouraging you to avoid alcohol and cigarettes. Medications are prescribed only when essential.

Minimally processed foods will supply you with the many important trace nutrients destroyed by excessive processing. Eliminating synthetic food dyes, flavorings and the antioxidant preservatives BHA, BHT and TBHQ from your diet means your baby will not be exposed to these chemicals.

Nutritionists debate the need for prenatal vitamins for everyone. But it is generally agreed that iron may be needed, especially for women who go into their pregnancies anemic. Look for a vitamin that is free of synthetic dyes. Folic acid is generally needed because of increased demands during pregnancy. Calcium needs are also increased and lack of it can exacerbate osteoporosis for the mother later in life. Four servings of cheese, milk, or yogurt each day will easily cover calcium needs.

Weight gain of about 25 pounds is expected during the entire pregnancy with the majority of weight gain in the last trimester.

Feeding your baby

After the baby arrives, breastfeeding is the best way to ensure optimum nourishment and decrease the risk of your child developing allergies.

Most babies fare well while nursing if the mother's diet is good and if she avoids gas-forming vegetables: broccoli, cauliflower and cabbage. If there is a problem it may be caused by liquid baby vitamins because these contain synthetic flavorings. If your pediatrician recommends vitamins, the pharmacist may be able to prepare a vitamin compound or recommend a natural liquid baby vitamin.

Most commercial baby foods are free of synthetic colors and flavors but contain starches to provide a uniform product. Using a blender or baby-food grinder with foods served to the rest of the family is a better choice and is less expensive. The baby's food should be prepared before seasonings are added so your infant is not encouraged to develop a taste for salt.

Barbara Hoffstein, R.D., has followed the Feingold Program for many years; she is a past president of the Feingold Association of the United States.

Baby vitamins

Most baby vitamins no longer contain synthetic dyes, but their synthetic flavoring can be drawn from thousands of chemical components that would be more fitting in Dr. Frankenstein's laboratory than an infant's diet.

A compounding pharmacist can make up many vitamins and medicines to your specifications. To locate one near you, call the Professional Compounding Centers of America at 1-800-331-2498.

Pediatric medication

Since most pediatric medicine - both prescription and over the counter - is dyed and flavored, the Feingold Association provides its members with a list of medications free of the offending chemicals. Your Feingold Association can provide the *Medication List* for you to give to your doctor or pharmacist or ask your doctor if the medicine can be prescribed in the uncolored adult form, with the dose adjusted to your child's weight.

In the nursery

A wholesome diet is not the only way to get your baby off to a good start in life. Today babies are protected against many once-fatal infectious diseases, but are exposed to hazards peculiar to our time. These include:

Diaper pail deodorizers - Limit exposure by keeping the diaper pail away from the area where baby sleeps or spends much time.

Perfumed diapers and pre-moistened wipettes - These can cause rashes and other problems.

Scented baby powders - Use any type of starch, such as cornstarch, arrowroot, or even potato starch.

Disinfectant sprays, cleaners, or deodorizers - In spite of what the TV commercials would have you believe plain soaps and fresh air are the best cleaners and deodorizers. If you want your room to smell like a bouquet of fresh flowers, we recommend you get a bouquet of fresh flowers.

Scented fabric softening strips - The chemicals in these can cause allergic reactions and/or behavioral problems in people of all ages. They are now available unscented. You can also use half a cup of vinegar in the rinse water to serve as a softener and deodorizer.

Formaldehyde - Do your eyes burn when you go into a fabric store? This chemical is often used to treat fabrics and give new clothes a crisp look. It's a good idea to wash baby's clothing and linens before their first use.

Avoid scented products of all kinds. Soaps, tissues, miracle carpet sprays, etc. The chemicals that provide the scent can be a serious irritant for the sensitive individual.

These suggestions are offered to you by Feingold parents ... who wish they had known these things when their children were babies. The extra effort you spend for your infant can pay off in a lifetime of benefits.

Our members write

Having a seven-month-old nursing baby has given me lots of time to sit and read. I've been a captive audience, so to speak. And so I escape - alone - to the library every few weeks and come home loaded down with more books on nutrition, natural cooking, and all the new "live longer" diets that have come along. My conclusion after all this reading is this: Why isn't the whole world a member of the Feingold Association? I have hardly read an author who does not advocate our diet. Most do not use the label of "Feingold" but they all say the same thing. Synthetic colorings and flavorings are bad for our health and can cause behavioral problems or worse yet, cancer in laboratory animals. Most authors also concur that BHA, BHT and TBHQ are harmful chemicals that are to be avoided.

When I sit in group meetings like PTA and church services I look around and wonder about the food that my friends are eating. What have the slick Madison Avenue advertising agencies persuaded all those mothers to serve their families? It truly upsets me to think that the pursuit of bigger profits has caused our country's food manufacturers to sell us all short on nutrition and good health.

Michael's success story

Today was a very hard day. Michael cried, whined incessantly, rolled around on the floor in a seemingly unending tantrum and generally tormented his little brother and everyone else in our household...all because the day before yesterday a well-meaning neighbor gave him a piece of candy. Tomorrow will be pretty much the same as today, but the following day will bring the departure of "Mr. Hyde" and the return of the happy, lively and relatively well-mannered 5-year-old we know and love.

Fortunately, today's behavior is a rarity, brought on by the mistaken belief that a piece of candy was safe - that is, free of artificial colors, flavors, and preservatives. Normally Michael is very careful about what he eats because, even at five years old, he realized that foods with these chemicals make him feel "funny."

Until two years ago the violent, irrational and often self-destructive behavior was not a rare occurrence. It was a day-in, day-out fact of life, which made him and everyone around him miserable. Crying jags, uncontrollable tantrums, headaches, learning difficulties, and a myriad of other similar problems were ruining his life and bringing me to the point where I no longer felt able to cope with the situation, let alone alleviate it. The next step would have been drugs...Ritalin for him, Valium for me.

We never thought it would be like this. Michael was a first child; he was wanted, loved, and considered a wonderful addition to the family. He came into the world unhindered by painkillers, bursting with a healthy vitality and immediately took to breast-feeding. Everything was fine, until the pediatrician gave him baby vitamins loaded with additives.

Michael's sunny disposition began to disintegrate rapidly. Crying, irritability, and sleeping problems became the norm. Subsequent check-ups failed to identify any physical problems. Perhaps it was just colic ... all day, every day? I finally began to suspect the vitamins and stopped giving them to him. I thought he was simply allergic to them.

All went well until Michael left the breast and joined the formula generation at about six months. He spent a good deal of the day crying for no apparent reason, had difficulty sleeping, refused to nap, and couldn't seem to relax or cuddle when being held.

Since Michael was our first child we had no other frame of reference for comparison to normal reactions at that age. We assumed his Jekyll-Hyde behavior was just a new stage in his progression toward toddlerhood. Unfortunately, by the time he was 14 months old, Mr. Hyde had pretty well taken over. The nice side of his personality rarely surfaced. We kept telling ourselves and each other that Michael was just hitting the "terrible two's" a little early. (I remember thinking that if this was a prelude to the two's, I wasn't going to last until three.) By the time he reached three, Michael's destructive behavior continued, and he spoke only a few rudimentary words.

Throughout this period the pediatrician assured me that he was "just all boy." It was only after I joined a mother's day out program (in an attempt to preserve what was left of my sanity) that I began to realize that there really might be something wrong with Michael. The program gave me an opportunity to observe other children his age, and the comparison was quite disturbing. During this period I spent a good deal of time locked in the bathroom crying, and when I wasn't there I was reading every book on child behavior I could find. Michael, of course, spent this time on the other side of the door howling like a banshee.

Some of the books I read alluded to the connection between diet and behavior problems, so I quickly singled out refined sugar as a possible culprit. After substantially reducing his sugar intake we noticed some improvement.

Then I saw Dr. Feingold on the Phil Donahue Show. Morning Break (a local talk show) followed with a discussion of the same subject. The mothers on the show seemed like intelligent, rational individuals who were really concerned for their children. As several of them told their stories, I realized they were describing my child! I had just had a baby, but the show was barely over when I loaded the kids into the car and headed for the nearest bookstore. Using Dr. Feingold's book as a bible I tried to purchase only pure foods. However, I had difficulty finding the right brands and sadly discovered that you can't believe everything that you read, especially product labels.

At this point I called the local Feingold Association and begged for help. They responded admirably. At the initial meeting I discovered that Michael was not alone with his problem and neither was I. The association provided me with a tested, up-to-date Foodlist, recipes, a monthly newsletter, the phone number of a program assistant to call for help and massive amounts of moral support.

I set to work with great hopes. A diary had to be started to track what Michael ate and the resulting behavior. The kitchen was cleaned out and restocked with foods from the Foodlist. And, I had developed a new attitude toward buying prepared foods. Within four days after the new regimen was fully operational, I was rewarded with a radical change in

Michael's disposition and behavior. Mr. Hyde gave way to a delightful, funny, and thoroughly loveable child.

The first six months saw several major setbacks, due largely to attempts to get by with brands that weren't on the list but had wonderfully reassuring labels. However, there was no doubt that the diet truly works. Michael's verbal skills grew at a remarkable rate. Within six months he went from barely understandable, single syllable words to discussions that included phrases such as "...Mommy, that isn't appropriate."

Today he's ... well maybe not today... but the day after tomorrow he will again be a sweet, funny, smart kid who is doing well in school, has a lot of friends and is a delight to be around. And that makes today a lot easier.

P.S. As for Dr. Jekyll, the 19th century novelist Robert Louis Stevenson's famous character, I think the poor doctor unknowingly stumbled on the formula for red dye!

Like father, like son

My husband had been a hyperactive child and while we were awaiting the arrival of our first child, I worried that it may be a little like its father. The baby was so strong and often thrashed violently inside me. But when Gabriel was born, he began breastfeeding and was a perfect angel.

Unfortunately, this stage was to prove short-lived. At three months, as I began introducing juices and other foods, Gabriel's temperament changed for the worse. But it was not until six months that we realized our son had a serious problem. By then he had become a terror, screaming for 2 to 3 hours at a time and only sleeping 4 hours a night.

By eight months, he was taking no naps and threw violent temper tantrums regularly. At times, Gabriel rocked methodically, beating his head against things. Twice he actually attacked us and clawed at our eyes while screaming, hitting, and kicking.

One day a friend told us about the Feingold Program. I thought, "a diet to help my baby? No way!" But for my friend's sake and because I had nothing to lose, I tried it. Wow! We wondered if Gabriel was all right. He slept for 17 hours. Soon his expression changed to a sweet innocent look instead of the half-glare I had been accustomed to. After several weeks, all of our son's symptoms disappeared and he became a calm, gentle child. Soon after seeing the dramatic change in Gabriel, my husband tried the diet. For the first time in his life, Rob was able to write a two- or three-page letter (a paragraph was the previous record). For the first time he was able to handle Gabriel, who was, of course, calm by now too. It wasn't long before my husband began to make major changes in his life, such as a more responsible job and a desire to go back to school.

When Babies Don't Sleep

Most parents of 3-year-olds would be very upset if their child woke up several times each night. For Marilyn, this represented a dramatic improvement in her child's sleep pattern. Marilyn wrote the following letter to the Feingold Association of Indiana.

Every night when our daughter sleeps 3 to 8 hours without waking up screaming, I thank you and all other Feingolders. For the first twenty months of life, Alice woke up every five minutes to 2 hours all night long.

My first indication that the cause might be artificial coloring came when she had a cold and I gave her Novahistine. The medication didn't make her sleepy, as it would my other two children. In fact, she was so wound up, it was 2 days before her arms and legs stopped moving. When she accidentally got some of my diet "grape" drink, and had the same reaction, I was sure it was the coloring. [Note: artificial flavoring and the synthetic sweetener could also have been irritants.]

I took everything out of her diet which listed coloring. But I actually changed her diet very little, and her behavior changed very little as well. I read everything I could on diet and hyperactivity, and followed the suggestions, but still without results. Then a friend gave me your address and I received the Foodlist, newsletter, and instructions.

Now Alice sleeps more soundly than ever, and for a longer time. She doesn't sleep "like a log" as do some children, but she and I sleep most of the night.

Behavioral Toxicology:

The adverse behavioral effects of chemicals

Bernard Weiss, Ph.D. is the Professor of Toxicology, Deputy Director, Environmental Health Services Center, at the University of Rochester School of Medicine in Rochester, NY. This article is based on his address to the 12th annual Conference of the Feingold Association.

Air pollutants, pesticides, fuels, solvents, and heavy metals are some of the toxic substances in our environment. The damage they cause is clear. The new science of behavioral toxicology came with the recognition that the harmful effects of environmental chemicals should also be measured by how people feel and function, not only by death and obvious damage.

The most vulnerable - "Dose is the key variable in toxicology," Dr. Weiss noted in his address to the Feingold Conference, "and young organisms will be affected at lower doses than the adult."

The youngest children are often at greatest risk, and the fetus can suffer severe effects from substances to which its mother is exposed. This was tragically confirmed by an episode of methyl mercury poisoning which took place in Iraq in the early 1970s.

Methyl mercury has long been used as a fungicide, and when the Iraqi government purchased 80,000 tons of grain, they requested it be treated to prevent spoilage. Instead of using the grain as seed for their crops (where the methyl mercury would not have caused harm) many farmers ignored the government's caution; they ground the grain into flour and ate it. This resulted in approximately 5,000 deaths and 50,000 cases of serious illness.

Effects on the unborn - Investigations into the poisonings showed that women who ate the grain during pregnancy delivered babies who suffered from retarded development. Even when the mother was not severely affected, the babies were. "One of the most sensitive targets of toxic metals in our environment is the developing brain," Dr. Weiss explained.

Subtle effects at low doses - Another well-known toxic metal is lead. Decades ago young children who consumed flakes of chipping paint were found to suffer from persistent hyperactivity, intellectual impairment and often retardation as a result of the lead poisoning.

Herbert Needleman, M.D., of the University of Pittsburgh, studied the harmful effects of lead by examining lead levels in the baby teeth of several thousand school-age children. (Measuring lead levels in teeth is a more accurate method than using blood samples because lead does not remain in the blood, as it does in the teeth.) The lead levels were then compared with the children's test scores. Those children with the lowest levels of lead consistently achieved the highest test scores.

Dr. Weiss explained the importance of Needleman's work: "Even in children who showed no indication of lead toxicity, there was a direct relationship between tooth lead and scores on intelligence and several other psychological tests." At low doses, far below the level at which one can detect obvious symptoms, toxic substances may cause harm. This was further confirmed by the work of David Bellinger, Ph.D., et al. Writing in the *New England Journal of Medicine*, Bellinger described a study testing 249 children from birth to age two.

Lead levels were measured at the time of birth and the babies were divided into three groups determined by the levels of lead found. Tests to measure cognitive development were started at 6 months of age and the infants were assessed at six-month intervals. "At all ages," Bellinger writes, "infants in the high prenatal exposure group scored lower than infants in the other two groups."

The researchers found that development scores consistently correlated with the level of lead exposure measured at birth. Bellinger concluded, "It appears that the fetus may be adversely affected at blood lead concentrations well below ... the level currently defined by the Centers for Disease Control as the highest acceptable level for young children." (*New England Journal of Medicine*, 1987; 316:1037)

The effect upon our society - Almost all of the babies in the Bellinger study came from upper middle class families, and even the high-lead group still had above average scores. A modest drop in test scores may not seem like a significant problem if you consider one child. But what are the implications for society as a whole? "All of our models of risk are based on the risk of individuals," Dr. Weiss explained, "but there is a societal risk as well that we have not taken account of."

He showed a graph that gave the current distribution of scores on a typical intelligence test, with 100 points representing the average score. Out of a population of 100 million, 2.3 million children will score over 130 points. But if the median score is lowered only 5 percent, to 95, the figures shift drastically. Only 990,000 will then score in the high intellectual range, and there will be a great increase in the number of children who will have to receive special schooling or be institutionalized. "In the 21st century that is a societal disaster!" Dr. Weiss emphasized. "The economic consequences are enormous. You can no longer talk about individual risk and set standards on that basis."

The case against food dyes - In 1985 the Committee on Drugs for the American Academy of Pediatrics published an article detailing a long list of known reactions brought about by the synthetic dyes ("food coloring") added to many drugs (*Pediatrics*, Vol. 76, No. 4, October 1985).

James Swanson, Ph.D., found that synthetic dyes impaired the learning ability of children. Researchers at Yale University reported that feeding dyes to newborn rats resulted in behavior that is "similar to attention deficit disorder with hyperactivity (ADHD) observed in children." (*Annals of Neurology*, Vol. 4, No. 2, August 1978).

The FDA study conducted by Weiss demonstrated that food dyes are capable of provoking hyperactive behavior in children, and that the youngest appear to suffer the greatest harm. Applying the principles of toxicology, we can conclude that if dyes have an obvious effect on some children, all children are at risk; and the developing brain of the very young is the most vulnerable target.

Assessing risk vs. benefit - When cavemen hunted dangerous animals for food and clothing they took risks in order to gain benefits. Coal brought black lung disease and polluted air, but it kept people warm in the winter. As our society became more complex, regulatory agencies were established to determine the risk vs. benefit of toxic substances and to decide which may be deliberately introduced into our environment, and in what amount.

Although dyes serve no essential nutritional purpose, they are added for marketing purposes to foods, beverages and medications consumed by most of our population, particularly children. For many years newborn infants were given vitamins which contained synthetic dyes even though the added coloring served no essential purpose. (They were very effective at leaving a permanent stain on linoleum countertops!)

And how many pediatric medications contain added dyes, synthetic flavorings, and so on? Nearly all of them. If the young child is vulnerable to the effects of these chemicals, then the sick youngster is at even greater risk.

Considering the risk - In his closing remarks Dr. Weiss quoted the late Phillip Handler, a famous biochemist and head of the National Academy of Sciences:

"A sensible guide would surely be to reduce exposure to hazard whenever possible, to accept substantial hazard only for great benefit, minor hazard for modest benefit, and no hazard at all when the benefit seems relatively trivial."

"Hyperactive" Adults

Who is this?

Excessive talking, tendency to interrupt
Nervous habits, such as nail biting, foot jiggling, etc.
Workaholic
Nervous, emotional, irritable
Erratic sleep patterns, difficulty getting to sleep
Distractible, tends to flit from one job or project to the next, seldom completing them; difficulty concentrating
Voice rises in pitch during a stressful situation
Has adult temper tantrums

It's the hyperactive adult. Long before most physicians recognized that hyperactivity was an adult problem as well, Dr. Feingold wrote, "As the troubled children pass through puberty they may experience a spontaneous alteration in their behavioral pattern, with a lessening of hyperactivity and aggression. This may occur with or without specific therapy (such as medication, behavior modification, reinforcement or dietary management).

"This spontaneous change in the behavioral pattern is frequently misinterpreted as 'growing out' of the disturbance. However, this is an illusion, since these children do not grow out of the problems. What on the surface appears as an improved individual, upon close study reveals a troubled person with deeply rooted psychological deficits, which prevent performance up to the level of mental competence."

Very few adults display the typical symptoms one associates with the term "hyperactivity." But behavior and learning problems don't disappear with the onset of adolescence, as Feingold families can testify. Difficulty in concentrating, trouble in sticking with a task, interrupting, nervousness and irritability are a few of the characteristics of the hyperactive adult.

Hyperactivity does not magically disappear with puberty

One of the classic symptoms of hyperactivity is the lack of impulse control. Researchers at the Robert W. Johnson Medical School in Piscataway, NJ have found a link between a chemical imbalance in the brain and an addiction to gambling.

They note that the lack of impulse control in the compulsive gambler may be due to a lowered level of serotonin in the brain. A four-year study indicates that EEG readings of the compulsive gamblers showed brain activity similar to that of children who have been diagnosed with ADD.

Some doctors believe that many hyperactive adults drink too much or turn to drugs in an attempt to relieve their symptoms. The combination of poor impulse control and substance abuse is a recipe for social disaster.

What does it feel like to have a reaction?

I am a 28-year-old Feingold adult...parents of hyperactive children often ask me what having a reaction feels like.

Initially, I feel my mouth and lips tingle and my eyes itch. I feel speedy (like drinking several cups of coffee) and sometimes feel cold. Occasionally I shiver. My mouth feels dry and I become very thirsty. Shortly thereafter, my skin starts to burn or itch.

Within an hour I become extremely irritable, impatient, easily frustrated and find it difficult to concentrate on one thing. I often feel extremely tired after the speediness subsides. When I awaken in the morning, I feel groggy and cranky (like a hangover). I am clumsy and find it difficult to focus on reading, and my handwriting and spelling deteriorate. I occasionally become forgetful, disorganized, and emotional. I don't like to be touched or feel penned in while having a reaction.

When I am not having a reaction I am well organized, efficient and anything but clumsy. Sometimes I am not aware that I am having a reaction until after I have become extremely cranky, or find myself unable to deal with what should be a routine problem.

Coping with someone who is having a reaction is not easy, but there are certain things I find helpful. I try not to put myself in potentially frustrating situations on those days, to put off chores that can wait, and just generally take it easy. I feel better when I am outside and active, and I try to be alone. I try to let the people around me know either that I'm having a reaction or that I'm out of sorts and encourage them to leave me alone.

A 35-year-old success story

Ron is a professional truck driver, and today he is a very cautious and careful driver, a far cry from the daredevil he was before going on the diet.

When hazardous weather conditions forced drivers off the road, Ron was the last to come in, and the first back out onto the highway. He had plenty of pent-up aggression and took it out behind the wheel.

Ron suffered from headaches, earaches, acid stomach, and needed to wear sunglasses (even when indoors) to protect his eyes from bright lights. Finally, he and his wife had "had it" and decided to give the Feingold Program a try. He said they got rid of 18 sacks of junk food. Not only did the diet work, but he also had the bonus of going from 220 pounds to 180.

Women are susceptible to these problems too, despite the pervasive belief that girls are not often hyperactive. In fact, as many women are affected as men, but because girls are less likely to exhibit the symptoms of physical overactivity, they are often overlooked.

Some statistics on the chemically-sensitive adult

Feingold member, Preston Edwards, M.D., gathered information from a questionnaire filled out by Feingold adults.

The purpose of the survey was to determine if he could identify a syndrome of symptoms that would help professionals pick out salicylate- and additive-sensitive adults. He hoped that this information would also help in the literature we produce for the public. Dr. Edwards is interested in this both as a physician, and as a result of his own personal problems with additives and salicylates.

Of the members responding, 80% were female. The survey showed a higher rate of reaction to additives than to salicylates.

The most frequent symptoms were: irritability, mood swings, loss of concentration, restlessness, compulsive doing, and poor sleep. These central nervous system symptoms represent an adult version of the Feingold child, or, more accurately, the adult Feingold syndrome.

The next most frequent set of symptoms was sinus congestion, headaches, fatigue, and muscle aches. These correspond very well to a medical syndrome of nasal polyps, sinusitis, asthma and hives known as the "aspirin idiosyncrasy reaction."

Less frequent reactions included skin rashes of all types, recurrent illness, sore throats, stomach pains, dizziness, diarrhea, wheezing and bladder irritation.

He found that 78% of the respondents were allergic to other foods, much higher than national estimates of 10-20% for the general population. There was a very strong correlation between a family history of food, pollen, and Feingold sensitivity, and the adult Feingold syndrome.

The length of the reactions varied from a few hours to weeks, but the majority lasted 2-3 days.

53% of the respondents said their problems started during early childhood. Another one third noted their problems began anywhere from age 7 to 45. Most of the Feingold adults apparently had a gradual onset of symptoms. But in those who could find a reason for the change that occurred, childbirth was the most common precipitation event.

Most people found out about the connection between their problems and additive/salicylate sensitivity through friends, by reading about it in publications, or in using the Feingold Program for a child. One fourth were put on the diet by their physician.

One out of four are sensitive to fumes of various types. Others mentioned MSG, caffeine, sulfites, and benzoates.

"We cannot really say how many Feingold children go on to become Feingold adults," Dr. Edwards noted, "but there certainly are some who have an inherited tendency to have a lifelong problem with salicylates and additives. We also do not know how many people outgrow their problems."

The aspirin triad

She is in her forties, and has recently begun to suffer from nasal congestion, recurrent sinus infections and nasal polyps. We'll call her Carol Smith - a fictitious name, but she exhibits some very real symptoms of aspirin idiosyncrasy reaction, or the "aspirin triad."

The nasal problems are the most common portion of the triad. The other two symptoms are asthma and urticaria (hives). Statistically, Carol has about a 10% chance of developing asthma and/or urticaria in the future. Some unfortunate people develop all three at the same time!

Carol's mother was able to tolerate aspirin when she was younger, but now experiences a life-threatening reaction with wheezing and shortness of breath if she takes any. And both women find they are allergic to other substances as well, including food additives.

Both are under the care of an allergist, and are among the estimated 1 to 2% of the patients in any allergist's practice who are aspirin-sensitive.

These women represent a very typical picture of the aspirin triad. It is considered to be hereditary, and can begin during early childhood; but it is most common in middle-aged women, and generally takes awhile to develop. The earlier it begins, the more severe the sensitivity is likely to be.

When the "hyperactive" child grows up

Nobody would have called Jerri a hyperactive child, but her mother always knew this daughter had "problems." Glancing through a diary kept during her early childhood, Jerri found that her mother came close to discovering the cause of these problems, but she didn't trust her instincts.

The mother wrote that Jerri, who was then a toddler, was having a bad day, "It might have been all the excitement at _____'s birthday party." Another entry: "She seemed to get grumpy and cry a lot. It must have been all that K--- A-- she drank yesterday." Although the family ate fresh foods grown on their farm, Jerri recalls a pitcher of [artificial beverage] was always nearby.

She excelled in her schoolwork and kept her behavior pretty well under control, but as she was growing up Jerri felt "like I was tortured inside."

It seemed to become increasingly difficult for Jerri to manage the internal chaos she felt. By the time she was in college her mood swings would run the gamut within a few hours, from euphoria to lethargy. This pattern repeated itself several times a day. Depression frequently enveloped her, and it just seemed like it was too much trouble to pick up a hairbrush. Even the good times were marred by the certainty that they would not last. She had close friends, but they could never predict how she would react to a situation.

Deep depression eroded her marriage, and every job she began ended in a paralysis of lethargy. "There was a time when I considered committing myself to an institution," she recalls. The depression intensified when Jerri began taking birth control pills, and she became suicidal. When she discontinued the pills, there was a lessening of the depression.

Jerri felt that her problems were the result of some external factor or factors. "I could sense that these mood swings and depressions weren't really me," and she experimented with many different diets and food regimens. Since her diet was then a "hippy" one of wholesome vegetarian foods, she didn't eat additives, but she consumed plenty of natural salicylates.

She sought help from all of the traditional sources - and the non-traditional ones too, but none of the doctors, counselors, vitamins or diets made much of a difference.

Jerri got her first clue to the causes during a trip to Japan in 1976. She had a drink of orange soda ("and in Japan, orange soda is really orange!") Within three hours she suffered a physical and emotional reaction so severe, it became obvious that the dye was to blame. "I figured I was sensitive to orange dye, so I avoided it...I drank green [sports drink] instead."

Two years later she read Dr. Feingold's book, *Why Your Child is Hyperactive*, and learned that other additives, as well as the natural salicylates, were causing the havoc she suffered.

Gradually, Jerri was able to determine her own individual tolerances. She's careful about what she eats, and infractions are rare. When they do occur, they aren't extreme, with the exception of synthetic dyes. Ingesting a dye will trigger an episode of crying and severe depression lasting from 24 to 48 hours.

Family members who recall an angry, volatile Jerri are astonished by the changes they've seen. "My closest friend tells everyone, 'You just can't believe the difference in Jerri.'"

A Feingold couple

"We had been on the Feingold Program for many years," Joanne told *Pure Facts*, "since my children were little. But they are grown now, and my husband and I didn't realize how far we had veered from the diet...at least not until a recent weekend.

"One Friday afternoon I had lunch at Wendy's and it included a Frosty. (Many years ago Wendy's Frostys were acceptable for Feingold families, but no longer are.) My husband, Bob, later recalled having a chocolate doughnut at work.

"We bickered all weekend long, and this is not the way we are! Then by Sunday evening I remembered the Frosty, and began to think back on how many additives have managed to slide into our lifestyle -- it was amazing how many small slips there were.

"The following day I went back to Wendy's and ordered the same meal, but minus the Frosty; and there was no reaction. By this time my husband had mellowed out too.

"Bob and I talked it over and decided it was time to come back home to Feingold. I have begun doing most of my shopping in Philadelphia at Fresh Fields. Even though it's a 45-minute drive it's worth the weekly trip. And Bob has gladly offered to pass up the doughnuts at work if I will pack one of Fresh Field's delicious natural cheese Danish pastries with his lunch.

"My weight has stabilized without dieting; I just eat good food. And we both have so much energy now. Instead of feeling washed out on the weekend we go places and do things we've wanted to do for a long time; in fact, we recently painted our house. I no longer find myself feeling disoriented, and can accomplish so much more.

"I have a reputation in my family for elaborate desserts; nothing has changed this holiday, except that now the treats are *naturally* good."

Help for the Very Sensitive

The chemically sensitive adult may be less visible than the hyperactive child, but the problems they face can be daunting.

What can you do when you are unable to tolerate nearly every food you try, when your skin breaks out or peels, and not dermatologist is able to help you? How can you normally when you are unable to travel because you cannot tolerate the chemicals found in hotel rooms? What do you drink when you cannot tolerate the water? How can you lead a normal life when you are very sensitive and those around you wear fragrances? Who do you turn to when your doctor doesn't believe you and it seems that nobody else has these problems?

While the chemically sensitive person is still dismissed by some professionals as the victim of a psychological disorder, thanks to the work of other physicians and many sufferers, this attitude is changing. Several government agencies now recognize MCS and EI (multiple chemical sensitivity and environmental illness) as valid disabilities.

NON-FOODS

They Can Trigger Reactions Too

The Feingold Program is a basic first step for some people.

Perhaps you see small improvements, but feel frustrated that you are not able to identify other culprits which appear to be triggering reactions, or to achieve a higher level of response. In this case, two possibilities to consider are: allergies (most commonly to milk), or sensitivity to other chemicals in your environment. Here is a brief list of some common irritants that can disrupt virtually any system of the body and can affect one's health, behavior, and ability to learn. (More information on carpeting, cosmetics, paint and perfume is presented in the next section.)

Carpeting- When it is new, most carpeting gives off strong fumes from the fibers and glues. In time, these chemicals gas out.

Cleaning products- If you have white vinegar and baking soda, you will be able to clean most surfaces in your home. For a comprehensive resource on non-toxic formulas for cleaning just about everything imaginable, consider the book, *Clean & Green*, by Annie Berthold-Bond (Ceres Press, Box 87, Woodstock, NY 12498). Your book store or health food store can probably order it.

Cosmetics- Fragrances and dyes are irritants in many products. Sensitive people may be unable to tolerate the powerful chemicals in nail polish remover and the glues used with artificial nails.

Dry cleaning- You may find your clothes retain a strong odor of the cleaning solvents. Try to air them outside until the fumes are gone. Some cleaners are offering nontoxic alternatives to the powerful chemical known as perchlorethylene.

Foam insulation- Mobile homes are particularly likely to be a problem if they contain urea-formaldehyde foam insulation since their size and tight construction concentrate the fumes.

Gas stove emissions- This isn't as potent a problem as kerosene heaters, but gas stoves are generally on the hit list for chemically sensitive families. If you experience symptoms that are especially noticeable in the kitchen, it's a tip-off that the gas stove could be the culprit.

You can test out your sensitivity by having the gas company disconnect the stove. For a few weeks, use a microwave oven, electric appliances such as a fry pan, toaster oven or portable electric burners. If you notice a significant improvement, then it's time to sell your gas stove and shop for an electric model.

Hair gel- Having trouble finding a product free of perfumes or other irritants? Did you know that you can substitute aloe vera gel? One member says she uses Lily of the Desert 99% Aloe Vera Organic Gelly; she says it isn't sticky and is as effective as gel.

Hand lotion- Highly sensitive people may want to try organic olive oil. Spread it on your hands and leave it for a few minutes; dab off the excess. It is not greasy and will leave your hands feeling soft.

Hotels and motels- Do you react to the bedding? Consider purchasing some barrier cloth and seaming it to make a piece large enough to cover the hotel bed. Spread it out, right on top of the bedspread, then place your own bedding on top for a restful night's sleep. Barrier cloth is made from untreated cotton that has been very tightly woven to insulate you from chemicals in the bedding or in the detergents used. For information on ordering barrier cloth, contact Janice Cottons at 1-800-526-4237.

Moth balls- In the book, *Healthy Homes, Healthy Kids*, the authors Joyce M. Schoemaker, Ph.D., and Charity Y. Vitale, Ph.D. suggest storing woolen clothes in a hot attic during the summer since the heat will kill all stages of the moth life cycle. (Island Press, (202) 232-7933, $12.95 paperback)

New clothing- Before you wear new clothing, wash it to remove the formaldehyde and other finishing chemicals. For extremely sensitive people, this is not sufficient. You may want to seek out "green cotton" (untreated).

Office machinery- Things such as copiers and printers can give off irritating fumes. Reduce the concentration by increasing air circulation (open a nearby window, or consider installing an exhaust fan).

Paint- Oil-based paint can give off irritating fumes, but so can latex. Major companies are developing new formulas that should be better tolerated.

Particle board- It is increasingly difficult to find furniture made from solid wood. The resins used in particle board contain formaldehyde, which "gasses off," releasing fumes that can be irritants. Some people find they can tolerate furniture made from particle board if all of it is painted with a sealant. Plywood may also be treated with formaldehyde.

Pesticides- Chemicals designed to damage the nervous system of insects are not likely to be kind to humans. Many mail-order companies provide safer alternatives.

Literature on alternatives is available from the Bio Integral Resource Center. For information send $1 to BIRC, P.O. Box 7414, Berkeley, CA 94707.

Printing ink- Printed materials may retain a noticeable odor for a long time after they have been printed. Some printers use soy-based ink, rather than petroleum based ones.

Scented products- Scented candles, incense, potpourri... you name it. If it smells, it can cause trouble for some people. Fragrance strips in magazines have received a lot of notoriety lately, since the encapsulated fragrances often break open during shipping.

Smoke- Cigarette smoke, fireplace and wood stove smoke, even food cooked over a grill, have been identified by Feingold members as irritants.

Vehicle exhaust- In high traffic areas, close the car windows and air-intake vents, and adjust the controls to recirculate inside air.

Water for drinking- Madison Plantation spring water is featured by Traditional Provisionals, a mail order business in West Virginia, calling themselves "purveyors of chemical-free food, clean water, and earth-friendly cleaning products." Their catalog includes organically grown meats and produce. For information, call (304) 725-6322.

Water for bathing- Another Feingold adult found that the softened water in her new home caused severe peeling of her skin. When she switched to untreated "hard" water the problem stopped.

This same woman tracked down the cause of severely irritated skin on her hands -- after many doctors were unable to help. She is extremely allergic to corn, and was reacting to the cornstarch routinely used on the inside of rubber gloves.

Resources for the highly chemically-sensitive:

- Chemical Injury Information Network, P.O. Box 301, White Sulphur Springs, MT 59645
- Human Ecology Action League (HEAL), P.O. Box 49126, Atlanta, GA 30359
- National Center for Environmental Health Strategies, 1100 Rural Avenue, Voorhees, NJ 08043

A Closer Look at Some Culprits

New carpeting

Highly sensitive people may be unable to tolerate the chemicals used in new carpeting, although most Feingold members need not be as cautious. There are many powerful chemicals that typically go into the process of manufacturing carpeting. The most potent of these appears to be "4-phenylcyclohexene," or "4-PC" -- the compound which gives new carpets their characteristic smell.

Debra Lynn Dadd, who has written extensively on environmental issues, notes: "While industry claims that animal tests show 4-PC to be harmless, an EPA risk assessment group predicted that it could create nervous system and genetic problems. We also point out the similarity between 4-PC and phencyclidine, which on the street is known as 'angel dust.' A Washington D.C. chemist working on the problem states: 'All in all we have a lot of reason to suspect that 4-PC is a pretty nasty chemical.'"

As the chemicals "gas out" of new carpeting, the smell will fade. In just a few days the residue of fumes will be reduced by about half. If you are planning to have carpeting installed it would be wise to try to allow it to air out as much as possible. Perhaps the retailer could unroll the carpeting the night before it is to be delivered. If it will be installed when the weather is mild, you may be able to keep the windows open. If you are moving to a new home, consider having the carpeting installed well before the move.

More about carpeting

One very sensitive Feingold member found a solution to her search for a new carpet she could tolerate. This is one of those happy stories than can take place in a small town, where folks all know each other. She and her husband went to a friend who owns a furniture store, and asked about the possibility of buying carpeting that had been stored long enough for the chemical fumes to have aired out. To everyone's delight, he found two rolls of carpeting that had been in his warehouse for six years! Both the colors and yardage were perfect, and our member had no reaction.

She wanted to avoid foam padding, so finding one that would not be irritating took a bit more detective work. They were able to locate padding made from compressed rag pieces encased in a plastic mesh. This type of product is generally used in commercial applications. It isn't as plush as foam, but worked out fine.

They also were shopping for furniture, and ended up buying some slightly used furniture from the storeowner's own home. All of the "new furniture smell" was gone.

Another option is to apply a sealant that will form a barrier and block the fumes. AFM Enterprises Inc. offers many products for chemically sensitive people. Their "Carpet Guard" forms a water and odor resistant barrier to carpets.

AFM also sells: cleaning compounds; bacteria, fungi and mildew control products; sealants for grout, tile, concrete, bricks, painted and unpainted surfaces; compounds to be used on metal roofs and heating and air conditioning ducts; waxes and polishes (including shoe polish); carpet shampoo; flooring, wallpaper and carpet adhesive; joint and spackling compounds, caulking and tile grout; polyurethane alternative; lacquer replacement; fire retardant for shingles; sealant to coat vinyl coverings in cars; and various paints, stains, primers, strippers and sealants. Contact AMF Enterprises, Inc., (800) 239-0321.

Cosmetics -- the Feingold Approach

The best approach for the Feingold member is to read labels, test each product individually, and watch for any reaction - physical or behavioral.

A common misconception about the Feingold Program is that it means "100% Natural." People are astonished to learn that our diet does not exclude all synthetic additives, sugar, or convenience food. Similarly, some women believe that following the Feingold Program means they must give up cosmetics. This is another misconception. Cosmetics are complex substances made up of ingredients from both natural and synthetic sources. The synthetic additives in cosmetics pose a problem for chemically sensitive people, as they can be absorbed through the skin; and many products contain added fragrance or chemicals that release fumes. Unlike food additives, we have very little clinical data or experience in dealing with cosmetics. But fortunately, they are required to list their ingredients. The Food & Drug Administration, which has jurisdiction over cosmetics, began requiring ingredient listing in 1976. (Most nations that regulate cosmetics, however, are far stricter than the United States. Many of the components in cosmetics manufactured in this country are not permitted in other countries.)

Regulating cosmetics

We've come a long way since women ate arsenic complexion wafers to poison the hemoglobin in their blood, and thus give themselves a fragile pallor...or have we?

Feingold members are often frustrated by what they perceive to be the FDA's (Food and Drug Administration) reluctance to adequately regulate food additives. But the situation with cosmetics is far worse. "Because cosmetics are not classified as drugs," explained dermatologist Dr. Kenneth Arndt, "no regulatory agency formally tests and certifies products prior to release on the market. Only in the event that a product creates a problem after distribution will it come under scrutiny for possible removal from sale." (*Harvard Medical School Health Letter*, 12/86)

Although the cosmetic companies conduct their own tests, critics contend that a $17 billion a year industry should not be self-regulating. Congressman Ron Wyden of Oregon compared FDA's authority over the industry to "a toothless pit bull guarding a multimillion-dollar mansion." (*The Human Ecologist,* Fall 1989)

Even if cosmetics were required to undergo testing, it would be very difficult to know what type of test to devise. Several thousand chemicals are used in cosmetics, in many combinations. And each person is likely to have his or her own unique sensitivities. Feingold Foodlists contain some cosmetics and other non-food products; we can offer broad guidelines, but members must ultimately depend on trial and error to find the brands they can tolerate.

Certified colors and uncertified colors

The colorings that are used in cosmetics can be divided into two categories: certified and uncertified (or non-certified). Certified colors are the petroleum-based dyes we generally refer to as "synthetic" colors. Feingold members must avoid these.

Their name comes from the fact that the Food & Drug Administration requires that every batch of the dyes be certified. Those that are approved for use in foods, drugs, and cosmetics are listed as "FD&C No. __." Those proceeded by "D&C" are permitted for use only in drugs and cosmetics. Lakes refer to the blend of insoluble materials and certified colors; they should be avoided.

Uncertified colors are permitted to be used without close government supervision. Annatto, caramel and beet powder are examples of uncertified colors derived from a natural source. But uncertified colors can also be synthetically produced. This is the case with iron oxide, which is found in nature, but is undesirable in this form because it can contain contaminants such as arsenic. The iron oxides used in many cosmetics are synthesized in laboratories and yield a purer product. It is a widely used coloring since it can be produced in shades of yellow, orange, red, brown, and black. Other uncertified colors found in cosmetics include titanium dioxide, manganese violet, ultramarine blue bismuth oxychloride, etc.

Dr. Feingold believed that uncertified colors were not likely to cause problems for our members. FDA regulations state that cosmetics which are designed for use in the area of the eye may not contain certified dyes. Another prohibited coloring agent is lampblack or carbon black (which is actually a form of soot) once used in eye makeup. It was found to be a carcinogen and has been banned. Today, mascara, eyeliner, and eyebrow pencil rely on iron oxide as their primary color source.

Eye shadow made with only uncertified colors is readily available, but select brands that do not contain BHT. Foundation, face powders, rouge, and blusher may use either certified or uncertified colorings, or a combination of the two. Look for labels which do not contain: "FD&C," "D&C," or "Lakes."

Fingernail polish

Nail polish is tolerated by some Feingold women. The synthetic dyes used are less likely to cause problems than the fumes released. Nail polish remover contains many irritants. The chemically sensitive person should limit her exposure to this as much as possible and use it only in a well ventilated area - or better yet, use it outdoors.

"Fragrance-free"

When a cosmetic advertises it is "hypoallergenic," "natural," and "allergy-tested" it is certainly worth investigating, but such terms are no guarantee. Generally they mean that the product is fragrance-free. (*FDA Consumer,* 11/86) But here's another problem. Even "fragrance-free" and "unscented" don't have to mean what they say. Since some of the chemicals used in cosmetics smell bad, small amounts of "masking fragrances" are added to disguise the odor. For example, castor oil is generally used in lipstick; and since it is found right under your nose, perfume is blended in.

Lipstick - real lipstick!

Of all the types of cosmetics in use, a suitable lipstick had been the most difficult for the Feingold member to locate. Now there are several brands made from natural pigments, and offering lovely vibrant colors. They look and function as any other lipstick; in fact you may have to check the label carefully to tell them apart from your traditional synthetically dyed lipsticks.

If you live near a well-stocked health food store, you may be able to choose your cosmetics there. But look carefully at the ingredients; some lipsticks sold in health food stores, which claim to be natural, are colored with the very synthetic dyes we avoid.

More than just a pretty face

There are some very practical reasons for using lipstick; it does more than enhance appearance. Unlike other parts of the body, lips do not have a protective outer layer of dead cells to help retain moisture. They contain no glands to supply oil, and have little melanin -- the substance that gives skin its color. Lips appear to be reddish because the tissue is so thin it is possible to see the underlying blood vessels.

Most Feingold members are able to tolerate Vaseline, despite the fact that it is petroleum jelly, and petroleum is a notorious offender for the chemically sensitive person.

The beauty business

Consumers aren't the only victims of the powerful chemicals used in cosmetics. Professionals who work with these compounds on a daily basis can experience severe reactions, and the professional may have even less information to go on than the consumer. Retail products must carry an ingredient label, but those that are sold to beauticians are not required to contain any ingredient listing.

Women no longer eat arsenic, and rouge no longer contains lead and mercury, but modern abuses can be found. The publication, *Emergency Medicine,* reported that a child was poisoned from drinking Super Nail Glue Off, a solvent for removing artificial nails. The manufacturer added purple dye and grape scent, along with the toxic chemical acetonitrile. To a child, it looks and smells like grape soda.

Feingold survival skills at the cosmetic counter

Actually, the Feingolder is well advised to steer clear of the cosmetic section of most stores, as it's generally located beside the perfume counter. They are not easy to avoid since stores love to place their perfumes -- a high-profit item -- at the main entrance.

When you shop for cosmetics, or anything that is applied to the skin, remember that much of what goes on your skin will be absorbed into your body. When you're new to the Program, avoid scents of all types if at all possible -- even ones that smell good. Later on you can test them out...if you're brave.

Paint

Fumes from paint (especially oil-based paints) can be very irritating for the chemically sensitive person.

For some individuals, these chemicals appear to be capable of causing violent behavior. Researchers at the Karolinska Institute in Sweden found a much higher incidence of violent crimes among prisoners who had earned their living working as house painters, car spray painters, and who were exposed to glues used in installing vinyl floors.

One New Hampshire firm has found a way to combine the advantages of oil-based paint with those of latex. Researchers at Micro Vesicular Systems, Inc. have developed a technique for encapsulating microscopic droplets of oil paint inside tiny sacs, suspended in water. When the water evaporates, the sacs break, leaving a smooth coat of pigment. Unlike traditional oil paint, this does not produce volatile fumes.

Solutions

"Our family has recently moved to a new house and need to paint my son's drab room. But he's extremely sensitive to environmental chemicals (not to mention food additives!) and I would like to find a brand of paint he will be able to tolerate. We are planning to paint in the spring so the room can be aired out before he moves back into it. He will be staying in another room while the work is going on, and I will keep the door of the painted room closed. Do you have any other suggestions?"

For the average Feingold member, these precautions would probably be enough; for the very sensitive person, however, avoiding a reaction can be far more difficult. The most obvious problem posed by paint is the odor it gives off when it is still wet. But there are other concerns for the highly sensitive.

Organizations such as the Human Ecology Action League (H.E.A.L.) offer this advice on dealing with paint. Long after paint has dried it "out-gases," that is, it releases fumes that may not be noticeable to most people, but can cause a reaction in the sensitive. After the paint has dried to the touch, closing off the room and circulating the air, by opening windows and/or using a portable fan, will hasten this process. (Don't use a central house fan, as it could circulate the fumes throughout the house.) It will probably take a few weeks before the process is fully complete. The ideal weather conditions for this are warm, dry air.

Chemically sensitive people try to make a paint job last as long as possible, so it's a good idea to have the wall as smooth and clean as you can before you begin to paint.

If you can, limit the painting to one coat, it will dry and cure more quickly. Paint with a high percentage of pigment content will probably cover the surface in one coat. Look for this information on the paint label.

Oil-based paints have a strong smell when they are being used, and require solvents for cleaning brushes. But once they are completely dry, they are not irritating and they are very durable. Latex paints are easy to use and not much affected by weather conditions, but they do contain preservatives (biocides, mold retardants, fungicides).

The Negley Paint Company offers low biocide/fungicide paint. Their address is box 47848, San Antonio, TX 78265.

Eco Design Company's Livos Non-toxic interior wall paint is an alternative to standard water-based house paints that may contain mercury and other toxic chemicals. They also offer non-toxic thinners, varnishes, shellac, adhesives, waxes, etc. To receive a catalog, call 1-800-621-2591, extension 103, or write to: EcoDesign Co., 1365 Rufina Circle, Santa Fe, NM 87505.

Sinan Company offers many types of paints, including children's art materials. They also sell plant-based cleaners, floor care products and polishes, wood primers, glazes and waxes. Sinan Co. at P.O. Box 857, Davis, CA 95617-0857; (916) 753-3104.

Major companies are responding to consumer's wishes

Benjamin Moore has a line called Pristine, and Glidden has its Spred 2000; both are free of the petroleum-based solvents that are such irritants for sensitive people. Sherwin Williams Dutch Boy Kid's Room paint contains fewer troublesome chemicals than typical paints. It has a latex base, and is free of lead and mercury.

Perfume! What is This Stuff?

It is a blend of as many as several hundred natural and synthetic chemicals, in an alcohol base. It is also a potential neurotoxin.

Synthetic ingredients are playing a larger and larger role in the manufacture of perfumes since the natural components can cost 1,000 times as much. Sensitive people can react adversely to natural oils in perfumes, but the synthetic components appear to be the most damaging.

One of the most disturbing developments in the manufacture of fragrances is the increase in the use of synthetic musks. Research conducted in the 1980s showed that a synthetic chemical called musk ambrette caused nervous system damage, weight loss and muscular atrophy in test animals.* According to a report by the Human Ecology

Action League, other chemicals which were tested yielded the following effects:

- Cyclohexanol - inhibition of motor activity, spasms, death, irritation of the upper respiratory tract and a narcotic effect when inhaled.
- Linalool - respiratory disturbances leading to death, narcotic effects.
- Methyl ethyl ketone - high concentrations caused unconsciousness, emphysema, congestion of liver and kidneys. In humans, this chemical caused marked eye, nose, or throat irritation, and numbness of fingers and arms.
- Eugenol - signs of intoxication.
- Musk ketone - deterioration of the liver.

Musk AETT- When it was shown in 1977 that this chemical caused permanent brain damage in test animals, the fragrance industry voluntarily stopped using it. Between 1955 and 1976 it was widely used as an ingredient in fragrances and as a masking fragrance in "unscented" products. Further research showed that when musk AETT was applied to the skin of animals it caused deterioration of the brain, spinal cord, and nerves. The initial reaction of the animals was hyperactivity, irritability, and a tendency to bite. This progressed to limb weakness, discoloration of internal organs and the nervous system, and degeneration of central nervous system neurons.

Although the industry has chosen to discontinue using musk AETT, it could still be legally used in fragrances since the Food and Drug Administration has not taken action to regulate it. While the FDA acknowledges that there are more and more reports of people reacting to fragrances, and the reactions may involve both the immune system and the nervous system, it considers the number of people affected to be very small.

*Spencer, Peter S, & Bischoff, Monica C. "Skin as a route of entry for neurotoxic substances". In *Dermatoxicology*, Francis N. Marzulli & Howard K. Mailback (eds.)(1984)(3rd ed.)(pp. 629-630). Washington, DC. quoted by Karen I. N. Stevens, in *The Human Ecologist*, Fall, 1990. To subscribe to the Human Ecologist, contact HEAL at P.O. Box 49126, Atlanta, GA 30359 (404) 248-1898.

Fragrances: who's in charge?

If you're sensitive to fragrances, you may have wondered about the regulations that govern their manufacture and use. In practice, there really aren't any.

The Food and Drug Administration is responsible for fragrances used in perfumes and personal care products, but manufacturers are not required to obtain FDA approval before using any such chemical additive in non-food products. (The exception is synthetic coloring, which is regulated.) Writing in *The Human Ecologist*, Louise Kosta notes, "Since cosmetic manufacturers are not required to clear fragrance ingredients prior to product sale, they do not. Extensive research on fragrance materials has been done by the industry, but, like fragrance formulas, this information is proprietary.

"Moreover, reports of adverse effects received by fragrance manufacturers from consumers need not be reported to FDA. Their participation in FDA's 'passive surveillance system,' which monitors cosmetics' adverse reactions, is strictly voluntary."

A Feingold mom writes:

"My seven year old daughter, Kathy, has a very devoted five year old boyfriend. Through this year I've been driven to eliminate more and more foods from her diet on the premise that Kathy is allergic to many otherwise permitted natural foods. Her seesaw behavior had me frantic. I was able to trace some reactions to cheating in school, but there were others I could not trace to food.

"Finally I decided she was allergic to five year old Wally! (He's a charmer, therefore his behavior was not the cause.) What I saw was that she was an uncontrollable stinker after playing with Wally. Anyway, one day I walked into the room they were playing in and was overwhelmed by the aroma! I asked Wally if he had aftershave lotion on. Wally, batting his doe eyes at me and a Mona Lisa grin on his face, coyly answered, 'Yest. My brothers get me ALL dressed up when I come to see my Kathy...and they get me to smell pretty.' I opened the windows wide. Then I threw Wally out (out the door, not the window) telling him Kathy was allergic to aftershave lotions, etc. He couldn't play with Kathy for 24 hours, until he bathed, and never when he uses any pretty smells. Things have quieted down in our house, as long as I do a sniff test on Wally before they play together."

OTHER PROBLEMS FROM FOOD ADDITIVES AND SALICYLATES

Dr. Feingold often said, "Food additives and salicylates can affect every system of the body." For more than two decades, volunteers have seen that he was right.

When Dr. Feingold presented his findings to the American Medical Association in 1973 he described an impressive track record of helping children who he referred to as "the failures of the medical community." Dr. Feingold's credentials were also impressive, and his techniques followed the best medical procedures: treat patients on the clinical level, gather information on successful techniques, and relate this to probable causes, using information found in respected medical journals. Since he was a clinician, it was his role to help a patient become well. The job of determining *why* a clinical technique works is the realm of the academician, or researcher. Dr. Feingold called upon his colleagues to begin the complex task of understanding what happens on the molecular level when a synthetically colored or flavored food enters a child's body, and why the result is often profoundly disturbed behavior or inability to focus. Very little has been carried out in this important area; there has never been a study of the Feingold Program as it is actually used.

Dr. Feingold called upon another group. He asked parent volunteers to provide the information and support which enables a family to find suitable food and test the program.

Most of the focus is on helping children with learning or behavior problems, but over the years we have received many reports of other family members experiencing unexpected benefits. The longer the Association has carried out our work, the more diverse the reports of other conditions responding to the Program. Dr. Feingold often told us that "any system of the body" can be affected by the additives we eliminate, but it still took us by surprise each time we learned of another condition which was helped.

While the research Dr. Feingold called for has not been carried out, work in related fields sheds some light on how symptoms that seem very different are interrelated.

Researchers at MIT have shown that nutrients in food can alter the functioning of the brain. Other researchers have demonstrated the effects that food dyes have on the brains of both animals and humans. Researchers and consumers report a wide range of negative effects from other additives, notably MSG and aspartame. Presumably, these additives also affect the chemistry of the brain.

Parents of "ADD" children often hear reference to neurotransmitters; these are chemical messengers that enable nerve cells to communicate with each other. The three neurotransmitters which are repeatedly associated with ADD are: serotonin, dopamine and norepinephrine.

Serotonin is called an inhibitor. It prevents us from doing things that are inappropriate or dangerous. In his book, *Tourette Syndrome and Human Behavior*, Dr. David Comings states, "Low levels of brain serotonin are associated with aggression, depression, violent suicide, alcoholism, arson, borderline personality, bulimia, and other impulsive behaviors. Low brain serotonin may also cause panic attacks." The Food and Drug Administration connects serotonin with migraine headaches, "Working with other chemicals, serotonin regulates blood vessel constriction and dilation. It can both sharpen and deaden pain." (*FDA Consumer*, Sept. 1992).

Another area where serotonin seems to play an important part is obsessive compulsive disorder, or OCD, when a person feels compelled to repeat an action over and over, and feels very anxious when they do not. Researchers at Brown University and Yale have found that drugs that increase serotonin can help OCD sufferers. "When utilized by the brain's neurotransmitters at normal levels, serotonin is believed to impart a feeling of certainty, so that people don't experience excessive doubt about what they think and do. If his serotonin level is out of whack, an individual may have no confidence in his decisions or actions, leading him to repeat actions over and over." (*Brown Alumni Monthly*, Dec. 1988).

The neurotransmitter, dopamine, is involved in the control of muscle movements, and may play a part in such disorders as Parkinson's disease and Tourette syndrome. The third important chemical, norepinephrine, is formed from dopamine, and helps regulate dopamine.

Considering how vulnerable the brain is to chemicals, it's no wonder the Program helps so many symptoms.

As the director of the Tourette Syndrome Clinic at the City of Hope National Medical Center, Dr. Comings has collected a wealth of information on symptoms which may be related to Tourette syndrome. They include: hyperactivity, ADD, dyslexia, obsessive-compulsive behaviors, conduct disorders, depression, mood swings, irritability, migraine headaches, short temper, anxiety, panic attacks, phobias, speech problems, sleep problems, addictive behaviors like alcoholism and eating disorders.

Comings has found that the Tourette patient is far more likely to have one or more of these symptoms. Apparently they are more closely related than they may seem at first glance. It would follow, then, that a technique which can help one of these problems (such as hyperactivity) might also alleviate depression or headaches, etc. in some individuals.

Because the Feingold Program asks the entire family to use the same foods, we hear of other problems that have responded to the change. Dad's headaches disappear, Mom is no longer troubled by PMS, and older sister isn't so distracted. The separate pieces of the puzzle begin to fit when you consider that foods and additives can affect brain chemistry, and that altered brain chemistry can result in a wide variety of symptoms.

Childhood Arthritis

I just wanted to let you know how thankful my family is for this diet, the work that goes into preparing the Foodlist information, etc. Thanks especially to Dr. Feingold and my neighbor who told me about the diet.

I have three children, ages 6, 5, and 3 years old. They have always been sick children, but my 5-year-old son was especially sick. Ever since Michael was 6 months old he would wake up crying, and there was nothing we could do except hold him.

At one year old, Michael would try to stand up after he had been sitting; but he would hold his leg and fall down, crying. We took him to a doctor to get an X-ray, thinking he might have broken or sprained his leg at some time. They said there was nothing wrong.

From then on the aches in his legs got worse, waking him up at night, screaming and holding his legs. Only aspirin and massaging his legs would put him to sleep. He also started having bronchitis and pneumonia or croup twice a month. One time when both the croup and leg aches were especially bad the doctors put him in the hospital. They ran tests for everything, including leukemia, cancer, and they ended up telling me that they thought it was all in his head and that he just wanted me to come into his room at night!

Well, this continued, and we changed doctors, and Michael was tested for everything again. By this time Michael was getting sick every time he got off the antibiotic. The doctors said to give him 3 to 4 baby aspirin every night for the leg and arm aches.

On Michael's 4th birthday -- one hour before his party -- his neck became stiff and he could not move it at all without screaming. We took him to the emergency room and the doctors said they could not find anything. Eventually the aches spread to his elbows, fingers and feet. He started to have swelling in his joints. It was so bad when he woke up in the mornings he could not walk and had to be carried.

The doctors diagnosed this as rheumatoid arthritis, and ran tests for it. The tests came back negative, but they said that in a young child it was often common to have negative results and still have arthritis. We were told that all we could do was to increase the aspirin to 3 or 4 in the morning and at night.

Michael became sicker, and became so sore it was painful to have anyone touch him. The huge bruises he got made it even more impossible to dress him. The pneumonia and bronchitis became more severe; and he had nosebleeds that were so bad, one day he hemorrhaged and we had to have his nose cauterized.

At our insistence, the doctors finally agreed to send Michael to a specialist at Johns Hopkins University, and at the same time they told us to put Michael on the Feingold diet because he was becoming hyperactive too. Well, to our complete surprise, the diet helped immediately. We discovered he is allergic to aspirin, and it was causing his coughing seizures. When we stopped the aspirin, the coughing stopped. We eliminated all other 'not safe things' and the leg aches stopped. It was one miracle after another and our children (whose illnesses had us to the doctors on the average of twice a week) have not been sick since April 28, 1980 -- the day we began the Feingold diet.

The only time Michael's leg hurts is when he goes off the diet. My daughter bedwets when she goes off the diet. One month later we were well into the diet when the day come for us to keep our appointment at Johns Hopkins. The doctor there examined Michael and told us he was a specimen of good health. By then we knew the doctor was not going to find anything wrong because we had already found the problem!

Our relatives and friends are amazed at how well our children are. For the first time in three years Michael is off aspirin, with no pain. Now I speak with my doctor only when he calls to check on how Michael is doing. (He's amazed!)

Needless to say, Michael's behavior has improved a lot. We had tried to encourage him to dress himself, but even at age 5 he found the whole thing too frustrating. He wouldn't even try to undress himself. We couldn't interest him in washing himself when he was in the tub. Two weeks after we began the diet he proudly announced that he had given himself a shampoo; and he now dresses himself with ease.

Asthma

Among the potential triggers for asthmatic attacks, the American Lung Association lists: food additives, azo dyes [the synthetic dyes eliminated by the Feingold Program] and benzoate preservatives [i.e., sodium benzoate].

The Food and Drug Administration has long required that Yellow No. 5 be listed by name on ingredient labels. This is due, in part, to their recognition of the danger the dye can pose for asthmatics.

More children affected

The incidence of asthma has risen drastically in recent years, particularly in children. Approximately ten million Americans suffer from asthma, and of that number, more than three million are children under the age of 18. In just four years between 1982 and 1986, the number of affected children grew by 25 per cent. Not only has the disorder become more common among children, it has increased in severity, particularly among black children living in inner cities. In 1987 the asthma death rate in East Harlem was almost ten times the national average. (Reported in the *New York Times Magazine*)

Deaths from asthma have doubled in the past decade. Since 1989 is the last year for which figures have been compiled, this toll could be far higher today.

Asthma disables children more frequently than any other condition, according to Miles Weinberger, professor of pediatrics at the University of Iowa College of Medicine. He notes that more than ten percent of all children now have, or have had, asthma and the greatest increase in hospital admissions for asthma is among 1- to 5-year-olds.

The rate of children being hospitalized doubled between 1970 and 1978, but innovations in medical treatment do not appear to have kept pace with the growing problem. In 1979 death from asthma for each 100,000 children ages 5-14 was placed at 0.1, but by 1985 that number tripled to 0.3 deaths. In people ages 15-24 the increase doubled from 0.2 to 0.4 deaths per 100,000.

A child who is exposed to second-hand cigarette smoke is at greater risk for developing asthma, and this is a particular problem if the mother or primary caregiver is the smoker. According to the Allergy Information Association of Canada, even the unborn child of a smoker may be harmed because a reduction of oxygen available to her can affect the oxygen supply for the fetus.

Asthma and allergy

Dr. Benjamin Burrows, a researcher at the University of Arizona College of Medicine, conducted a study of 2657 people and concluded that all types of asthma are allergy-related. His findings challenged the long-held belief that there were allergic and non-allergic types of asthma. It was reported in the *New England Journal of Medicine,* March 1, 1989.

Although statistics lend themselves to various interpretations, professionals who work in this field are clearly alarmed, and the problem is being reported by other countries as well.

Canada's Centre for Disease Control reports similar troubling statistics. Among people between ages 15 and 34, there has been a 163% increase in asthma-related deaths. They also note the greatest increase has been in deaths among asthmatic women. Canadian epidemiologist, Dr. Donald Wigle, suggested that "environmental factors such as food additives or air-tight office buildings containing irritating pollutants may be increasing the rate of fatal asthma attacks." [Note: an epidemiologist is a scientist who uses statistics to identify potential causes for health problems.]

The British medical journal, *Lancet,* noted a startling increase in asthma among that country's school children. Between the 1940s and 1980s the number of asthmatic children tripled. The *Lancet* reported: "Environmental agents -- including traffic jams, industrial and domestic pollutants, ventilation plants, tobacco smoke, natural allergens and food additives -- can help to provoke bronchial hyper-reactivity and so provide the background conditions for the development of asthma."

Other suggested triggers

An often-mentioned trigger for asthmatic attacks is sulfur dioxide *(Journal of Allergy & Clinical Immunology* 1985;76;40-45) and the various sulfur-based preservatives. Sulfites have been used not only in salad bars, wines, and some convenience foods, but have been added to medicine for asthmatics.

Research at the Royal North Shore Hospital in Sydney, Australia points to MSG (monosodium glutamate) as a potential trigger.

Dust mites, animal dander and cigarette smoke can be even more potent irritants if they are found in air tight homes, schools or offices.

A few years ago the *New England Journal of Medicine* described artificial flavoring in toothpaste as a potential cause of bronchospasms in some asthmatics. [In addition to artificial flavoring, toothpaste typically contains dye and saccharine, both petroleum derivatives which Feingold members report as triggers for asthmatic attacks.]

FDA cautions asthmatics

The Food and Drug Administration lists many different potential triggers for asthmatic attacks. These include exercise, respiratory tract infections, a wide range of environmental irritants, both at home and in the workplace, as well as certain drugs and food additives.

The list of intrinsic asthma "triggers" goes on and on, including aspirin and other anti-inflammatory drugs such as ibuprofen (Motrin, Advil, Nuprin) and indomethacin (Indocin), and the food and drug coloring tartrazine yellow (FD&C Yellow No. 5). FDA requires that this dye be listed on the ingredient labeling of all foods and those drugs taken internally in which it is used, to alert the 47,000 to 94,000 asthmatics the agency estimates may be sensitive to it.

FDA is also concerned about the group of chemicals known as sulfiting agents that can cause serious problems for an estimated 5 percent of all asthma sufferers (*FDA Consumer*: Jan. 1995), and as many as two-thirds of asthmatic children (*The Harvard Medical School Health Letter*).

Finally, the following dyes used in medicines were noted by the American Academy of Pediatrics Committee on Drugs as being bronchoconstrictors:

Red No. 2
Red No. 3
Red No. 4
Yellow No. 6
Blue No. 1
Blue No. 2

[*Pediatrics,* October 1985]

Editor's note: When a dye, such as Red No. 2 or Red No. 4, is banned from use in foods, that does not necessarily restrict its use in medicines.

Asthma medication can backfire

There appears to be a growing concern that the use of bronchodilators actually poses a serious threat for asthmatics. When the medicine is inhaled, relief can be fast, giving the impression that the crisis is past and lulling the asthmatic into the belief that he can remain where he is. The medicine opens the airways, exposing the already sensitive lungs to even more of the irritant.

Women at high risk

A study presented at the 1990 World Conference on Lung Health questioned the connection between the practice of prescribing sedatives and tranquilizers, sometimes in combination with antihistamines, and the increase in deaths from asthma. The Public Citizen Health Research Group reported that women are twice as likely to be given prescriptions for these additional drugs than men, and their death from asthma has increased twice as fast.

Like many other childhood afflictions where the cause is not understood, parents seeking help may find themselves blamed for their child's problem. Incredibly, a past president of the College of Allergists was quoted in the early sixties as saying, “One of the commonest types of juvenile asthma is caused by an overprotective, domineering mother...the best treatment is a ‘parentectomy’ -- separating the child from his mother.” *(Allergy Quarterly)*

Althea’s story

In the literature, an increasing number of articles are being published about asthma; they indicate through scientific study that the incidence and mortality rates of asthma are increasing at an alarming rate. The medical community has not identified why this is happening.

The medications and technologies are also growing in number, complexity and cost in an effort to relieve this life-threatening and debilitating condition. Many times the patient has to look beyond accepted medical treatment and find what works for him.

During my early Feingold years, I worked as a nurse practitioner in a large Southern California HMO’s Walking Well Clinic. In my department we were encouraged to develop a limited practice of patients whose stable medical problems needed only monitoring. Althea fit into this category and came in regularly for general check-ups, blood pressure control and asthma management.

The asthma had plagued her since childhood and was by far, her most serious problem. In the early 1950s when Althea was a young married with two small children, she was told to move away from the East Coast if she wanted to see her children grow up.

In the early 1950s asthma was, in general, a mystery to the medical community. The treatment for asthma and its severe complications required a long, arduous recovery.

As I got to know Althea, I developed a real respect for this no-nonsense lady who had learned to live with her debilitating condition. She used many medications and adapted to the many limitations the asthma placed on her lifestyle.

On smoggy days Althea stayed home in her air-conditioned house, venturing out only in the cool mornings. The in-house confinement lasted from February to July; it greatly hampered this baseball-lover's trips to Angels or Dodgers Stadiums where she dearly loved to go and cheer her favorite team. When a really important game was scheduled, Althea would take her pills, puff her pipe (as she called the inhaler) and attend the game anyway, often paying the price with an acute asthma episode.

Althea came into our clinic from time to time with acute bronchitis. She required antibiotics, refills for her inhalers and medications, but had a demeanor that said, "Let me out of here, I'll be just fine." She had managed her asthma most of her life, and since she recovered successfully from acute episodes the physician/mentor I worked with did not question her judgement and self-care. On one of her regular appointments Althea came in, sank into the chair and declared her frequent headaches had become more severe and were now constant, and I was to fix it. She admitted to having headaches for years, but never mentioned them before because she hated taking more pills and there was nothing we could do about them anyway. Her face was pale with dark puffy circles under the eyes. Her usual sparkle was gone. She was wheezing more than usual and her blood pressure was mildly elevated. The clinical picture she presented was of allergic response.

In those days my Feingold energies and information were focused on children, but I was aware of the food allergy-headache relationship, and started Althea on a testing program for wheat, milk, eggs, chocolate and nuts. The foods were tested one at a time, and when she tested nuts, the different varieties were introduced one at a time.

On Althea's follow-up appointment she still had constant headaches and was discouraged with her detective work, reporting no response to any of the categories of food. The one exception was a definite increase in symptoms when she ate almonds, which she did almost daily. Almonds...salicylates...it rang my Feingold bell! Trying (unsuccessfully) to contain my excitement, I explained the implication of her detective work and gave her the information on the Feingold Program.

Althea was very serious about feeling better and implemented the necessary changes in her diet so successfully that by using the diet, along with a change in medication she became headache-free within a short time.

The other benefit for Althea was a dramatic improvement in her asthma. Whenever she let the diet slip, her headaches returned and the asthma worsened. Encouraged by the improvement, she identified other offenders and further refined her eating and life-style. Althea continued to improve her health and quality of life. Within a few months she was so delighted by her new freedom from symptoms, this gutsy lady took a 6,000 mile automobile tour of the United States. Even more remarkable, the trip took place during the months of May and June, when she previously would have been locked in her air-conditioned house.

All along the planned route, friends and relatives had a doctor standing by for the medical emergency (Althea) that was expected to pull into their driveway. Except for puffing on her pipe in humid Texas and Florida, the trip was a healthy, grand success that would have been impossible in the pre-Feingold days just a few months earlier.

Many years of asthma took their toll on Althea's lungs, and she ultimately moved out of the Los Angeles smog to the clearer air of the Arizona desert. She lives an active semi-retired life that includes a data entry job she works at out of her home. The only asthma medicine she needs is her pipe as long as she follows her diet.

The scientific work continues, in an effort to identify causes and find better treatments for asthma. If you are suffering from this difficult condition, or watching your child's life being disrupted, while you wait for a medical breakthrough, you may be losing valuable time and the opportunity for a better quality of life.

Colleen Smethers, R.N.

Autism - the Invisible Prison

Can the Feingold Program help an autistic child? Volunteers are cautious not to offer false hope, but some parents report a significant reduction of their child's autistic symptoms.

The autistic child doesn't interact normally with other people, and may even be unable to relate to his parents. Development is slow in many areas, including speech, comprehension, and social skills. An autistic child may behave in bizarre ways as a result of a need to obsessively repeat behaviors or an extraordinary sensitivity to stimuli such as noise or lights. This condition is estimated by the National Institutes of Health to occur in about five out of every 10,000 births and affects boys four times as often as girls.

Some children exhibit autistic symptoms to a lesser degree and may be labeled as "autistic-like." The child who has been diagnosed as hyperactive or ADD may have some autistic characteristics. (Parents of chemically sensitive children often report they have an unusual sensitivity to noise, light, or touch.)

Autistic children often have obsessive/compulsive traits. This all seems to indicate that rather than being separate conditions, these various behavior disorders may be related, at least in some children.

Background

In the 1940s many doctors believed that autism was the result of a cold, rejecting mother and the diagnosis was considered a life sentence. Within the past few years these ideas have been challenged, and significant contributions to the understanding of autism are coming from parents and from the affected children.

Mary Callahan's book, *Fighting for Tony,* is an account of her successful struggle to deal with her son's devastating condition. Mary, who is a nurse, discovered that Tony's autistic behavior was due solely to a severe milk allergy.

Judy Barron and her son, Sean, co-authored the book, *There's a Boy in Here*. (This book and Mary Callahan's are both published by Simon & Schuster.) Judy used a different approach. She persistently refused to allow Sean to divorce himself from reality. It took years of effort on Judy's part, and at age 16 Sean began to leave his autistic isolation.

Son Rise

Barry Neil Kaufman has dramatically related this approach in his book about his child, *Son Rise*, and his second, *A Miracle to Believe In.* The newest book, *Son Rise – the Miracle Continues*, incorporates his original work, plus greater detail of the program that transformed his profoundly autistic son, Raun. Suzi and Barry Kaufman rejected the advice of an impressive array of "experts" who foretold a dismal outlook for their toddler.

Rather than extinguish their son's behaviors, the Kaufmans joined him -- with relish and enthusiasm. They were rewarded with an insight into the world of the autistic child, and gained an understanding of, and respect for, why the child behaves as he does.

By entering into Raun's world they were able to design approaches to invite him into theirs. Their success is no less than dazzling. Today Raun is a bright, articulate young man who has recently graduated from a competitive college with an impressive academic record, and a zest for life. Even as a child, his gentle wisdom surprised those around him, and often educated the adults who had sought to teach him.

The Kaufmans followed their hearts, first in their work with Raun, and later in the establishment of a pastoral retreat where one can challenge not only the limitations of autism, but of life itself. This philosophy teaches that an event is negative only if we perceive it as such; they believe Raun's autism was an opportunity, not a tragedy.

The author writes, "Instead of trying to discourage what others judged as our son's weird and inappropriate behaviors, we joined him lovingly and respectfully, jumping fully into his bizarre, unpredictable, and fantastic world. Unexpectedly, what began as a journey to find our son became a journey in which we found ourselves." Kaufman describes this philosophy in detail in his book, *Happiness is a Choice*.

Feingold parents will see many familiar experiences in this book. Following one of a number of professional evaluations he writes, "After the evaluations, we were left with ample diagnoses and test scores -- but no help."

The Kaufman's retreat, called the Option Institute, is located at 2080 South Undermountain Road, Sheffield, MA (413) 229-2100.

Allergy

In an address to the Feingold Association, Dr. C. Kotsanis an otolaryngologist and allergist, pointed out that allergy is defined as a "hyperactivity of the immune system." Your immune system evaluates every substance that comes into your body; this includes pollen, foods, synthetic chemicals, etc. Those things perceived as harmful are attacked by the white blood cells. The white cells then release histamines, which can cause various unwanted side effects.

Digestion

After food has entered the stomach it must be digested, or broken down into small particles. Bacteria and enzymes digest the food and prepare it for absorption into the bloodstream by way of little finger-like projections in the intestines. When the intestines are healthy, a layer of mucus -- or "mucosa" -- which lines it, keeps undigested food inside. But when the intestines have been damaged by things such as parasites, abnormal bacteria, fungi, or overuse of antibiotics, the mucosa can't effectively seal in the contents, and particles of undigested food can escape into the bloodstream.

If food leaves the intestines before it is completely digested, it will be identified by the white blood cells as the "enemy" and the cells will then try to destroy it.

Nutrition

Dr. Kotsanis emphasized that in order for the body to work as it should, all of the systems need to be given the necessary raw materials in the form of nutrients from healthful food. The brain needs these nutrients to create chemical neurotransmitters, which affect our behavior and ability to think. These same nutrients enable our immune system to function well, and allow cells to be created and repaired. In other words, the foods we eat are the ingredients for our body's chemistry -- they create us and determine how well we function.

He described an in-depth study he and his staff conducted with autistic children, in which he measured many different factors. Dr. Kotsanis found that every one of the autistic children was sensitive to food dyes, some foods, and molds. Most of them had abnormal flora in their digestive system, and most had an overgrowth of yeast. More than half had evidence of parasites. The diets of all of the youngsters were very deficient in vitamins and minerals -- falling well below the RDA in most cases.

A look at the foods these autistic children ingested was of particular interest to Feingold families. If you analyzed their dietary intake on the basis of calories, percentage of carbohydrates, etc., it looked fine. But a closer look showed a diet of highly processed/junk foods. For most children, their only vegetable was French fries! Even those children who ate better food had trouble with digestion, leading to deficiencies. The first approach Dr. Kotsanis took was to have the families of the autistic children eliminate food dyes; this is the advice he routinely gives to parents of ADD children as well. Then, the various deficiencies that had been identified were treated. Only after these problems had been addressed did the auditory training begin.

Auditory enhancement training

Many children with autistic symptoms are extremely sensitive to sound. They may hear sounds that are not normally detected by the average person, or may experience pain from what we consider to be normal noise levels. The simple technique of auditory enhancement training proved to be very effective for all of the children in the study. The child hears a filtered, special sound through headphones; the session lasts about 30 minutes, and is given twice a day for ten days. With this combination of nutrition and auditory training, Dr. Kotsanis was able to achieve a better than 70% correction rate, with all of the children benefiting to some degree.

Sound of a Miracle, by Annabel Stehli, describes a technique that helps the autistic person who is extraordinarily sensitive to certain sounds. Her new book, *Dancing in the Rain*, is a collection of stories by parents of children who have benefited from auditory integration training. It is available from the Georgiana Institute.

Many doctors, including C.A. Kotsanis, M.D practice this therapy. He believes that autism is a form of a learning disorder, and differs from ADD (attention deficit disorder) primarily in degree.

Of all the children he works with, Dr. Kotsanis considers autistic youngsters to be the most difficult, but he reports excellent results over the past several years with a multi-faceted treatment program combining allergy, nutrition, and auditory training.

Contact the nonprofit Georgiana Institute for the name of a qualified professional in your area. Phone (860) 355-1545 or e-mail georgianainstitute@snet.net; www.georgianainstitute.org.

The autistic child sees the world differently

The National Academy for Child Development helps autistic children by identifying which of the senses are operating incorrectly and developing therapy to accommodate this.

When an individual has an extreme sensitivity to noise, light, touch, etc., he will adjust his behavior to avoid the discomfort this sensitivity can bring. If you have a severe headache you will behave differently and will be far more sensitive to noise that when you feel well. Your sense of touch is different when your skin has been sunburned.

The National Academy for Child Development (NACD) believes that the child who displays "autistic" behavior is often one who has experienced an injury to one or more portions of the brain. (The term "injury" is used in a broad sense, and does not necessarily refer to a blow to the head.)

When a child is "hypo-auditory" or extremely sensitive to sound, the NACD states, "He is bombarded with sound. As we attempt to talk to such a child, he not only is hearing our distorted voices, but a buzz from the fluorescent light overhead, the conversation in the next room and the traffic outside. The greater the quantity and volume, the more difficult the interpretation. Depending upon the degree of the problem, such children will act confused, increase their activity level and degree of disorientation as the volume increases, or simply, turn off auditorially just to survive."

Hypo-central vision and hyper-peripheral vision

Many autistic children avoid direct eye contact and see things "out of the corner of their eye" rather than looking directly at objects. The child with "hypo-central" vision does not see well by looking straight at something. And the term "hyper-peripheral vision" refers to the ability to see well with peripheral vision, to see objects when one is not looking directly at them.

Treatment

The treatment program developed by the NACD would be tailored to the child's area of brain dysfunction. In addition to a variety of approaches, they stress the importance of nutrition and have long supported Dr. Feingold's work.

A child who has extreme sensitivity to noise, plus vision distortion, would spend much of his day in an environment designed to compensate for these sensory dysfunctions. He would use earphones so that only one sound is heard, and background noises eliminated. The room designed for such a child is dark so peripheral vision would not be used. In this room (called a "blacklight room"), the only colors that are visible are white or fluorescent. The child's central vision is stimulated by using fluorescent toys. According to the NACD, many "autistic" children respond immediately to this new, non-threatening environment.

The parent's role

The NACD believes that parents are the child's best teachers. The programs are designed to be taught to parents, who then use them in their own home. Experienced coaches meet with the families on a regular basis to assess the child's progress and offer additional recommendations.

The Academy treats children with a variety of problems, and believes its program can also enhance the lives of "normal" or "gifted" children.
For more information contact the NACD, Inc., P.O. Box 380, Huntsville, UT 84317-0380, phone (801) 621-8606.

NACD's perception of the "autistic" child follows the neurological/sensory model. A child who has been labeled as "autistic" is viewed not as an emotionally disturbed child, or as a child with a psychiatric problem, but as a child with sensory dysfunction whose abnormal behavior is a reflection of abnormal perception.

Helping Quinn -- a child who is *not* autistic

Quinn's grandmother, Carole, supported her daughter-in-law's search for answers, and came up with a solution for providing this little boy with his heart's desires.

Quinn's behavior was always erratic and very emotional, always on the destructive side. His mother, Leslie, was told he would grow out of it, or she could try drugs, and find special schools for him when he was old enough. But the advice they were being given was sorely lacking, and Carole was fairly certain Quinn was autistic. His eyes were always darting around the room and he would flip his hands around each other in a very confused fashion. If another child were in the room, he would hurt him. Quinn is a big boy for his age, and his twin sister is very tiny and often on the receiving end of her brother's behavioral outbursts.

On the children's second birthday, Quinn was confused and angry, and his actions became more pronounced as more children and adults came to the house. To call the evening a "disaster" was an understatement, and Leslie was at her wit's end. Afterward came a series of chance meetings with people, plus a doctor who suggested the Feingold diet, although he was unclear of the details of it. Leslie wanted to try diet, and had to do a great deal of research to locate information on it. But she persisted and the diet evolved into a way of life. As a result, the family was rewarded with a pronounced change in Quinn, who went from being non-verbal to talking. His body movements were now under *his* control, his eyes were steady, and the erratic behavior was replaced by normal 2 1/2 year-old behaviors.

To celebrate the twins' third birthday, Carole made a Stage One cake, and for the first time Quinn could eat the same food as everyone else, including the icing. It was great! Not only could Quinn enjoy the food and the people, but he did just fine in the atmosphere of confusion -- a disaster the previous year. There was not one mishap (with the exception of his sister upstaging him a few times).

Carole writes, "Thank you to the Feingold Association for giving me my grandson. We may have lost him in a maze of drugs and special schools if not for you."

Fragile X syndrome and autism

Fragile X syndrome is a chromosomal abnormality that is believed to affect about ten percent of autistic males. Allan Reiss, director of behavioral genetic research at the Kennedy Institute of Johns Hopkins University, suggests that since fragile X is genetically based, the same may be true of autism. Many people carry the defective genes, but do not exhibit any of the symptoms. Males are more likely to have pronounced autistic type symptoms or retardation. Female symptoms are usually milder.

Rebecca's story -- dealing with extreme sensitivity

She likes music, Barbies, patent leather shoes, her friends and chocolate. She is helpful with her two younger sisters, considerate and patient. We've also been on the Feingold Program for almost three-and-a-half years now. Why, you might ask, with such a wonderful child, so calm and patient that she sits in synagogue with her father for two and a half-hours every Saturday morning, would you have her on the Feingold diet?

Well, sometimes we also forget. We hadn't had a reaction in almost two years. The mere thought of it evokes terror in all of us, Rebecca included. You see, Rebecca isn't merely "hyper;" she becomes what the "experts" call autistic tendencied. What this means to us is that our perfect, beautiful daughter, if given a microgram of Yellow 5 or TBHQ, et al, becomes autistic. Unfortunately, last week we were forced to re-experience the nightmare of life with an autistic child.

We knew something was wrong when Rebecca began weeping inconsolably at 8 am. When she tried to speak, she sounded as if she had marbles in her mouth. No question here! By 10 am, she was curled up in the fetal position, squawking like a chicken, dumping the sleeping baby from her bed, tearing at her own flesh, and later running out the front door onto our busy street.

Finally, at 11 am, our neighborhood pizza parlor was open so I could call Sammy, the owner, to ask him what he did different this time. He said "nothing, just like always: unbromated flour crust (whole wheat to boot!), tomato paste, spice and tofu."

"No, Sammy" I pleaded, "SOMETHING was very different. I'm living with an autistic child today, when you saw I had a normal girl yesterday."

"Oh yeah," says Sammy, "the tofu tasted bland so I sautéed it in butter flavored oil, but I swear it's kosher."

"Yes, of course it's kosher," I responded, "the Rabbi sees to that. Unfortunately, nobody polices your claim to be 'Natural' the way they police your sign that says you're kosher. This oil has TBHQ in it! I'll take my tofu bland the next time please!"

Well, here it is, five days later. The reaction finally ended! My daughter spent 5 days in the house in front of old musicals on video (Oklahoma!), I didn't know what else to do with her. My husband had to stay home from work on Friday because she was too dangerous to the other two children and needed one-on-one supervision.

Sammy from the pizza store was kind enough to call several times to apologize. (I'm more sorry than he is, I'm sure.) My only regret is that we didn't videotape her under the dining room table, curled up, crying and squawking while trying to hit me and my three-year-old with a stick. Who would have believed THAT was Rebecca?

Maybe, if I could just flip on the video every time someone criticizes me for being food-neurotic, or overprotective for homeschooling, or every time my mother tells me that I need psychological help because I imagine my daughter to be chemically sensitive... But they would only think she is acting, because that couldn't possibly be Rebecca!

The Autism Research Institute

A pioneer in the search for treatment is Dr. Bernard Rimland, director of the Autism Research Institute. The institute provides information on current developments in the diagnosing and treatment of autistic children, as well as literature on controlled studies. You can request a "Parent Package" which includes a diagnostic checklist, sample of the informational newsletter and much helpful information. Write to ARI, 41872 Adams Ave., San Diego, CA 92116. The ARI is a nonprofit organization; please enclose a $5 donation to defray costs.

Parents are also playing a crucial part in the search for causes of autism. The keen observations of a Leominster, MA mother has led to the discovery that the polluted air and water generated by a factory in their town has resulted in the birth of an extraordinary number of autistic children. Even when a parent has been away from the town for many years, their children are at high risk. The closer the citizens lived to the factory site, the higher the incidence of autism. A TV documentary on the community included an interview of the mother who traced her autistic child's condition to the town's industrial pollution. Ironically, one scene showed her frosting a brilliantly colored birthday cake for her child.

Notes on Autism

Some parents of autistic children report that those behaviors lessen when they avoid synthetic chemicals. Other parents note that the child behaves normally while on the Program, but that an infraction results in behaviors characteristic of autism.

Dr. Feingold's comment that this diet "entails no risk, no harm," and the observation of many professionals that "it's worth a try" seem especially appropriate for the parent facing the devastation of autism.

For the child who is not comfortable in our world, and whose body may already be suffering from the effects of toxic chemicals, what is to be gained by exposure to the non-essential synthetic chemicals added to foods?

My son, Michael

Linda didn't want to believe her son was autistic. Michael didn't display all of the characteristics of autism, but he had so many that the prognosis looked bad.

From day one he had been extremely hyperactive, had numerous allergies, ear infections, poor sleep habits, cried frequently, seemed always to be agitated, and resisted being held.

It was futile to try to comfort this little baby, who stiffened his body so that it was rigid and hard. By age two it was clear that Michael's language was not developing. He would later learn to speak, but could only repeat what he heard. If he were asked, "Would you like to go outside, Michael?" his response, "Would you like to go outside, Michael?" was a code for saying "yes."

When a preschool teacher tried to coax him down from climbing up a bookcase, he echoed her words, "No, no, Michael, please come back down!" with a tone of anguish that seemed like his body had taken on a will of its own.

Michael's future looked hopeless, but his parents refused to give up on him.

The family's exhaustive search for answers was as distressing as their child's problems; Linda was blamed for everything. Since she was 29 when he was born, her doctor reasoned that Linda had "spoiled him rotten" and her refusal to accept the verdict indicated her refusal to accept reality. Some people told her she was overprotective while others blamed her for neglect.

Linda recalls a team of child developmental specialists who spent two and a half hours in a room with Michael. They went into the room prim and proper, and emerged later in a state of disarray, with the psychologist's blouse hanging part way out of her dress-for-success skirt. The recommendation Linda received was "Michael was retarded below age 2; the couple should institutionalize him, go home, and have another baby."

But this little boy had some remarkable strengths. His memory was phenomenal and when he was only three he could identify his favorite records just by their titles printed on the label.

Linda agreed to try medication. The first day was wonderful; the three-year-old could sit in a chair, and could look at his mother. The second day he sat in the chair, but that was all he could do; the little boy stared straight ahead with a vacant look. On the third day of Ritalin, Linda described him as a "raving maniac." Other drugs were tried, but Michael "freaked out" on them. (He was already on a heavy regimen of drugs to control seizures, asthma and allergic reactions.)

He was a super-hyperactive child -- off the charts!

In the preschool designed for learning disabled children, four-year-old Michael continued to operate in a frenzy of activity. He had the autistic traits of rocking, twirling and walking in circles. Linda saw he was trying to fit in, but was too agitated, stiff, and simply too busy to do so. His own negative behavior seemed to be very upsetting to him. He seemed impervious to pain, and it was as though his mind was too far ahead of his body and the body was unable to catch up. A professor of pediatrics at the University of Oklahoma had a scale of 1 to 10 for rating hyperactive children -- number 1 was normal behavior and 10 was the most severely hyperactive. He rated Michael a 13! Another doctor observed Michael in his school. Less than ten minutes passed when the diagnosis was "autistic." At the urging of the preschool teacher, the physician stayed to watch him for a longer time. The diagnosis was changed to "mildly retarded," and then later "really bright." The final diagnosis was a sincerely befuddled "I have no idea!"

Linda's mother had heard of a doctor from California whose treatment for hyperactive children was generating a lot of controversy. It was the mid 1970s, and *Why Your Child is Hyperactive* had just been published. After much searching, Linda located the book and decided that after trying everything else she would do this as well. At least there could be no harm from it -- that proved to be wrong.

Michael had a severe reaction to medicine, and appeared to go through a withdrawal when synthetic additives were removed.

Michael's reaction to the Feingold diet was terrible! Nearly two decades later, Linda recalls the nightmare she went through after she removed the synthetic additives from Michael's food and medicine. He went from a "13" to a "20;" the experience was horrible. Linda now believes that he was suffering from symptoms of withdrawal. (This is the opposite of what most families report, but underlines the importance of parents staying in close touch with their physician. They had changed doctors and Michael was now under the care of a sympathetic professional.)

Linda and her husband had committed themselves to give the Feingold diet a 100% effort for 30 days, and persisted through several weeks of Michael's destructive behavior. Linda reasoned that patients are told to give medicine a 14 to 30 day period before it may work, and felt the same could be true of a dietary change. But her patience was wearing thin; there were only 2 or 3 days of the 30-day trial left, and Michael had shown no improvement.

It was a snowy day, shortly before Christmas, and Linda took her son out to play in the snow. The phone rang, and she went inside briefly to answer it. When she came back outside Michael was nowhere to be found. Linda searched frantically, expecting he had climbed over the fence and taken off, so it was a shock to discover him lying on the ground, in the snow, with his eyes closed. Alarmed, she called his name and shook him. Michael opened his eyes and said "tired," then closed them again. Linda had never seen him tired. She carried him hurriedly into the house, searching for evidence of a blow to the head or other injury, but could find none. She changed him into dry clothes and took his temperature, but Michael slept through it all.

Two-and-a-half hours later he was still sleeping when Linda rushed him to her pediatrician's office. The doctor knew Michael well, and feared head trauma. The office was filled with crying children, with the exception of one who slept peacefully on Linda's lap. After a 1-1/2 hour wait, the pediatrician went over Michael "with a fine tooth comb, checking for everything!" Finally a smile came over the doctor's face, "Linda, Michael is asleep." "Come here," he told her, "I want you to feel his leg." She pressed her finger into the soft flesh and was startled that it was not characteristically rock hard. "What's wrong?" she asked anxiously. The doctor gently explained, "Honey, that's the way he's supposed to feel. I don't know if it's the diet you're on or a miracle, but this child's muscle tone is normal."

His little body had never really been relaxed before.

It was the first time Michael had experienced a restful sleep. He slept for a long time and then all night long.

The next day when Michael came home from school he willingly sat on Linda's lap and listened to a story without her having to hold him there. She took him for a walk and didn't have to hold on to him. "That night my husband and I sat in astonishment as we watched our son sit down quietly and eat his dinner. We didn't dare talk about what was happening for three days. It was as though doing so would somehow break the spell."

Similar wonders were taking place in the classroom as well and it was several days before Michael's teacher dared to say anything. "He can sit, he can listen to instructions," were the heavenly words Linda heard, and the two women hugged from sheer joy. Within two months of beginning the diet, his hyperactivity went from a 13 to a 3. The seizures stopped after a year on the diet, only to return after an infraction.

The first infraction was a memorable event caused by a red sucker. The nightmare came back in full force and it was a week before the calm child returned. Another time Michael had a drink of Dr. ------, Linda relates, and he didn't know where he was. She found him in his bedroom, disoriented and acting spacey. He cried and hugged her, begging her to take him home.

Since his verbal skills were still limited, Linda had not said anything to Michael about their change in foods, and she assumed he had no idea he was on a diet. But the next time Linda's brother came to the house, and Michael saw his uncle holding a bottle of Dr. ------, the four-year-old said, "Uncle Kenny, Dr. ------ makes you wild and crazy."

Michael figured out a lot about food additives and their effect. He said that red suckers make his head hurt real bad. Other foods "make his stomach dizzy." He was extremely careful not to put anything in his mouth unless it came from his mother, grandmother or teacher. Today, at age 21, Michael still sticks completely to his diet.

The adults didn't realize how much Michael understood.

He attended a public school and graduated with a C average. Teachers who read Michael's history tried hard to avoid having him in their class. A few weeks later, they fought to keep him from being transferred out. He was invariably the hardest working and best-behaved student, and was eager to win their approval.

At Michael's high school graduation Linda ran into the doctor who had told her she had created all of her son's problems. There were no apologies.

The pediatrician who first told Linda her son was sleeping normally has kept track of his patient to this day. He tells parents about Michael and that diet is an option to consider for their child. Professionals have expressed their appreciation to the family for having opened the door to so many other children. They are not as quick to put limitations on any child and are open to trying new techniques that may be unproven, but cause no harm.

Today Linda describes the son she was advised to give up as "loving, responsive, bright, curious, wonderful, and a great kid."

Autism, Intolerance, & Allergy

A growing body of evidence suggests that in many children with autistic symptoms the observable abnormalities are linked to biochemical intolerances, allergies or metabolic errors.

The cause of autism is unknown, although it's clear that it is a biological disorder involving the brain. There are no conclusive medical tests at present. The diagnosis must be based upon observation of the child's behavior, thus the parent observation and intervention is critical in the diagnosis and subsequent treatment of autism.

One way to study the child's system is to examine the entire way they react to various stimuli, including foods and various chemicals they ingest.

For a number of years the European medical community has been researching allergies/intolerances as it applies to autism. In 1994 Brenda O'Reilly came over from England and spoke to both the University of North Carolina (UNC) and Duke University. Brenda is the parent of an autistic child, and coordinator of an autism support group in England; she has been exploring this topic for a number of years. She presented information by Dr. Rosemary Waring of Birmingham University.

At the FAUS Conference Brenda described the problems the autistic child faces:

They can't get rid of naturally toxic compounds, including their own metabolic waste products. These chemicals then react with one another and create other compounds that may be very toxic to them. Food exacerbates the children's autistic condition. Dr. Rosemary Waring found a possible link between certain foods a child eats and behavior.

Dr. Waring reported, "So far the children we look at who tend to be allergic to food lack or have low levels of a particular enzyme, and this enzyme ought to detoxify some of the amines and phenols present in foods."

Since the enzymes don't detoxify these amines and phenols, the food gives the children a "high" and causes them to have bizarre behavior. Dr. Waring says autistic children seem to crave the foods that affect them the most.

Enzymes, gluten, casein

The medical community in Europe is looking at several different problems with autistic children including the enzyme deficiency and urinary peptides, i.e., gluten, and casein antibodies. Gluten is found in wheat, oats, barley, rye, barley malt; and casein is found in dairy products.

The enzyme that appears to be lacking is called phenol-sulfotransferase-P; as a result, children have a problem processing foods such as cheese, chocolate, bananas, apples, as well as other foods containing phenols and amines. [Additional information on this is available in the book *Food Chemical Sensitivities* by Robert Buist, Ph.D., 1988, Avery Publishers.]

When symptoms begin

Brenda noted that the children in Dr. Waring's study generally developed normally for about 18 months to 2 years. Then they started to regress, to lose speech, eye contact, and the ability to play. Boys are most vulnerable, and for every girl who displays autistic symptoms there are four boys.

Removing the offending foods does not "cure" autism, it just helps to alleviate symptoms.

Brenda's son

Although she had a normal pregnancy with her autistic son, Allistair, Brenda did have a respiratory infection, was treated for high blood pressure, and took medicine for pleurisy while breast-feeding. The baby developed normally until about age two, at which time he changed abruptly, first with hyperactive behavior, then he began to regress, and rarely slept. His eating habits also changed abruptly. He wanted only a few foods -- those that brought on the hyperactive behavior. (The autistic child not only tends to crave those foods, which are poorly tolerated, but many of them begin to eat a variety of non-food substances, such as dirt; this practice is called "pica.")

When she told her doctor that certain foods seemed to make Allistair hyperactive, Brenda was labeled a neurotic mother, and the doctors she consulted would not believe there was a problem. Other doctors would later confirm Brenda's observations, and one told her that a child's allergies are likely to worsen before the autistic symptoms begin. It also appears that a child is likely to change "handedness" before the onset of the autistic symptoms, and that these children tend to come from very allergic families.

Serotonin

Brenda's extensive reading of medical journals suggested that some autistic children tend to have high levels of the chemical neurotransmitter serotonin in their brain. When Allistair's serotonin level was measured it was found to be five times the normal level for a child of his age. Some metabolites of serotonin are similar to that of the hallucinogen LSD, and a close look at the autistic child will show many similarities to the person who is "high." An acquaintance who had experimented with drugs in the 1960's observed Brenda's son, and told her "That kid is tripping out."

Studies conducted on autistic children show they excrete a chemical called bufotenin -- a psychoactive substance that breaks down from serotonin. If the enzyme deficiency means that the autistic child is unable to get rid of serotonin properly after it is used this may be the reason he behaves in strange ways.

This theory is further supported by research conducted in the 1970s. It study found that 80% of the children checked were excreting bufotenin without being given any foods that contain serotonin. Japanese researchers found that 100% of the children tested excreted it.

Using diet for autism

By using a very limited diet, Brenda has helped to reduce her son's extreme behaviors. He is nowhere near normal, and is non-verbal, but he is much easier to live with, and seems to enjoy life more. The foods that have been removed from his diet include milk, yeast, chocolate, salicylates, corn, carrots, and synthetic additives.

Unlike the Feingold Association's ADD program, a dietary program for autistic symptoms is likely to take a long time before results become apparent. Brenda recalls that it took a year before she saw the full impact of the dietary changes on Allistair. In fact, it is typical that the child will become worse for the first two to four weeks. Brenda and other parents report that it appears as if they undergo withdrawal as their "fixes" are removed, and their body starts to rid itself of the substances that have built up in their system. Despite the experience of parents, scientific exploration of the link between autism and allergy is still in its infancy. The first improvement Brenda noticed was that her son began to sleep through the night.

Major food offenders

A variety of foods may trigger adverse reactions in susceptible children and adults. The worst offenders are wheat, cow's milk, oranges, tomatoes, chocolate, cheese, and sugar, and many have adverse reactions to medications.

The body gets rid of phenols when they attach to sulfates, but Brenda's son didn't have enough sulfates to accomplish this. The normal range of sulfates in a person's body is between 2.1 and 11.6; low normal is 1.5; Allistair has only 0.17. People who suffer from migraine headaches also have low levels of several enzymes necessary for the sulfates to work. Brenda found that many of the mothers in her parent group suffer from migraine headaches. The fathers of the autistic children typically have allergies such as hay fever, or skin rashes, and allergy sufferers also have low sulfate levels. If both parents fit this category, the children are at high risk of being deficient in this important chemical. One of the functions of sulfates is to line the gut wall to keep unwanted substances from getting through the gut and into the blood stream.

Physical reactions

Autistic children have an excessive thirst, as though they are busy trying to get the substances out of their body, to flush them out. Sulfates break down the molecules into much smaller parts so they can be more easily excreted.

Parents have observed that from 10 minutes to 2 hours after eating the child will exhibit a behavioral change. This is often accompanied by physical symptoms such as partially red ears, dilated pupils, excessive sweating, red cheeks, and constipation.

Sulfur

Brenda explained that normally the body can change sulfur into sulfate and then excrete it. "We think autistic children are unable to add oxygen to sulfur (to convert it into sulfate). In addition to antibiotics, many antipsychotic drugs contain sulfur, and this doesn't work with children with this problem. Sulfur is also found in foods, particularly cabbage, onion, garlic and egg yolk."

Food intolerances and ADD

Brenda continued, "Many of these children are not so much *allergic* as *intolerant* of foods. They probably have a metabolic problem or biochemical problem where they cannot handle the substance in food when the food is broken down and digested. We also give them digestive enzymes and that does help."

Autism is a physical illness that presents itself as a mental disorder.

"We can do all these interventions and they do help to alleviate some of the symptoms, but the child still has autism. There is such a varying level between the children; some are so severe we just can't do anything, and some, we think, get right back down into ADD and ADHD. So there's a whole spectrum of children who probably have the same problem. That's why we are working with the Feingold Program. With autistics we think there's something else as well because there is something making them go so far into this that they're losing their brain function."

Is there an ADD/Autism connection?

Dr. Waring has done a preliminary screening on 5 children with ADD/ADHD and has postulated that due to their low sulfate levels, a connection may be present, and that further investigation is needed. Brenda suggests, "So it might well be worth checking your children for this problem, either with us [through blood and urine samples shipped to England] or when the testing program is up and running here in the United States. I don't think this is the whole answer to autism or hyperactivity. I think it's one part of it. But whether this problem is caused by another problem further up the chain, we don't know. This is what we hope to find out with research."

Testing for enzyme deficiency is needed in the US

The parent support group brought Dr. Waring to the U.S. to address doctors at Duke and the University of North Carolina about her research. She told them "We need to find funding for proper medical research, and develop a testing protocol." She applauds Dr. Bernard Rimland for his ongoing efforts, specifically the Defeat Autism Now conference he organized earlier in 1995, which brought together scientists from around the world.

The goal of preventing autism

Brenda believes that once the syndrome of autism is better understood testing will be routinely done on newborns, just as it is done for PKU. If this were to come about, then parents could be given early notification and the child's diet could be restricted in an effort to prevent damage. Perhaps these children would be able to reintroduce those foods at a later time. [This is the case with the PKU syndrome, and also with the children using a high-fat diet to treat seizures.]

Brenda summarized, "Autism is a physical illness that presents the mental disorder, and it starts in the gut, because your brain doesn't exist by itself. Whatever you eat must affect the brain because you use what you eat to make the brain function."

Bedwetting

Enuresis is a common reaction to additives/salicylates according to the reports we receive from our members.

One woman described her very sensitive 6-year-old son: "Within three days of beginning the diet, his bedwetting stopped. So did the screaming and out-of-control behavior. He is a particularly sensitive child, and some reactions have been brought on by Dad's after-shave lotion, red apples (he can handle golden delicious apples if they're peeled), raspberry, and any kind of pineapple (fresh, frozen, canned, juice, etc.).

"One of the worst reactions came after his Dad gave him one piece of raisin bread toast. Within ten minute he went 'bonkers' and the reaction lasted for three days!"

Another member wrote, "Our son did not want to be on the Feingold diet. He felt sorry for himself and made remarks that he was being cheated. As he realized that his father and I were dedicated to this diet and the help it could bring him, he slowly began to show less defiance. Of course, sticking with the diet resulted in improved behavior, and this helped to make our point clear. But the biggest benefit it brought him personally is the fact that now he no longer wets the bed.

"Being 8 years old with no friends, in trouble at school, working on Mom and Dad's nerves at home, bullying his little brother, being loud and obnoxious, were no small problems to deal with. But he has always considered the bedwetting to be the worst of his problems. He had even reached the point where he was having problems staying dry during the day. This always happened on high stress days. A check-up by our doctor identified nothing physically abnormal with his urinary tract. The doctor then gave us medication and a booklet to try to build his bladder's holding capacity. This was no help; in fact, it made the problem worse. (It's interesting to note the medication was bright red.)

"Now our son can go camping with the scouts, or stay overnight at the home of a friend. He no longer complains about the diet, and he certainly doesn't feel deprived."

Staying dry -- Melissa's triumph

"While the children were involved in their gymnastic class, I overheard three of the moms talking about a special diet. One mother was particularly enthusiastic about this food regimen, and described all the problems her daughter had, and how many of them have cleared up.

"As a scientist, I was very skeptical; it sounded a lot like wishful thinking. But as a mother I knew Missy had problems that didn't seem to have any logical answer. She suffered from a chronic runny nose and rashes, she bruised easily, often looked anemic, and the skin on the bottom of her feet was constantly peeling. She had major temper flare-ups that didn't seem to be related to any reasonable cause.

"But of all the problems Missy endured, the worst was the enuresis. At age five, she still was unable to stay dry during the day, although she did not bedwet.

"Doctors visits and tests didn't give any clues. I had set up an appointment to see a urologist, but knew that on the first visit he would just ask me to keep a food diary. That was something I could do before our visit, and perhaps get a head start on some sort of solution. So I began to keep a log of the foods Missy ate. I remembered the one mother at the gym saying that the natural salicylates caused her daughter to have sleep problems, so when Missy wet about three hours after she had grape juice, I made a note of that. A grilled cheese sandwich (with very YELLOW cheese) brought on uncontrollable wetting within one hour.

"The next time we went to gymnastics, I went up to the mothers and said, 'Talk to me!' I wanted to learn everything I could about the Program. Using what information I had, the wetting stopped in three days. I was shocked!

"But there were setbacks; I didn't tell my husband for a long time that I had made changes in Melissa's diet, and so he gave her unallowed foods. Finally, I told him and received the expected reaction. They were on their way out for the day and when I asked him not to feed her certain foods, his reaction was 'Garbage!' They came home after two hours. Missy was experiencing a major reaction, and my husband said, 'I'll do anything you want!' So, with that, our family began the Feingold Program.

"I had a lot to learn. A new shirt, which was never washed, resulted in uncontrollable wetting. The wrong toothpaste brought a wet bed. And then there was the time the baby sitter thought my homemade play dough looked too plain, so she added some yellow dye to it!

"The longer we stayed on the Program, the better I was able to identify the smaller, more subtle reactions. Certain shampoos set her off, so did scented fabric softening strips, and I got rid of the aerosol spray used for dusting and polishing furniture. It wasn't so bad, since there's a safe substitute for nearly everything.

"The anemic look, bruising, rashes, etc. are a thing of the past, but the happiest news of all is that my daughter can now be dry all the time. I didn't scold her for wetting, and she never said much about it, but her disposition was getting increasingly gloomy as she got older. She had been a very easy-going child, but by age four I could see the problem taking its toll. "It was so hard for her; she pretended not to care, but felt really worthless. She got angry too easily, and would even bite people. Once we found the reason, I apologized to Missy for not having been able to help her. Needless to say, she feels good about herself now, and has her sunny disposition back.

"Missy is a real stickler about her diet. She knows exactly what she can eat, and doesn't have any desire to cheat. I often think about those mothers at the gymnastic class, and about how lucky it was that I happened to hear them talking about the Feingold Program. How many other children, and their families, are suffering needlessly?"

Leah

"Leah was never diagnosed as a hyperactive child, but she did seem to have a very short attention span and at age 8 still had a bedwetting problem. She was placed on Tofranil for this and the drug did stop the bedwetting. However, she complained of an inability to sleep soundly. At this point we discontinued the drug and began to experiment with the Feingold diet. Within a matter of days the bedwetting stopped and each time she has wet the bed since it can be directly traced to something eaten the previous evening which was not additive-free.

"In addition to ceasing the bedwetting she also improved at least one letter grade in each of her subjects. At the end of last year's school year, her teacher expressed to me pleasure in Leah's improvement. She said when Leah entered her class she seemed unsure of her abilities, but by the end of the school year she had shown the most overall improvement of any of her students. I am sure there are probably thousands of children like Leah who don't appear to have any real problem, but who could be greatly improved with an additive-free diet."

Studies on bedwetting

The connection between enuresis and allergy is not new; G.W. Bray described the role of allergy in *Archives of Diseases in Childhood* in 1931.

More recently, researchers in England have addressed the fact that children labeled as hyperactive seem to be more likely to suffer from enuresis. Egger, Carter, Soothill and Wilson have conducted various studies in which hyperactive children are placed on highly restrictive diets. As a result, the majority of the children experienced a significant improvement in many areas, including enuresis.

In the May 1992 issue of *Clinical Pediatrics*, Egger et al. published a study titled, "Effect of Diet Treatment on Enuresis in Children with Migraine or Hyperkinetic Behavior." The authors wrote, "Twenty-one children with migraine and/or hyperkinetic behavior disorder which was successfully treated with an oligoantigenic (few foods) diet also suffered from nocturnal and/or diurnal (daytime) enuresis. On the diet, the enuresis stopped in 12 of these children and improved in an additional four."

The work of Kaplan et al. in Canada also suggests children with behavior disorders are more prone to suffer from various physical problems, including enuresis.

Childhood Depression - The Quiet Epidemic

This is a true account. We substituted the name "Betsy" to protect the privacy of our young subject.

Another Thanksgiving Day was drawing to a close, ushering in the joyful but hectic weeks of preparation for Christmas.

Given a choice of before-bed snacks, our 7-year-old daughter selected a slice of applesauce cake and milk. Expecting to share the moments with everyone present, she was understandably disappointed when her grandfather asked her to eat somewhere else because the table was being used for a card game.

She did not protest, but left the room rather solemnly and without her food. I followed her into the living room and found her lying face down on the sofa, quietly crying.

"I wish I had a gun!" she said resolutely, yet with sadness in her voice.

When I asked if she wanted a toy gun she told me no, a real one.

"Why?"

"Because I want it to happen," she sobbed.

Worried, but not wanting to make matters worse by reacting with panic, I questioned Betsy calmly about her feelings. Had they started recently?

"No, I've been having these feelings for a long time. I tried to make it happen before," she said, and her words sent a shock wave through my body.

A little coaxing soon brought her mood up, but in the weeks that followed there were many other emotional upsets that triggered tearful admissions that, for Betsy, life was a hurtful existence.

Her gloom seemed to accelerate as the weeks went by. My husband and I discussed each sign of depression and each incident of obvious emotional turmoil in detail. We knew that children who talk about suicide should be taken seriously. Betsy told us that she had tried to take her life at least three times. Although she obviously had never gone far enough to do actual physical harm to herself, it was clear that she was preoccupied with the notion of ending her life, and that she was experimenting, at least in her mind, with ideas on how it could be done.

I once broke a light bulb. She offered to help me pick up the pieces, but I refused her help, telling her she might be badly cut. "Could you die from being cut on a piece of glass like that?" she questioned.

"No," I told her, "Not unless you were cut in a bad place." Her reply sent a chill down my spine. "You mean like a place that goes bump-de-bump?"

Once, at my office, she asked if the building had a stairway to the roof. I asked why she wanted to know.

"I was thinking I could jump," she replied quietly.

Little upsets more and more often became major threats to her well-being and ego. Once, during a particularly frightening encounter with the demon that had robbed her of her self-confidence, she confessed to being afraid of me, looking at me wildly as though I were some stranger not to be trusted.

Even her small works of art brought home from school had taken on a macabre appearance. I remember a chalk drawing done on black construction paper. The only objects on the paper were three graveyard headstones. Each bore the initials of one of us. Each time her emotions ran rampant I tried to dig deeper into her feelings. I did not want to let go of the idea that showing her my concern and how much we both loved her would overcome her fears and help her to cope with her doubts. But my efforts were to little avail.

I asked if she thought she might feel better talking to someone else about her problems.

"Yes," she answered.

"Who do you think could help?"

"A psychologist," she said without hesitation. The precociousness of her reply did not surprise me. Vocabulary and communication had always been Betsy's strengths, and we marveled at her youthful awareness and outstanding memory. Impressing other two- and three-year-olds with words like "ferocious" had been easy for her. But now she talked of "feeling strange inside" and "being afraid." The ferocious beast that haunted her small body could not be conquered alone.

The weeks of sessions with the pediatric psychiatrist went by slowly, and we became restless with the snail's pace with which such therapy must proceed. We were at a loss to understand what had suddenly overcome our bright, articulate, gregarious little girl. Within a short period of time Betsy became uncooperative with the doctor. We grew impatient. Eager to find an alternative, or at least an adjunct to the counseling, my mind was almost constantly occupied with thoughts of what could be done.

Perhaps that is why I recalled a girlfriend talking about a kind of food program that had been helpful in improving her children's behavior, attitudes and moods. I had listened politely, questioned her, and had even spoken to a couple of pediatricians about the possibility of our daughter showing evidence of this hyperactive syndrome. But I was told that hyperactive children are destructive, out of control, terrors to live with, and unable to function very well.

And besides, they reassured me, hyperactive children were almost always boys. None of these adjectives fit our daughter. Or did they? Oh sure, she had always been very active and had slept very little as an infant. She would not sit to ride in a stroller, making shopping trips exhausting chase scenes. But young children always have more energy than their parents can tolerate. I believed she was just a normal, frisky toddler.

Had I fallen for all the cliches? The issue here was not hyperactivity, but depression; a feeling of hopelessness severe enough to make our only child want to cease to live. If there was any chance the Feingold diet could help her through this and restore her emotional stability and tranquility, I had to at least try it.

My husband was skeptical and Betsy was distressed. "I don't want to be on a special diet. I just want to be normal!" Her words were like needles, piercing me throughout.

Despite her initial objection, Betsy was remarkably cooperative. Only six days after beginning the diet I saw the first visible signs that something was changing. That evening, just after dinner, our daughter put her head in my lap and fell asleep. She took a nap, that's all, just a nap. This is something most parents take for granted, but it was the first time I can remember Betsy being calm and at peace.

We began to observe other changes as well. She no longer showed a low tolerance for frustration, poor concentration, inability to accept small disappointments - all symptoms listed in the *Feingold Handbook*.

The change in Betsy's personality has been dramatic. From the moment I first noticed the obvious improvement in her mood and physical control, to this day, Betsy has not looked backward. Our child's depressions have become only a bad memory, for us and for her.

The day following her initial change to serenity our 7-year-old announced that she did not ever want to go off the Feingold diet. She hasn't.

Depression

"Clinical depression" is the name for the persistent disabling condition of joylessness that affects an estimated 30 to 40 million Americans. It is believed to be a major cause of suicide.

While depression is not new, the age group affected by it has dropped dramatically in the past few decades. The National Institutes of Mental Health notes that prior to World War II depression typically affected people in their 50s. Today it occurs most often among 25- to 44-year-olds.

Another startling statistic is the increase in depression among young children. It has only been within the past ten years or so that therapists have recognized the existence of childhood depression. One estimate of the number of cases of childhood depression in the United States is 400,000, or close to 2 percent of children ages 7 to 12. The frightening statistics on teen-age suicides have attracted national attention. Five thousand teen suicides were reported in 1986 -- a 300 percent increase over the previous three decades.

While the victim of depression is twice as likely to be female as male, the American Academy of Child and Adolescent Psychiatry reports that the male risk for suicide in the U.S. is between three and four times that for females. In other words women are at greater risk of becoming depressed, but men are more likely to translate it into violent action.

At least 25,000 Americans take their own lives each year.

The psychiatric profession now recognizes that biochemistry plays a role in depression. The profession's DSM III manual (list of symptoms used to diagnose mental disorders) has been updated to include seasonal affective disorder (SAD). In this case, depression is connected to the reduced exposure to light during the winter months. In other words, psychological factors are not the sole cause of depression. Biochemical influences are being recognized and investigated by the scientific community.

After World War II

World War II is a turning point for many statistics. It signaled a sharp drop in the age at which depression is likely to start. It also marks the point at which behavior problems in children gradually began to rise to epidemic proportions.

Dr. Feingold noted, "The first half of my almost fifty years as a physician were spent as a pediatrician. During this pediatric experience I had exposure to thousands of children with a great variety of ailments. Yet

I had no recollection of a high frequency of hyperactivity and behavioral problems through all these years." But in the years following the end of World War II, the use of synthetic food additives increased dramatically. They continue to increase, as do the problems of hyperactivity, depression and the incidence of suicide. Is there a connection?

The mentally or emotionally disabled child and adolescent

As many as 14 million U.S. children under the age of 18 may be suffering from mental illness according to a study conducted by a committee of the Institute of Medicine. Estimates ranged from a low of 7.5 million (12 percent) to the high of 14 million (22 percent). The problems identified by the committee included: depression, autism and hyperactivity.

Depression in the very young

This is being seen more and more frequently, and in children of increasingly younger ages, according to John C. Pommery, M.D., in an address to the American Academy of Pediatrics. It is difficult to diagnose in the child because depression can manifest as behavior problems.

Hereditary factors

Researchers have found evidence of hereditary factors in individuals who suffer from depression. Other research indicates that there may be a hereditary component in suicide.

Dr. John Mann of the Cornell University Medical Center reported that suicide victims tend to have an abnormality in the production and use of serotonin, one of the many chemical messengers brain cells use to communicate. Serotonin abnormalities have also been suggested in hyperactive children.

Finding help

Parents seeking help for their emotionally disabled child or adolescent may find that most services are designed for adults and their families. But the need for programs to serve adolescents is critical.

The time when parents become aware of the need to seek out help is generally the time when the family is in crisis. This makes it particularly difficult to locate and evaluate their options.

Professionals who are highly qualified in some areas are not necessarily the appropriate resource for a child or teenager. And for-profit treatment centers may not inform families how severely limited insurance coverage is.

Where to look

A central resource for the problem of adolescent emotional disabilities was established at Portland State University (Portland, Oregon) in 1984. The purpose of the Research and Training Center is to improve services for mentally/emotionally handicapped children and their families.

The Center has funded projects to develop statewide parent organizations. These model groups will serve as prototypes for other parent-run support groups. The Center publishes a National Directory of Organizations Serving Parents of Children and Youth with Emotional and Behavioral Disorders. This directory lists organizations that provide services.

Parents of children in crisis need immediate guidance and support. They can contact the Research and Training Center on Family Support & Children's Mental Health at Portland State University, P.O. Box 751, Portland, OR 97207-0751 or can call (503) 725-4040.

The role of nutrition in serious mental disorders

"In the treatment of insanity, while admitting the underlying neurotic predisposition, it is universally acknowledged that diet is a potent aid to recovery."

(from the February 1, **1896** *Journal of the American Medical Association*)

The things we eat can affect us physically, and can affect the way we behave. In his landmark book, *Why Your Child is Hyperactive*, Dr. Feingold described a patient who experienced both physical and behavioral reactions (hives and belligerence) after consuming certain foods, food additives and aspirin. Once he identified the trigger for hives, and removed them, the physical symptoms disappeared and her behavior normalized. This is the approach being taken by a minority of psychiatrists who treat the puzzling collections of symptoms labeled "schizophrenia."

In her book, *Natural Healing for Schizophrenia and Other Common Mental Disorders*, Eva Edelman has done an outstanding job of making a very complex topic understandable to the average reader. She does not intend for this book to be a do-it-yourself guide, but rather an invaluable educational tool for those who have loved ones suffering from various mental disorders.

Ms. Edelman describes the contributions of pioneers like Abram Hoffer, as well as the late Carl Pfeiffer and Roger Williams whose work was based upon the concept that the brain requires nutrients to function well, and if some of those nutrients are deficient, the brain will not work properly.

Most psychiatrists today treat mental disorders like schizophrenia with drugs alone, but how can they ignore nutrients, Edelman asks, when nutrients are "the raw materials from which the brain creates its neurotransmitters, the chemicals which communicate messages from one nerve cell to another?" Not only do nutrients create beneficial chemicals in our brain, but they also help to protect it from harmful chemicals.

In the early stages of schizophrenia, the book notes, "Most patients experience difficulty concentrating, learning and remembering, problems making decisions, and a lack of motivation." How many people with these symptoms are routinely being labeled ADD and placed on drugs, with no consideration of the possible causes of their symptoms?

While schizophrenia is believed to occur, typically, in people between the ages of 15 and 25, it can show up in children. Some of the symptoms are the same as those seen in youngsters diagnosed as hyperactive: temper tantrums, fears, bedwetting, nightmares, and learning difficulties. Some children who are successfully on the Feingold Program have night terrors and/or hallucinations when they react to an infraction of food additives.

Natural Healing for Schizophrenia, second edition, is available from Borage Books, Eugene, OR; (541) 683-8720. www.BorageBooks.com.

Our foster child

When the case manager told me the child I would be taking into foster care was "hyperactive" I knew we were the right family. We had followed the Feingold Program for almost five years and I conducted monthly meetings for our local chapter.

But then we learned the rest of the story, and it was grim. Ruthie was seven, but mentally was only about nine months old. She was non-verbal, never sat still, banged her fist to the side of her head, ground her teeth constantly, was abusive to others and could not be left alone for even a second.

Her natural mother reported that she banged on windows and television, she took off her diapers and smeared feces all over the walls...and the list goes on.

This behavior classified Ruthie at what is called level three. (Level one is the highest functioning.) A level three child had never been placed in a private home, but the state was initiating a pilot program and Ruthie was a part of it.

We saw the behaviors that had been described to us, only worse. In addition to having a baby, a 3-year-old, and a teenager, I provide full time day care in my home.

Ruthie's only interaction with the children was walking up to them and banging them with a toy, or grabbing their hair, knocking them a few times and then walking away -- still holding on to their hair.

With constant love, consistent behavior corrections and the Feingold diet, our foster child began to change. She learned to go up and down the stairs with only verbal direction; she was toilet trained during the daytime hours -- wearing underpants, not diapers. She stopped grinding her teeth; the banging of her head stopped; she began freely hugging and kissing both the members of our family and the children in day care. She played, and learned to work the busy box toys; she listened and responded to verbal directions and she was able to make and keep eye contact.

The change in Ruthie was so dramatic the pediatrician who followed her since birth could not believe it was the same child.

She stayed with us eleven months until a change in jobs forced us to move to another state. Ruthie's natural mother would not permit her to come with us so she was placed in another home and a different school. She was much easier to place this time since she was now functioning at level two! In her new home there was no attempt to keep Ruthie on the Feingold diet and her behavior quickly deteriorated. I am told that she is classified at level four, with behavior far worse than before. She now bites herself and others, wears diapers all the time, and has had diarrhea for nearly a year. She is black and blue from her elbows down, and on her thighs as a result of pulling and biting herself. The state has been unable to find anyone who will take Ruthie, so the only recourse left is institutionalization.

Ever since we were forced to give Ruthie up, we have fought and prayed to bring her back into our home, but placing children across state lines is one thing the bureaucracy hasn't been able to deal with -- so far. But we are not giving up.

Meanwhile, our foster child will never know this, but she has helped many other children. Her remarkable change demonstrated to all those involved in her care how effective the Feingold Program is for these youngsters.

In my efforts to have Ruthie placed here in Michigan, I have come in contact with many professionals who have expressed an interest in learning more about the Feingold Program. Two area doctors are now referring patients to our association for help.

This month I will be speaking to a support group for families of children suffering from mental retardation. I hope our experience will encourage them to consider the influence diet has on the behavior of their children.

How does Feingold fit in?

Can food additives and salicylates contribute to the behavior problems of children/adolescents with mental or emotional disorders? Based upon Dr. Feingold's clinical observations and the experience of some member families, the answer appears to be "yes," at least in some cases.

Since there currently is no way to predict who will benefit from the Feingold Program, the same trial period used by anyone testing the program would be a suitable test for the hyperactive child suspected of having an underlying mental/emotional disorder. For a youngster under close supervision the test would actually be simpler.

Many Feingold parents would dispute the inclusion of "hyperactivity" as a mental or emotional disorder. This certainly does not fit the child who behaves normally on the program, and becomes hyperactive only when exposed to synthetic additives or salicylates. On the other hand, it is typical for the child suffering from a mental or emotional disorder to have hyperactivity as one of the most noticeable symptoms. Thus, some include hyperactivity itself as a disorder.

The dark memories

Through my teen years I was placed on a variety of mind-altering drugs. It was a terrible experience.

All five of the kids in my family had the reputation of being "wound up." My parents were always shooing us out because if we were inside we would get "into things." My behavior in school was not a problem; I did well and got along with my teachers. But social interactions with the other children were difficult for me. I was called a troublemaker and non-conformist.

Since I was overweight, I was given diet pills (amphetamines) when I was about eleven years old. (That was back in the days before the FDA banned them for weight control.) Then, a few years later, I took Ritalin; I hated taking it, and the drug didn't have any effect on my behavior. Other drugs were tried: Stelazine and Thorazine are two I can remember, but there were others.

Looking back, my behavior was not very far out of line before I started on the amphetamines. But I believe that these drugs, as well as the others, were causing me to behave inappropriately. When I was on them I didn't feel like myself. It was like I couldn't control myself; I'd do things and not understand why. Now I can look back and see that these drugs were mind-altering substances.

My brother and I were both seeing a psychiatrist -- the one who gave us the Ritalin. I told him I didn't like the drug, I didn't like the way it made me feel, but everyone said it would help me, so I took it. My brother would put the pill in his mouth, and then spit it out when nobody was looking but I was the one who did what I was told. One day I decided that if I took all of my drugs at once, then I would get rid of them and wouldn't have to take them anymore. My "overdose" was considered a suicide attempt, and I found myself in a psychiatric hospital. (State law required this.)

The ward I was in was made up of just teenagers, and all of us were pretty heavily drugged. At times I was taking three different drugs simultaneously. I hated the way I felt; I knew this wasn't the real "me," and repeatedly asked the doctor to let me stop the medications. Finally he agreed, but took no steps to phase out the dosage. They were simply stopped -- cold turkey. The withdrawal was as bad as being on the drugs. I would alternate between being very depressed, uptight, lethargic, and then manic (having excessive energy). None of this was recognized as a result of the withdrawal; I was made to feel that everything was my fault.

While the hospital was not the horror chamber we sometimes hear about, it was a depressing place. There was no freedom; we had to be where we were told, doing what we were told. Most of the patients went through a cycle that started with resistance. Eventually, it would become apparent that this didn't do any good, and the patient would learn how to play the game. The goal was getting out, and we learned what we had to say and how we had to act in order to get it.

After almost a year I got out of the hospital. My new doctor wanted to put me in a halfway home, but I returned to my home instead. As soon as I could, I left home, got a job and went back to school. My goal was to become a mental health associate. I felt I could make a difference in the system, and that I understood how to provide better care to people in need. Instead, I became a wife and mother.

When my son was four years old, I began hearing about a diagnosis of "hyperactivity." (This came as no surprise.) His doctor gave me the choice: Ritalin or diet. There was no way I was going to subject my little boy to drugs, so we began the Feingold Program four years ago. We truly are a "Feingold family" as my husband and other children need the program as well. We are quite salicylate sensitive, and when I overdo them, or otherwise go off my diet, I end up with a headache. On the diet, I'm a much calmer person; and I've found that the ringing I used to have in my ears has disappeared.

Writing this story is a form of therapy for me. For many years I blocked the sad memories of my year in the mental hospital. If you had asked me a few years ago, I would have sworn I never had that experience.

I guess I still believed everything was my fault, just as I had always been told as a child. Then, while I was attending a Feingold conference, and listening to the speakers talk about our troubled children it all came rushing back. It was very painful to acknowledge what had happened, but I'm relieved that this demon is out in the light of day and I can deal with it now. I'm not yet ready to give you my name; maybe that will come with time.

Developmental Delays

Developmental Delay Resources (DDR) is an organization formed in 1994 by four exceptional women. These professionals had been seeing an alarming increase in the number of children who were being diagnosed with problems of all types. The purpose of DDR is to introduce parents and professionals to the role of nutrition, immune system problems, and sensory processing dysfunction in the acquisition of developmental delays such as learning disabilities, speech and language problems, ADD and autism.

Their first major project was a survey of nearly 700 children, indicating a disturbing link between children with developmental delays and the amount of antibiotics they had taken. The children typically were developing normally in their first year of life, but had more health problems as they grew. These youngsters had more ear infections and negative reactions to immunizations, compared to the other children surveyed.

The DDR is located in Maryland, but holds conferences and workshops throughout the United States. Their address is 4401 East West Highway, Suite 207, Bethesda, MD 20814, (301) 652-2263.

Sensory integration therapy

A person who experiences the world differently is going to behave differently. If one or more of the senses is slow to develop, it will be difficult for a child to advance.

Patricia S. Lemer, M.Ed., NCC, Executive Director of the nonprofit Developmental Delay Resources, described sensory integration dysfunction at a conference of the Feingold Association.

Dr. A. Jean Ayres conceived sensory integration theory. It's based on the premise that when information is processed by the senses either a motor or behavioral response is the result. Whereas educational and medical interventions often treat the output, what should be treated is the

the problem with how the input is being processed. If the input is abnormal or is not being processed properly then the output is going to be abnormal. The more abnormal the processing of the input, the more abnormal the behavior or the motor response is.

Over time, disorganized output can eventually result in developmental delays. For Feingold children, who are affected by something physiological such as food, nutritional, or environmental factors, the body's ability to process that sensory information may already be impaired.

For some children, being touched is an upsetting experience.

The **tactile system** (the sense of touch) is the only sense that is fully developed at birth. This is why we can use touch to calm an infant or child. The tactile system has two ways of responding: it has a protective mode and a discriminatory mode. The protective is the more primitive of the modes, where a touch is perceived as an assault. As the tactile system develops it becomes more discriminating. We are able to feel whether the sensation is hot or cold, whether the touch is light or heavy; we can discriminate whether the touch is reassuring or threatening.

The senses of touch, hearing and seeing are all related.

Children who have sensory integration problems have difficulty telling the difference between a touch that is a gentle nudge and one that is threatening. Their systems are in the protective mode rather than the discriminatory mode much of the time. This is called "tactile defensiveness," which can result in inappropriate reactions. What happens to such a child who gets pushed in line at school? He may strike back at the kid who touched him because the brain of the tactilely defensive child perceives he was hit, even though it might have been just a light touch. That light touch set off the protective mechanism in his brain that says, "I got hit. I'm going to hit back."

Tactile defensiveness is not just on the outside of the body. When there is tactile defensiveness in the mouth the child may have feeding problems or reject foods that are gritty or have unfamiliar textures or tastes.

Tactile defensiveness can also relate to hearing and vision. If a child's sense of touch is not functioning properly the other senses may not be able to develop appropriately. The sense of touch is more primitive than the visual and the auditory system. If there are tactile problems the child's ability to move up the ladder of development and use higher level of sensory integration will be affected. He/she may not be able to look and listen normally. If that tag in his shirt is driving him crazy, paying attention to what the teacher is saying will be difficult. How many of you cut the tags out of your kids clothes? How many of your kids can't wear their socks unless that seam is exactly right? This is tactile defensiveness.

[Note: Try turning the socks inside out so the smooth side of the seam touches the child.]

Occupational therapists use a technique of brushing a child's skin with a special brush to help normalize the information the skin is taking in and develop more normal tactile responses.

The **proprioceptive system** deals with the information that is coming in through the muscles and joints. It is what allows you to sit in uncomfortable chairs for a long time without leaning on the table, without falling off. Your body's muscles are giving information to your brain that they are okay. This system allows you to feel comfortable with gravity.

The child who has problems in this area needs to have deep pressure applied to the muscles; the way to get that is by moving. A child whose muscles aren't giving the needed feedback will wiggle and squirm until he/she feels secure, and can then pay attention to what is being taught. Proprioception is one of the systems most closely related to good self-control.

The **vestibular system** controls balance and is physiologically located in the inner ear. So what happens when a child has ear infections? The child's vestibular functioning will be affected. The vestibular system, like the tactile system, is already developing in utero. It's not as mature at birth as the tactile system, but a child knows when he's balanced and unbalanced and can detect motion. That's why kids love to be rocked. Rocking is calming because it stimulates the vestibular system. When a mom is required to stay in bed during pregnancy, the infant does not get the vestibular stimulation it would if the mother were moving around.

A child can have both a hypo and a hyper-reaction to the vestibular system. Kids who get motion sickness are having an overreaction; others may crave motion and vestibular stimulation. Both of these reactions are at the abnormal ends of the scale. What sensory integration therapy does is help a child tolerate a certain amount of movement, but not crave it.

The vestibular system is also involved with bilateral coordination – getting both sides of the body to work together. It is connected to several important aspects of brain function: the language center of the brain, eye movements and to the digestive tract. That's why people sometimes throw up when they have too much vestibular stimulation.

Muscle tone is related to the vestibular system. Kids with low tone need continuous vestibular stimulation. They have trouble sitting still and staying alert at the same time. If you watch them during the day, they gradually fade, slouching down in their chair and may eventually slide off!

A good teacher will know when it's time to start working those muscles to increase that tone. If you have a mini trampoline at home, it's a great thing to have your child jump on it for a couple of minutes before going to school. If the teacher is willing, have her put a mini "tramp" in the classroom to give the restless student a break; that will make it easier for him to pay attention. Many tutors are using trampolines to help kids with memory skills such as learning the alphabet or number facts. The rhythm of jumping enhances the ability to pay attention and remember facts.

The sense of touch, which involves our largest organ, the skin, is the first to develop and is fully functional at birth.

Hierarchy of development – Look at it like the rungs of a ladder; the bottom rungs (basic sensory channels) lay the foundation for development, and each rung provides the basis for the next steps above it. The top two rungs (cognitive and perceptual skills) are what is taught in school.

When you have a child who is being treated academically or behaviorally and you approach the problem from the top down, it doesn't work. You have to work from the bottom up and also from the inside out because you have to teach the system how to monitor itself, how to organize itself and contain itself in an automatic way, rather than structure it from the top. One of the things that occurs at the top is self esteem; everyone talks about self esteem, as though we can hold it in our hand, like "we're going to increase his self esteem." Unless you move up the ladder, unless your body feels comfortable with gravity, unless you feel healthy, there is no way you can work on self-esteem from the top down. All the behavioral and emotional components can be related to one of these lower level sensory processes.

Developmental Hierarchy

Cognitive skills	Writing	Imagination
	Spelling	Visualization
	Reading	Self esteem
	Capacity for abstract thought & reasoning	
Perceptual skills	Organization	Speech & language
	Attention	Concentration
	Visual perception	Auditory perception

Fine motor coordination	Speech & language Eye-hand coordination Controlled oculomotor skills	
Gross motor coordination	Balance Motor planning Oral motor	Visual motor integration Bilateral integration Lateralization Body percept
Innate reflexes	Tactile comfort Sucking reflex	Eye movements Gravitational security
Basic sensory channels	Tactile Auditory Vestibular	Visual Kinesthetic Proprioceptive

Physiological reactions that can interfere with the development of the higher senses include: nutrient deficiencies, immune system dysfunction, chemical sensitivities, inflammation, and allergies.

Ear Infections

"Mommy, did you have tubes in your ears when you were young?" The Feingold mom thought her child's question was silly until she stopped to think about it.

Most of the children on the block suffered from chronic ear infections -- all but two families: hers and the family with the reputation as "health nuts."

Feingold parents frequently report that one of the benefits of the program is that their children's ear infections either stop or are greatly reduced. Some new information suggests a connection between the increased use of food additives and a dramatic increase in chronic ear infections.

Dramatic increase

Susan M. Schappert, an epidemiologist at the National Center for Health Statistics, found that the number of doctor visits for ear infections in children under the age of 2 increased a whopping 224% between 1975 and 1990. Why? Some suggest it is because more young children are in day care centers where they are exposed to infection. But this doesn't seem to be a valid reason since the number of older children suffering from ear infections has risen as well.

Otitis Media

This is the name for middle ear inflammation. The typical symptoms include earache, pressure and a feeling of blockage in the ear, muffled hearing, sometimes accompanied by a fever. Pre-schoolers are the most vulnerable and the problem is greatest in the winter and early spring months. Otitis media is the most common ailment after colds. The Food and Drug Administration reports that "half of all children will have an ear infection before their first birthday, and nearly 90 percent by age 6."

Ear infections account for 30 million doctor visits per year at an annual cost of about $2 billion for diagnosis and treatment with antibiotics, according to the Otitis Media Advisory Council.

Antibiotics

The commonly used antibiotic, amoxicillin, has generated heated debate among doctors. While it is accepted as a treatment for acute ear infections (accompanied by a high fever and a painful earache), most physicians also use it to treat chronic inflammation of the middle ear (otitis media).

Writing in the *British Medical Journal*, Dr. George G. Browning notes, "...in most children antibiotics make no difference to the outcome in either the short or the long term. More than 85% of the children will be pain free within 24 hours irrespective of whether they have been treated with an antibiotic or not." *(Br. Med. J. 1990:300 1006-1007).*

Another blow to traditional treatment was struck by Erdem I. Cantekin, Ph.D. from the Children's Hospital of Pittsburgh. He was part of a team investigating the effectiveness of antibiotic treatment for ear infections. Writing in the *Journal of the AMA*, Cantekin found that amoxicillin "is not effective in the treatment of persistent asymptomatic middle ear effusions [fluid build-up] in infants and children." He concluded,. "recurrence rates were significantly higher in the antibiotic-treated group than in the placebo group." The article claims that children who take amoxicillin for chronic ear infections are up to six times more likely to have a return of the symptoms than children who took a placebo *(JAMA, Dec. 18, 1991 - Vol. 266, No. 23).*

Both Cantekin and Browning point out that European doctors use far less antibiotics for ear infections.

Dr. Charles Bluestone, the primary researcher for the Pittsburgh study, came to a different conclusion, writing that the use of antibiotics "increases to some extent the likelihood of resolution" of the chronic ear infections.

What followed was a battle where Cantekin was accused of unethical practices, and dismissed from his job. Bluestone, in turn, was criticized for accepting $260,000 from the pharmaceutical company SmithKline Beecham and $3.5 million in research grants *(JAMA editorial, 12/18/91).*

The Feingold perspective on ear infections

The practice of adding synthetic dyes and artificial flavorings to pediatric medicine is hard to justify. The experience of our member families, along with the critical reports noted above, suggests that these additives in antibiotics could play a part in triggering a child's next episode of otitis media.

If your child takes medication of any kind, try to obtain it in an uncolored form. The Feingold Association's *Medication List* will be helpful, and your doctor or pharmacist can assist you in locating a suitable product. If you are unable to find what you need, consider contacting the Professional Compounding Centers of America for the name of a compounding pharmacist near you. The number is 1 (800) 331-2498.

Please Note: Unlike otitis media, acute ear infection is a serious condition that can cause damage. Always consult your physician in the case of illness.

Allergies, sensitivities and ear infections

An allergic response can cause swelling of tissues in any part of the body. The same may be true for chemical sensitivity. When the swelling occurs in the Eustachian tube it blocks this canal, preventing fluid from draining out. As fluid builds up in the middle ear, it provides a fertile breeding ground for bacteria and infection.

Other potential offenders

Milk - Some doctors report that milk allergy is a likely trigger for ear infections. Allergy, particularly to milk, is not unusual among Feingold members, and this would be worth investigating if your child continues to have ear infections. Milk sensitivity can also trigger behavior problems in many children.

Smoking - The child who is exposed to cigarette smoke is nearly three times as likely to suffer from persistent otitis media, and when more cigarettes are smoked the child's risk increases even further. This data was reported in the *Journal of the American Medical Association* by researchers at Seattle's Children's Orthopedic Hospital and Medical Center *(JAMA 249: 1022-25).*

Eye-Muscle Disorders

Strabismus

The pregnancy was normal, the birth fast, and we had another little boy. Since we had a little fella only a year-and-a-half at home, we thought how nice it would be to have built-in friends.

All seemed to be fine until Marty was about 4 months old. The crying started and it did not stop. My pediatrician even commented on the fact that she could not examine him. At about 8 months he seemed to be frustrated at the fact that he could not communicate with me and would scream at me over something like a balloon in the store.

At 15 months he was extremely proficient in speech and ordered the entire household to be at his command. The stress caused by this crying and demands was taking its toll on our family. We could not have friends in nor could we take this baby anywhere.... If we finally got him to sleep, the slightest noise would wake him up and the crying would start up again. This crying continued long after his second birthday; the poor baby was begging for help. He never awakened NOT crying until he was almost 4, even on Christmas.

When Marty was 2-and-a-half I started the long trek for a doctor to help me, even to listen to me. How can any reasonable person tell you to BE FIRM with a baby that hasn't slept in 30 hours? We both needed help so badly. I now began to think "allergies." The first allergist told me to take him for an enzyme study at a university hospital. The hospital was not interested because he did not have diarrhea, but told me if it were an enzyme problem it would take care of itself at puberty. I cried -- I couldn't go on for ten more minutes much less ten years. After spending thousands of dollars, this summarized his medical report: "An important key to improving Marty's life is to reduce biochemical stress as much as possible."

Just after Marty turned 3 I noticed his left eye turning in. In a way I was relieved -- I was sure he had a tumor. The doctors, my family, my friends could no longer say that I had spoiled this child. *I* could not make his eyes cross, after all. Maybe a medical answer would be imminent. Finally, there would be answers to weeks without sleep, incessant crying, and violent rages. I braced myself for the worst. No matter what the diagnosis, any answer would give me hope that something would be done for him. I was desperate. A well-respected eye doctor, highly recommended, found no problem. His eyes continued to turn in. Six months later he was given glasses for farsightedness.

Months went by and the children in Marty's class could all print their name on their Valentine cards. Marty couldn't. Now a teacher sees a problem and another door is opened for me. She did tell me to seriously consider holding him back a year from kindergarten.

Like a miracle I met Feingold parents who helped me to get Marty on the diet 100%. We had previously eliminated the colors and flavors, but not the preservatives and salicylates. We started the diet 100% on January 25. Soon his eyes were no longer crossed. In March we had his eyes thoroughly examined, and glasses were no longer needed. That August he was tested by the school district. He was not below normal in anything and was above average in many things. We are having no problems in kindergarten. He is doing beautifully.

Marty's eyes still cross if he is on a reaction -- if he eats any food with a forbidden chemical additive. We feel the salicylates were the greatest offenders. We can only imagine what the little head must feel like, when these [salicylates and] chemicals are powerful enough to make those eyes cross.

Nystagmus

This is a condition where the eyes rapidly, involuntarily vibrate, making normal vision impossible.

Dr. Feingold learned about the effects of diet and nystagmus from one of the families using the Program. He found that removal of additives and salicylates was essential, and that benzoates -- both naturally occurring and synthetic -- were also major offenders. Benzoates are found in some foods, such as cranberries, and are used as a preservative (sodium benzoate).

Hives: The Start of the Feingold Program

In his book, *Why Your Child Is Hyperactive*, Dr. Feingold described how he devised the K-P (Kaiser Permanente) diet, for the purpose of treating aspirin-sensitive patients who suffered from hives. The use of the diet to help children with behavior and learning problems was a later development.

The first person to use what the media later called the "Feingold diet" was not a hyperactive child. It was a woman in her forties. Dr. Feingold wrote: "In the summer of 1965 a woman entered my office in the allergy clinic of the Kaiser Permanente Medical Center. She was suffering from acute hives. Her face was swollen, mainly about the eyes. An eruption of the skin, giant hives can be moderately painful and unsightly to the point of the grotesque. She looked, and obviously felt, miserable.

"I read the medical history of this patient, examined her and tested her for allergy. Since the tests were negative, I concluded that artificial food colors and flavors might be involved.

"Food additives had been a causative factor in previous cases of hives that I had seen. I immediately placed her on a diet to which she quickly responded. The skin condition vanished within seventy-two hours."

from *Why Your Child Is Hyperactive*

Studies on hives

The Journal of Allergy & Clinical Immunology reported the results of a single-blind study which explored the role of food additives as a causative factor in asthma and urticaria (hives). The study involved a total of 34 subjects. Seventeen of them suffered from chronic urticaria, 14 from asthma, and 3 had both.

Yellow dye (tartrazine) and aspirin were the worst offenders in provoking hives; sulfur dioxide presented the greatest prob1em for the asthmatic subjects.

Source: "Value of Oral Provocation Tests to Aspirin and Food Additives in the Routine Investigation of Asthma and Chronic Urticaria." Genton C, Frei P, Pecoud A. *Journal of Allergy & Clinical Immunology* 1985;76 (1);40-45.Vol. 10, No. 10

Researchers in Britain documented the connection between food additives and hives in a double-blind study that took place at the Paediatric Allergy Clinic, St. Mary's Hospital in London. Reporting in the October 18, 1986 issue of *The Lancet,* Supramaniam and Warner found that more than half of the children tested developed symptoms of hives and/or angio-oedema (swelling of the skin) when challenged with food additives.

Forty-three children who responded to an additive-free diet were challenged with artificial food additives in a double-blind study, and 24 of them reacted to one or more of the additives. (Feingold members will be surprised to learn that aspirin sensitivity was detected in only one of the subjects.) The children ranged from age 3 to 14. Twenty-four reacted to one or more of the additives, but none of the children reacted to them all.

One of the surprising discoveries was that an extremely small dose of just 1 mg. was sufficient to trigger a response in some of the children. (This type of extreme sensitivity was later observed by Rowe & Rowe, reporting in the November 1994 issue of *The Journal of Pediatrics.*) In contrast, the Egger study of diet and hyperactivity used 150 mg. of tartrazine for a period of one week *(The Lancet, March 9, 1985).*

This extreme sensitivity confirms what Feingold parents have long known: Grandma's protest that "just a little bit won't hurt" isn't necessarily so.

The researchers go on to say, however, that the patients were carefully monitored in the hospital during the challenges, and some of the symptoms may have gone unnoticed in another setting. But for some of the subjects, their sensitivity was so keen, the authors noted, that it could have been dangerous to challenge them with the 150-mg. dose.

The additives tested were:
Tartrazine (Yellow No. 5)
Sunset Yellow (Yellow No. 6)
Amaranth (Red No. 2 -- banned in the U.S.)
Indigo carmine (Blue No. 2)
Carmoisine (a red dye not used in the U.S.)
Sodium Benzoate
MSG
Sodium metabisulphite
Aspirin

More than half of the children reacted to one or more of the food additives.

Hives and stress

Deborah never had any reason to be concerned about food additives and salicylates -- until she was 32. That was a very stressful time in her life: a divorce, move to a new home, a new job -- and hives! "Horrible hives, body welts," Deborah told *Pure Facts.* Itchy, disfiguring hives were appearing every other day, accompanied by fatigue.

She sought help from four different dermatologists in the San Francisco area. "These were highly respected doctors," she said, "top men in their field, and they told me they were sorry. 'There is nothing we can do.' One of them gave me an antihistamine (bright blue pills), but not one said anything about aspirin sensitivity or about a change in diet.

"My boyfriend finally persuaded me to see his doctor - the head of the department of internal medicine at the University of California/San Francisco." Through his efforts Deborah learned about the Feingold Program. "I began the Program in April and within three days the hives were gone. My boyfriend is so excited about the change the diet has brought for me. He is on it himself, feels great, and tells everyone about it."

Deborah hasn't been eager to try adding back salicylates. After two years of suffering from hives, she is enjoying feeling well, and finds plenty of food to enjoy on Stage I (non-salicylate list). Even the smallest infraction (dye especially) brings a return of the hives, and a bad case can take as long as seven days to go away.

Although she did not have a history of the childhood behavior problems typical of many Feingold adults, Deborah noted that she experiences behavior changes (as well as the hives) when there is an infraction. She becomes very tense, irritable, uncoordinated and accident-prone. "I'm a tense wreck!"

As assistant manager of a tennis-health club, Deborah has no difficulty staying on the diet at work. Those around her have been very interested, and she has provided them with information about the Program.

Letter from a child

"I get giant hives from an artificial color, called tartrazine, Yellow dye #5, and also from some artificial flavors. The pediatrician told me that the giant hives could kill me! In fact I have had to go to the hospital several times because of giant hives in my throat, and they gave me shots of adrenaline. I know that the Feingold diet can save my life because there are so many foods that have artificial colors and flavors."

Timmy, Age 11

Nasal Polyps

Chad went on the Feingold Program to support his son, but it turned out that his own response has been even more dramatic. He used to suffer from painful nasal polyps.

"Suffer" certainly is an appropriate word for anyone afflicted with nasal polyps. These are nodules that form in the cavities behind the nose and adjacent to the sinuses. They are little sacs that develop by themselves or in groups, and a single polyp can become as large as a grape. There isn't much extra room in this area, and as these growths enlarge and multiply they prevent drainage and put pressure on the adjacent organs. The result is a feeling of heaviness and intense pressure, with painful, pounding headaches.

Treatment usually begins with antihistamines, decongestants, and possibly allergy shots. In severe cases doctors prescribe steroids to help shrink the polyps, and then perform surgery to cut them out. Since the surgeon is working in an area where there are so many vital organs, it is necessary for the patient to be able to respond to instructions. Because only light sedation is used, the procedure is quite painful.

A few weeks after the family began using the Feingold Program, not only was his son doing well, but Chad began to see a big difference in how he felt. The pressure, the headaches, nasal congestion, and of course the polyps somehow seemed to be connected to the ingestion of certain food additives and salicylates.

The doctor who had been caring for Chad, an eminent allergist and ENT specialist, was astonished. "You were one of my worst patients," he exclaimed, "what have you done?" Chad replied, "Have you ever heard of Feingold?" Yes, the doctor had, but had never paid much attention to it. "I need a copy of this diet," he told Chad, "we might become famous over this!"

Chad may or may not someday become a footnote in a medical text. For now, just feeling good is enough.

Seizure Disorders -- Does Diet Play a Role?

"My name is Brewer and I don't eat additives." Brewer's mom explained that this is the way her 8-year-old son introduces himself. These eight years have been difficult for the family. Not only did Brewer have the classic symptoms of the ADHD child, but he also suffered from several kinds of seizures.

"He was always active and getting into everything," recalls his mother, "and if he had a seizure while he was up in a tree, it meant a fall. He always seemed to be bloody." The Feingold diet improved his behavior "about 100%" according to his mom -- so much that most people refuse to believe that Brewer has ever been hyperactive. The diet has not had any effect on the seizures, however; that is under control through a combination of surgery and medication. But Brewer's mom is enthusiastic about the help the Feingold Program has provided. "When you have a child with a problem as serious as seizures," she told *Pure Facts*, "the last thing you need is to add in hyperactivity."

Another family's experience

Carrie was an impossible baby. The youngest of four, neither her mother, who is a teacher, nor her father, a physician, were able to comfort or control her.

The seizures started slowly, and by the time Carrie was eight they had her parents and pediatrician gravely concerned. A ten-day hospital stay, countless tests, and consultation with experts in several fields did not yield any answers as to why Carrie had seizures. They found only that the neurological signs were not there.

While the tests indicated "nothing wrong," the truth was that everything was wrong; Carrie's destructive behavior created havoc in the family.

"Out of sheer desperation" the family tried the Feingold Program. (A day of picking -- and eating -- apples resulted in the worst episode ever. Salicylates would be found to be a major offender.) Within two weeks of beginning the Program, Carrie's behavior became normal and she has not had a seizure since. In her case the seizures were strictly "psychomotor" episodes. Today she is an honor student in college.

Seizures -- another aspect of the problem

Stewart is not our "Feingold" child but he needs the diet as much as his younger brother.

Following a severe viral infection, our 12-year-old son had a seizure. The doctor put him on Tegretol, and he seemed to do quite well on the medication. When the white tablet was changed to pink, I knew synthetic dye had been added, but wasn't too concerned since it's our 10-year-old, Michael, who is on the Feingold diet.

The seizures were under control, but Stewart wasn't. He had always received top grades in school; he really liked it, and thrived on the competition. It was clear that he would be going on to the top academic high school in our area. Suddenly, he began to bring home failing grades; he was getting into trouble in school; he became very loud, walking into things, and began slurring his words.

Maybe it was a "slump," maybe it's just his age. (Stewart was now 13.) My husband and I tried to make sense out of this drastic change, as did his teachers and principal. Testing by a psychologist brought a chilling message. Our son had developed a "permanent learning disability," she told us. We had better forget any thoughts of an academic education and look for a skill he could be trained in. She also suggested we have his neurologist put him on Ritalin. (This was totally out of the question. Michael had a terrible time with it.)

Driving home, Stewart asked, "Mom, do you think I'm allergic to the red dye in the pills the way Michael is?" No. I was sure this wasn't it, but the next time we saw the neurologist I asked him. "No." He didn't think so, but did not entirely rule out the possibility.

I wanted to pursue Stewart's hunch, and tried to obtain a month's supply of the uncolored Tegretol so I could test it, but nobody seemed to understand what I was trying to do. I called the manufacturer, doctors, and pharmacists. When I called the Philadelphia College of Pharmacy they informed me the medication is available in the white generic form and told me where I could obtain it.

Stewart began using the uncolored medication on a Monday. Tuesday afternoon I was at the school and saw his homeroom teacher. "I can't believe the difference in this child," she told me. "Up until now he was so fidgety, touching everything and everyone; I thought he was just being 13-years-old."

A few days later his English teacher sought me out and had a similar story. "I don't know what's going on, but Stewart is unbelievable. For months he has been sitting in my class staring into space...as though he had no interest in anything. Today he had his hand raised for every question."

At the end of the week our "permanently learning disabled" son won the class spelling bee!

"Reaction Reported to the Dye in Tegretol"

The August 1988 issue of *Archives of Neurology* published a letter from Ivan S. Logan, M.D., or the Department of Neurology at the University of Virginia. In it, Dr. Logan described the symptoms experienced by an adult patient, diagnosed with epilepsy, who had been successfully treated with Tegretol. After the manufacturer changed the medicine by adding red dye, the woman reported that within a few hours of taking the dyed pill she began feeling "uptight, tenseness of the scalp, feeling veins and arteries popping out from the skin, coughing, dry heaves, and a crawling and itchy feeling in the skin, but without rash."

Dr. Logan experimented with use of both undyed and dyed Tegretol, and found that the symptoms could be replicated when the dyed pill was used. He also noted that, "Anecdotal reports of altered clinical status associated with the introduction of the new Tegretol tablets have also recently appeared in the epilepsy lay press."

Seizures, Tegretol and dyes

The child who suffers from both seizures and hyperactivity faces a difficult choice.

For many years the treatment of choice for most of these youngsters has been Tegretol (carbamazepine), available in an uncolored white tablet. When the synthetic dyes (Red No. 3 and Red No. 40) were added to the drug, families following the Feingold Program were alarmed. Although carbamazepine is available in the generic form, some parents have said that this is not identical to Tegretol, and cannot be used with success by all children.

More recently a liquid form of Tegretol has been introduced, but it is unacceptable because it contains Yellow No. 6 and "flavoring." *Pure Facts* spoke with a physician representing CIBA Geigy, the company making Tegretol; he insisted that adding dye to this drug is essential in order to gain a child's cooperation. This is despite the fact that the bottle used would be brown, so the only time the child would see the liquid would be when the spoon went from the bottle to his mouth.

What can a parent do?

You may want to consider finding a "compounding pharmacist" to help you get a form of the carbamazepine which duplicates Tegretol, minus the added dyes/flavorings. One compounding pharmacist explained that the reason families were not successful using the generic was that the strength is permitted to vary significantly.

To obtain the name of a compounding pharmacist in your area call the Professional Compounding Centers of America at (800) 331-2498.

A Good Night's Sleep

A Feingold adult relates a connection between additives, salicylates, and sleep disturbances.

Denise began the Feingold diet way back in 1972, a year before Dr. Feingold first introduced his program to the American Medical Association. Her aunt had learned of Feingold's work and had successfully used the diet with her son. Denise's mother hoped it would help her daughter to sleep normally.

She was an impulsive child, and often seemed to be lost in her thoughts, but for Denise the most troublesome thing was being unable to fall asleep at night. "I remember being in bed for hours, and would ask 'Mom, how do you go to sleep?'" she recalls.

Seventeen years later, Denise still sees the difference foods and salicylates make -- both in her sleep and in her 3-year-old daughter's behavior.

Sweet dreams for Katie

We have been on the Feingold diet for 1 year now. From the time our daughter could walk, until she was 22 months old, her naps lasted only 45 minutes; after that she took no naps at all.

Every night it took Katie well over three hours to go to sleep. Then we had night after night full of night terrors.

We stayed home most all the time because Katie was always running on a destructive course. If we were where there were toys and lots for her to do, she would check it out for a few minutes then would be gone checking out the building and whatever else she could find. Usually she just ran and DID -- not to be mean, but because she totally couldn't help herself. My Mom found an article on your diet and thought it sounded like there was help. I was so glad to receive your information so quickly.

Katie was to the point that she could no longer even do a puzzle without crying and saying "I can't, I can't." She couldn't sit to do anything.

After 3 days on the diet she asked to do puzzles. She took out her most frustrating puzzle, the one she just takes out one piece and quits. Well, not that day. She sat calmly and hummed a song and did the whole thing, plus all her other puzzles. I said, "Katie, how would you like to cut something out?" and she did it!

Needless to say her night terrors are gone and she goes to sleep in about 10 - 15 minutes most nights. She still is a pretty wound up little girl, but I feel there is hope. I used to feel like I would crack, and end up with an ulcer. We are very good friends with our doctor and he knows Katie and us so well; he has helped a lot in all our healing.

I am very lucky to have such a supportive husband and we all work together. Our little boy doesn't have the problem and neither does my husband, but I know I do. There are many foods that cause me to have trouble sleeping. My Mom wishes she had known about the Feingold Program long ago.

I know our problem wasn't as extreme as some, but it has worn on us so we thank you for all your help and we do spread the word.

Narcolepsy and sleep apnea

Narcolepsy (an inability to stay awake), sleep apnea syndrome (the periodic cessation of breathing while asleep), depression, irritability, excessive fatigue, headaches -- these are just some of the maladies and discomforts which adults have reportedly eliminated or brought under control by going on the Feingold Program, says Jack J., a long-time adult member and volunteer who had been diagnosed as having severe sleep apnea syndrome.

Jack first learned of the Feingold Program in 1978 when he saw Dr. Feingold on the Phil Donahue Show. He was home at the time "being a house-husband," he says. "Because my condition included an inability to concentrate and make decisions, I had to quit my job as a mechanical engineer two years earlier."

His condition was so severe that a tracheostomy had been performed on him in hopes of alleviating the problem. The tracheostomy did not help. "But," he says, "within five days after eliminating synthetic colors, flavors and preservatives, I was a whole different person."

Jack returned to work and has helped many other adults with problems that might be caused by synthetic chemicals. "There are a lot of people around who could simply be better than they are now, but these chemicals get in the way."

He has heard success stories from other adults, many of whom started on the Program because of a hyperactive son or daughter. But, they say, their efforts were doubly rewarded when they found that their own physical or mental difficulties were eased by the elimination of certain synthetic chemicals.

"One woman wrote that her husband became violent, with an uncontrollable temper when he went off the diet," Jack recalled. "Another woman says she no longer feels her usual rush of anger after being on the diet for only three days. And a member in Florida wrote about becoming depressed, mean and grouchy after drinking two glasses of fresh orange juice (a salicylate).

"We have no real scientific evidence as to why these offending substances trigger such a wide variety of adult problems," he says. "All we know is that they do for some people. We don't even know how many people are involved, although we suspect that the number is considerable.

"Considering the nature of some of the ailments that have responded to the Feingold Program (and by this I mean sleep apnea syndrome, narcolepsy, petit mal seizures and numerous cerebral problems that have been reported) it's a good layman's guess that the central nervous system is affected by these offending substances. In fact, I would not be surprised by any neurological dysfunction responding to the Feingold Program."

Jack noted that many people are also affected by environmental factors (newsprint, tar, pesticides, gas appliances) and by such substances as sodium benzoate, MSG, corn syrup and even brown sugar, which is not routinely eliminated.

For any adult considering the Feingold Program, Jack says, "there is everything to gain and nothing to lose but some effort, but each individual must determine for himself if the program is the answer for his unique problem."

Crib death linked to sleep apnea

Sleep apnea syndrome is a condition where the sleeper snores loudly, sometimes gasping for breath. Breathing ceases for at least ten seconds, and often longer, and these episodes are repeated many times throughout the night. It is believed to affect several million Americans, most of them men.

According to the Food and Drug Administration (FDA), "The loudest snores come from those who experience seriously disturbed breathing during sleep. Some victims may not breathe at all for three-quarters of their time asleep. Breathing pauses have been recorded for as long as three minutes. Four minutes without oxygen can result in irreversible brain damage. Alcohol, sleeping pills, and tranquilizers can make sleep apnea worse."

The FDA further notes, "Autopsies suggest that sudden infant death syndrome (SIDS) may be caused by repeated periods of inadequate oxygen intake brought on by respiratory abnormalities such as sleep apnea, though other factors may also be involved."

SIDS

Additional support for the connection between adult sleep apnea and SIDS was published in *Pediatrics* magazine in 1988.

The work of a Norwegian physician, Torleiv O. Rognum, indicates that these babies die as a result of lack of oxygen. The researchers found that the bodies of infants who had died of SIDS contained large amounts of a chemical called hypoxanthine. Earlier work shows that the body's production of this substance rises when it is deprived of oxygen for long periods of time.

SIDS is responsible for the death of between one and two of every 1,000 infants before their first birthday.

Sleep disorders and salicylates

Sleep is supposed to be a restful experience, but for Gloria, sleep was exhausting. Shortly after falling asleep her heart would begin to beat irregularly. "I would suddenly awaken and find myself sitting bolt upright, or even standing beside the bed, feeling short of breath and wondering what hit me."

Gloria began to notice a pattern, with severe sleep attacks occurring after she had eaten tomato sauce, an apple, strawberries, or pineapple (a trace salicylate). Stripping furniture with chemical solvents also caused an attack.

She described her experiences: Then I began to experience more severe problems. I had been painting the house, and the following morning the right side of my face went numb. I experienced slurred speech, dizziness, blurred vision, and constant fatigue. I felt like I had been hit in the head with a rubber mallet.

All of these attacks occurred within one hour of eating, but I couldn't find a correlation. I was also doing decorative painting almost every day with oil-based paints. I asked every doctor if this could be a factor. No one knew.

I visited many doctors in my search for relief. The drugs I was given brought a host of severe reactions, including a full scale Meiners attack, which is best described as a wide awake nightmare.

The cardiologist put me in the hospital for a two-week stay. Then I was given more drugs, and found to be intolerant of all of them. (The sleeping pill was red.)

"I remember feeling like I had spent the night fighting for my life."

When I left the hospital, I went on a diet recommended by the hospital's nutritionist. It was basically a weight control diet with fruit three times a day.

My attacks became worse than ever. I had difficulty breathing and felt like I was coming apart at the seams. My doctor said I was suffering from anxiety depression. He said the drugs were not causing my problems because "only people who read books have side effects."

I ended up in church next Sunday asking God for a clue. On Tuesday I made an appointment with an allergist because I knew I had attacks after eating.

I no sooner told the allergist I was having a sleep disorder problem when he leaned forward in his chair and said, "I know what's causing it; you have anxiety depression." So-o-o I said "let me describe my symptoms."

The allergist told me he didn't deal with food allergies as he had his hands full with pollen. (We live in the pollen capital of the world.) But as I was walking out the door he ponderingly said, "Maybe you are intolerant to salicylates in foods." The word struck like an arrow piercing my brain...I can still feel the sensation. My first clue. (I later went back and thanked him for that word.)

But at the time I felt like I was at another blind spot in the road. I was in tears by the time I returned home and found my sister on the phone waiting to talk with me. I told her what I had learned so far and mentioned the foods I had identified as causes. When the conversation, and my crying, had ended I learned that my niece and her friend were in the next room and heard my phone conversation.

They came into the kitchen and my niece's friend said, "You know you sound as if you have the same problem as the hyperactive children I teach. Some of them can't tolerate salicylates."

Voila! My second clue. SALICYLATES! That wonderful word spoken twice in one hour. She told me about Dr. Feingold's book, and I was at the bookstore an hour before it opened.

Within three days there were no more irregular heartbeat attacks when I slept. That was August of 1984 and I've been able to see a correlation between the attacks and heavy use of household cleaners, oil-based paint, and natural gas. That explains why I would become so irritable or have an extreme exhaustion spell after cooking a big meal. I have not felt that way since I turned the gas off and began using my electric skillet and microwave oven.

Much love and my thanks to everyone at FAUS.

What is Tourette syndrome?

Tourette Syndrome (TS) is a neurological disorder characterized by involuntary muscular movements and one or more vocal tics.

These multiple tics usually begin when the patient is between the ages of 2 and 16. Males are afflicted about three times more often than females. For information, contact the Tourette Syndrome Association, 42-40 Bell Boulevard, Suite 205, Bayside, New York 11361-2820. Phone: (718) 224-2999.

Alternatives to medication for Tourette syndrome

The Tourette Syndrome Association (TSA) has long received reports of non-drug therapies which have helped families deal with TS. The Alternative Therapy Network, which functions independently from the TSA, collects information on techniques that have been used by those dealing with TS.

One of the popular alternatives is diet management, which, while not yet proven as successful for Tourette syndrome as it is for hyperactivity and attention deficit disorder, has helped many families. Sheila Rogers, who heads the network, says, "Most of the information we have received relates to diet control, nutritional supplementation and environmental allergy therapy. A high percentage of those with TS appear to have allergies and/or sensitivities to foods and chemicals in foods, as well as to chemicals in the environment."

To receive information on the network and its excellent newsletter, *Latitudes*, or to share your experiences, write to: Sheila Rogers, 1120 Royal Palm Beach Blvd., #283, Royal Palm Beach FL 33411 (561) 798-0472.

The Alternative Therapy Network marks the first systematic effort to collect information on the effectiveness of non-drug therapy for TS. Ruth Bruun, M.D., former chairman of the TSA Medical Committee, writes, "It has generally been acknowledged that TS and tics may actually encompass a variety of different disorders with different causes. Therefore, certain treatments may be valid only for some patients. Other treatments, which may be only mildly effective in most patients, may be effective in a patient with mild symptoms or may be effective as an adjunct to one of the standard medications.

"Medications produce their effects by altering the rate of formation and release in the brain of certain neurotransmitters (chemical compounds which carry messages from one nerve cell to another). Since certain nutrients are necessary as building blocks for the manufacture in the body of these neurotransmitters, it is logical to assume that these nutrients may also have an influence on behavior. It has been demonstrated, for example, that a meal which is rich in lecithin (i.e., one containing eggs or liver) may elevate the level of choline in the brain and thus cause an increase in the amount of the neurotransmitter, acetylcholine."

Genetic basis for Tourette syndrome

Tourette Syndrome was long considered to be a psychiatric disorder, but is now believed to be the result of an inherited gene. While boys are most likely to exhibit the symptoms, particularly tics, girls are more likely to have obsessive-compulsive behaviors. It is still not clear how these various pieces of the puzzle fit together, and what part diet may play.

Another trigger for tics

Some children develop tics after they have had a bout with strep, according to researchers at Brown University School of Medicine and Memorial Hospital of Rhode Island.

When a child has an infection, the body creates antibodies to fight it. A strep infection appears to stimulate a form of antibodies that affects the neurotransmitters, which in turn, can trigger tics and a wide range of symptoms (hyperactivity, ADD, obsessive-compulsive disorder, etc.).

If your child has had a strep infection, which is followed by any of these symptoms, you may want to refer your pediatrician to the following article and consider the appropriate tests and treatments. The citation is: "Antineuronal Antibodies in Movement Disorders," by Louise S. Kiessling, M.D., Ann C. Marcotte, Ph.D., and Larry Culpepper, M.D., MPH, *Pediatrics* Vol. 92 No. 1 July 1993.

TS and ADD/ADHD

David Comings, M.D., is director of the Tourette Syndrome Clinic in Southern California, and author of *Tourette Syndrome and Human Behavior*. Dr. Comings noted that the individual with TS is very likely to also have one or more other problems such as hyperactivity, attention deficit disorder, dyslexia, conduct disorders, mood swings, migraine headaches, panic attacks, speech or sleep problems, or addictive behaviors.

Dr. Harvey Singer, director of the Tourette Syndrome Clinic at Johns Hopkins University, says that 50 to 60 percent of TS patients also have ADHD (attention deficit hyperactivity disorder). One of the most controversial aspects of treating such people is that some of the medicines used for these conditions can bring on or worsen the TS symptoms.

Some doctors say that the drug, Ritalin, can cause the symptoms to appear in a child who is predisposed to having TS. They do not use the drug if there is a family history of tic disorders. Other doctors contend that such a child would eventually have the tics and other symptoms anyway, and the Ritalin just causes them to appear sooner. This is very different from the information provided by Ciba-Geigy, the manufacturer of Ritalin. The company has published a warning in the *Physician's Desk Reference*, "Ritalin is contraindicated...in patients with motor tics or with a family history or diagnosis of Tourette syndrome."

Ritalin and tics: one child's story

"In the May issue of *Pure Facts* there was an article about children who use Ritalin in addition to the Feingold diet, to better control themselves. My husband and I also had to make that decision. Our son had been on the Feingold diet for two years, but needed additional measures to successfully meet the expectations of full day kindergarten. We started out on 5 mg. of Ritalin, and by the time he was going into first grade the dosage had been increased to 20 mg. According to the *Physician's Desk Reference*, Ritalin dosage should not exceed 60 mg. daily.

"He was having problems paying attention at the onset of first grade, so his doctor increased the dosage by another 5 mg.

After the increase in Ritalin our son started to have multiple, persistent, involuntary motor and vocal tics.

"Before we started the medication, my husband and I asked about side effects. We were assured the most serious side effect he would probably experience was a stomachache. We were also given some papers for further information. One section mentioned that a serious side effect that may occur is TS symptoms. If that happens, medication should be stopped immediately, and the symptoms should stop. It also stated that if the symptoms do not cease, your child had TS since birth, and the Ritalin simply caused the symptoms to emerge sooner. He said they would have eventually emerged a few years later if not on the medication.

"After the increase in Ritalin, our son started to have multiple, persistent, involuntary motor and vocal tics. We stopped the Ritalin, but the symptoms became worse. These involuntary vocal tics increased up to 40 times per minute. He was not able to function at school; he basically could not function at all.

Our doctor initially told us that our son had TS from birth, but later admitted that he was never "born" with it, that the Ritalin had caused it.

"Before all this happened, we had heard of a center which treats ADHD. No medication is used, only vitamins, minerals and amino acids according to excesses or deficiencies in certain blood levels [the Carl Pfeiffer Treatment Center in Naperville, IL].

"In four days of treatment his symptoms decreased dramatically and by the fifth day he only had TS symptoms periodically. It took another two months before they were gone completely. The doctors at the center did not know that the nutrients would help get the Ritalin out of his system. Its primary purpose was to lower his histamine level. Thankfully, it did both.

"Today his blood levels are much closer to normal range. He has been on this program for six months now and is much better behaved and more focused than he ever was on Ritalin. Our son remains on the Feingold Program, but we are able to be more flexible as he can tolerate more kinds of foods."

FOOD ALLERGIES

If you are completely on Stage One, but still having problems, consider food allergies.

"Any compound in existence, natural or synthetic, has the potential to induce an adverse reaction in any individual with the appropriate genetic profile."

Ben F. Feingold, M.D.

Dr. Feingold, who was an allergist as well as a pediatrician, recognized that an individual could be sensitive to, or allergic to, virtually anything. In developing the "K-P Diet" (now known as the Feingold Program) he focused on just a few substances: synthetic food dyes, synthetic flavorings, three antioxidants, and the temporary removal of "salicylates." He narrowed down the focus to these -- not because they are the only, or even the most important items to avoid -- but because his many years as a clinician taught him that they are major offenders for many people.

A brief history of allergy

1905 Francis Hare, an Australian physician, published *The Food Factor in Disease,* after connecting migraine headaches with food.
1906 Dr. Clemens Von Pirquet, of Vienna, Austria, coined the word 'allergy' to describe an adverse response to substances which don't affect most people. Dr. Feingold later studied with Dr. Von Pirquet.
1908 A child whose allergy to eggs provoked asthmatic attacks was successfully immunized by the English doctor, Schofield.
1912 A New York doctor successfully duplicated Schofield's work.
1917 Food allergy symptoms reported in the *Journal of Urology.*
1921 "Food Allergy as a Cause of Abdominal Pain" was published by W.W. Duke. He followed with similar articles connecting allergies to bladder pain and Meniere's Syndrome.
1931 *Food Allergy: Its Manifestation, Diagnosis & Treatment* by Albert Rowe was the first book on the subject.
1942 Arthur Coca, M.D. published *Familial Nonreaginic Food-Allergy.*
1951 Rinkel, Randolph and Zeller published *Food Allergy.*
1958 English psychiatrist Richard Mackarness connected obesity with food allergy.

1962 This is the year of Rachel Carson's *Silent Spring* and Dr. Theron Randolph's *Human Ecology & Susceptibility to the Chemical Environment.*
1973 Dr. Feingold's book *Introduction to Clinical Allergy* was published.

"Allergy" vs. "sensitivity"
The reaction most Feingold members experience to certain additives and salicylates is not an allergic reaction, Dr. Feingold believed.

He considered it a pharmacologic, or drug-like response, and felt that it was dose-related. This means that the "hyperactive" child is simply more sensitive than his peers -- that he has a lower tolerance for some chemicals. The reaction one experiences from a sensitivity to additives can "mask" itself as an allergic response. So the more familiar reactions such as hives, rashes, or respiratory problems could be the result of food additives, not pollen or your pet cat.

"Allergy is an inherited constitutional disorder involving the immune system," Dr. Feingold wrote in *The Feingold Cookbook*. "Intolerance to food additives and salicylates is not an immunological disturbance. Therefore, it is not allergy. It may clinically simulate allergy, but the two are not identical.

"Skin tests for food allergy are not reliable and therefore are not recommended. Skin tests for intolerance to food additives have no value."

A true allergic reaction involves the body's immune system. But the reaction most people have to additives is a pharmacologic (drug-like) one, and is dose-related. This means that Johnny may become aggressive from a single sip of synthetic "fruit" punch, whereas Tommy may have to drink an entire glass before we see his behavior change.

With an allergy, Jenny reacts to one bite of wheat bread, while Julie can eat any amount and is not affected at all. For this reason many individuals will have a negative reaction to a chemical such as a synthetic dye, provided the dose is large enough; but only some individuals are bothered by wheat.

Dr. Feingold wrote, "Allergy commonly does not cause hyperactivity, though in some individuals it may. Allergy usually produces the opposite clinical pattern, one of lassitude, fatigue, tiredness - actually hypoactivity."

He advocated testing for food allergies the same way salicylates are tested: by using an elimination diet. By first removing the most likely offenders (additives and salicylates) you should have an easier time identifying any food allergies.

If you suspect you have an allergy, be wary of food additives.

Feingold volunteers sometimes hear a parent say, "My child has allergies, but I don't think the additives bother him." Our experience suggests that the child who is allergic is the most likely to be affected by additives. These observations are supported by a study reported in the *Journal of Allergy and Clinical Immunology* (78:1039-1046, Nov 1986). Moneret-Vautrin wrote, "Intolerance to food additives occurs most often in people with food allergies, in asthma patients with nasal polyposis and drug intolerances, and in people with chronic urticaria (hives)."

More and more people are suffering from allergies.

The Allergy Information Association of Canada reports a drastic increase in the number of people who believe they suffer from allergies. In 1970 it was estimated to be 3% of the population, and today it is more than 30%. This increase is too great to be accounted for solely by better methods of detection.

One explanation is offered by Sweden's Dr. Bengt Bjorksten. He cites the factors that set an individual up for allergic reactions. The first is one's genetic inheritance, followed by exposure to pollutants which can irritate the respiratory system and make a person vulnerable to the other factor: the food, pollen, animal, etc. which comes their way. This theory is supported by researchers in Japan. They found that the number of people who suffer from cedar pollen allergy (as prevalent as our hay fever allergies) is about 5% in rural areas, but over 13% in urban areas where the air is polluted (*Annals of Allergy*, Vol. 58, April 1987).

Substituting the word "synthetic food additives" for pollutants (and many consider the two to be interchangeable) suggests an interesting way of looking at the problem of allergies. Perhaps the powerful chemical additives make an individual more vulnerable to foods and environmental irritants.

Do you outgrow allergies?

Another comment Feingold volunteers question is, "He used to have allergies, but he outgrew them." (Milk is often mentioned as the culprit.) Professor Eric Gershwin, an allergy specialist at the University of California-Davis, says, "Once allergic, always allergic." The child who had allergies does not outgrow them.

"Symptoms may moderate over time," he notes, "but the potential for an allergic reaction -- once the right set of circumstances pops up -- is always there." In his book, *Introduction to Clinical Allergy*, Dr. Feingold described this. Just as the symptoms of hyperactivity may change as a child gets older, the same may be true for allergy. What appears to be "outgrowing" the allergy is just a change in symptoms.

How should you test for food allergies?

Dr. Feingold believed the only reliable technique for identifying food allergy was the time-honored elimination diet. (Remove the suspect food(s) briefly and observe any change. Then reintroduce them one at a time and watch for reactions.) He cautioned parents against having their children undergo scratch testing for food allergies. However, he did believe scratch tests are useful in identifying allergies to pollen, grass, etc.

Fine tuning your success on the Program

Once a child or adult responds to the Feingold Program, it is often helpful to go further and consider other foods and/or chemicals that may be adversely affecting one's health and/or behavior. The Feingold Association often receives requests for help with other problems such as food allergies and environmental sensitivities. A brief description of some of these potential problems is covered in the *Feingold Handbook,* but the association encourages members to seek assistance from a professional and/or the appropriate support group.

Don't overlook the possibility that environmental irritants may affect you or your child

Lynn Murphy, Feingold member/allergy sufferer, advises parents to be especially careful to limit exposure to additives, salicylates or allergens during the season when the pollen, etc. is at its worst. A child who can tolerate tomatoes or milk most of the year may not be able to handle these when the ragweed is in bloom. As with many aspects of the Feingold Program, re-read your *Handbook*, pay close attention to changes in your child, and trust your own judgement.

Seeking help for allergies

Our association networks with other groups in many related fields. Some of these resources are described in this book and in Feingold newsletters. Information may also be found in the reference section of your library or through a self-help clearinghouse. For information on self-help groups in your area, you can contact the National Self-help Clearinghouse, 33 West 42nd Street, New York, NY 10036. (212) 840-1259.

Selecting and preparing food to accommodate the needs of an allergic family member can be very difficult -- and makes the Feingold Program look simple!

The most likely offenders.

It is not unusual for the Feingold member to be allergic to one or more foods, with milk appearing to be a common offender. Dr. Feingold counseled his patients to first give our program a try, and if there was no response, or partial response, to then seek help from a physician trained to deal with allergies. He advocated that the patient test for suspected allergens by temporarily removing them and keeping a diary of foods eaten, noting any change in behavior or other symptoms.

Which foods are the worst culprits?

More than 90% of food allergies are caused by six foods, according to Neil S. Orenstein, M.D., of the Harvard Medical School. These are: corn, eggs, milk, yeast, wheat and soy. Many of these are hidden in processed foods, making it very hard to identify them. Allergy to grain, especially wheat, is difficult to deal with; and for the individual who must avoid several grains, it is even harder.

Symptoms of allergies

In her book, *The Impossible Child,* Doris Rapp, M.D., describes some of the many symptoms that could be an indication of an allergy. A few of these include red patches on the cheek or "fire engine red" ears, circles under the eyes, and the "allergic salute," where the child uses the palm of the hand to rub his nose upward, eventually leaving a wrinkle near the tip of the nose.

Another physician who has published a great deal of information to help parents in detecting allergies is William Crook, M.D. A good book on the subject is *Solving the Puzzle of Your Hard to Raise Child.*

Parents have found another good resource - particularly on recipes for allergic children - in *How to Improve Your Child's Behavior through Diet* by Stevens and Stoner.

Allergic irritability syndrome

Kids who behave like brats and seem to get colds all the time may actually be suffering from allergies, says the American College of Allergists, which has even coined a new term for the condition: "allergic irritability syndrome." As many as 10 percent of American children may have allergic irritability syndrome, says allergist Dr. Gerald L. Klein in the organization's publication, *Annals of Allergy.*

PART FOUR
THE COST TO SOCIETY

The Kellogg Report - a Landmark Study

An estimated 15% of American young people exhibit obvious learning and/or behavior problems, and current methods of treatment are not working. Nutrition, lifestyle choices and the state of our environment hold solutions to many of the crises that beset our society. This is the conclusion of the mammoth *Kellogg Report: The Impact of Nutrition, Environment & Lifestyle on the Health of Americans* by Joseph D. Beasley, M.D., and Jerry J. Swift, M.A. The Institute of Health Policy and Practice, 1989, The Bard College Center, Annandale-on-Hudson, NY 12504. Funded by the Ford and W.K. Kellogg Foundations, the seven year project asks, "Could the learning and behavior problems of the young today be due to deeper, biological factors not adequately addressed by current psychology or medicine?"

Causes and a plan of action

The report goes further, addressing the issues of chronic illness in people of all ages, and deteriorating living conditions in third world countries. It explores reasons for these crises and offers action plans to reverse them. Modern medicine, the authors contend, attempts to use outdated models for current health problems. The formula that was so successful in controlling infectious diseases is not appropriate for dealing with the health problems Americans face today. "The chronic conditions which challenge us today -- from hypertension to learning disabilities -- do not respond to the simple formula of 'identify the cause and eliminate it' that works for infectious diseases."

They call for a new medical paradigm, a new frame of reference, which recognizes our individual differences and health requirements, and looks at the total lifestyle of the patient. "Many who readily accept the link between diet and heart disease, or other chronic physical conditions," they note, "find it hard to imagine that nutrition could have a direct and determining effect on human behavior and personality dysfunctions."

A narrow view of nutrition

When diet is considered, the medical approach is generally to single out one factor, such as cholesterol content of food, and to zero in on this as the single cause, much as physicians did when they identified a single cause of an infectious disease.

Unfortunately, there are many factors that work against the formulation of a new health paradigm. Most of our nutrition education comes from food advertising. The estimated $10 billion spent to promote brand name products is one hundred times the amount spent for nutrition education. "The National Cancer Institute has traditionally spent less than 1% of its funds on nutritional research. This is all the more amazing in light of the statement by Dr. Gio Gori, Deputy Director of the Institute, that about 60% of cancers in women and 40% in men appear to be related to diet."

Government, medicine and business

During the past decade, FDA efforts in the area of nutrition have been directed toward restricting the sale of vitamins and minerals, while critics charge that unsafe drugs are being ignored by the agency. "Drugs are foreign to the body," the authors point out, "while nutrients, on the other hand, are essential to the body.... The body stores up nutrients for future needs; it eliminates drugs as fast as possible."

While good food is slowly gaining recognition as a vital component of health, it is being increasingly subjected to nutrient-destroying processing.

"In America...never in history has such an astonishing and continuous abundance of food been produced year after year, not merely for farmer's own families (now less than 4% of the population) and the nation as a whole, but for countries around the world.

"At the same time, thanks to the modern food processing industry, never in history have nutrients been so systematically and massively destroyed or discarded...as during this golden age of nutrient discovery and technological. Neither the Food and Drug Administration nor the American Medical Association are likely to contribute to a solution." The authors charge both "have abandoned their earlier stands and joined the food-production industry in lauding the volume, variety, and value of today's food supply."

They also note the problem of conflicting interests in other areas. "Regulatory agencies and university researchers are closely tied to the food industry. In one year studied, almost half of the leading officials at the FDA had previously worked for organizations the agency was attempting to regulate."

Medicine, USA style

Changes are even less likely to come from the medical schools. What the authors describe as tunnel vision in medical training begins with the pre-med curriculum, requiring an overwhelming number of science courses, to the virtual exclusion of the humanities. The result is a greater degree of specialization in a progressively narrow area. "Many researchers," Beasley and Swift contend, "along with physicians and lay people who take an interest in the subject, see nutrition playing a primary role in human health that the more conservative bodies and those who follow their lead regard as unproven, unwarranted, and possibly dangerous."

The National Cancer Institute and American Cancer Society come in for criticism as well for having a "stranglehold" on cancer research, and for preventing Nobel laureates like Szent-Giorgyi and Pauling from gaining funds to do research on the connection between diet and cancer.

The patient who feels merely unwell or anxious is likely to be brushed aside. Only when the complaint becomes a full blown observable disease is he given treatment, and it is often a radical treatment. Similarly, insurers are notorious for failing to cover small preventive medical procedures, but pay for major surgery.

Freud believed that "the mental is based on the organic" but few psychiatrists consider the diet/behavior connection. In true silver bullet tradition, the prescription pad is generally the first weapon whether the patient is an anxious adult or a hyperactive child.

Beasley and Swift wrote in 1989, "If we assume the prevalence of learning and behavior disorders is indeed about 15% of all school children then the learning and behavior disordered population comes to about seven million youngsters!"

The authors point out that medical pioneers have historically been ignored or harassed by their peers, and only after their death have their discoveries been integrated into medical practice. Dr. Feingold is certainly in distinguished company.

Schools in Crisis

Aggression, throwing books and desks, cursing and kicking teachers, threatening them with pens and stealing their wallets. Is this the high school "blackboard jungle"? No, it describes children as young as five in Ontario elementary schools.

In a series of articles published in the *Toronto Star*, Louise Brown described the efforts of educators in the province to deal with very young, uncontrolled students.

Some schools have special "behavior classes" for children who are considered a threat to others. The class size is kept small - no more than eight children - with a specially trained teacher and aide. The *Star* reports that 6,000 children in Ontario have had to be placed in such classes. Educators are calling it a "toxic situation, a behavior crisis" in the schools.

The Federation of Women Teachers Association of Ontario has organized a buddy system to try and stop new teachers from quitting in their first year. The colleges are being faulted for failing to prepare their graduates to teach in such an environment.

Puzzled professionals look at the problems besetting elementary schools - not just in Ontario, but throughout North America. Where do they assign the blame? As always, the culprits are: parents, poor families, rich families, TV, and society in general.

Nobody wonders about what these children have eaten for breakfast, if indeed they have eaten at all. No thoughts of what is served in the cafeteria, or what their parents will eat for their lunch and how this might affect the way they treat their child.

Meanwhile, researchers in Alberta reported the effect of synthetic food additives on hyperactive pre-school children (Kaplan and associates, 1989). And to the east, in the province of Ontario, distressed teachers and principals puzzled over the unexplained behavior of more and more children.

Dr. Feingold addressed the issue of delinquent behavior many years ago. Feingold parents have found a vital piece of the puzzle. How bad must it get before those who search for solutions will listen?

Violent Behavior in Children

Once again a child uses a handgun to kill another at a Washington, DC high school. In Lehigh Valley, PA, residents are shocked to learn of two families where teenage children have killed their parents.

For a few days alarmed officials in Washington appear on the evening news, speaking with authority and determination, vowing to take action. Committees of 'experts' will gather to conduct the predictable hand wringing, talk about poverty, drugs, guns and lack of accountability on the part of the young. They will discuss conflict resolution and call for more money to be spent on more programs, and after brief coverage in the local newspapers the issue will fade until another child with another weapon guns down somebody else.

The Lehigh murders were not generated by poverty or abuse; these teen offenders came from families trying hard to provide moral and spiritual guidance. When a youngster seems to run amuck, despite a family's best efforts, we all seek out the reasons why.

Drugs, alcohol, gangs, hate groups and media violence still don't get to the core of the problem: why is one child so vulnerable to influences that do not have the same fatal effect on his peers?

Eastern Pennsylvania is the home of the Toughlove movement, where parents use strong measures to force their children to be accountable for their behavior. But, while Toughlove has often been a Godsend and has turned around the lives of many children headed for disaster, it still does not provide answers for why one child is so much more vulnerable than another.

The 14-year-old Washington youngster was only one of many who had a gun in his possession on that January day, but he was the only one to use it. Unfortunately, many children carry guns, many find themselves in potentially explosive situations, and chances are that many are tempted to use a weapon. But most of them don't give in to the momentary impulse...why?

As for the teenagers who killed their parents, children in every community become enraged with their parents at times, and have access to weapons, but in nearly every case, they restrain the impulse to act out their anger.

Expert committees would do well to change their focus. Instead of searching for answers in outside influences they should take a closer look at the children themselves -- both those who are able to control their impulses and those who are not.

Diet, hyperactivity and ADD

The Canadian Centre for Justice Statistics points out that the typical teenage offender is a hyperactive male, with learning problems, poor social skills and low self-esteem. These are typical characteristics of children who benefit from the Feingold Program, but when the suggestion is raised that highly processed junk food could play a part in antisocial behavior, one generally hears that possibility dismissed, with a reference to the famous "Twinkies defense." This is the story behind it.

The Twinkies defense revisited

In November of 1978 a former city Supervisor in San Francisco, Dan White, killed another supervisor and the city's mayor. The media used the information that White's diet was primarily composed of junk food, and created the "Twinkies defense." It is a sarcastic reference to the claim that one is not responsible for his actions since his behavior is influenced by eating junk food.

Unfortunately, this presents a simplistic picture, that of a single snack changing an otherwise normal person into a murderer. We all know that most people eat junk food without becoming homicidal.

But this all-or-nothing scenario distracts from a more realistic one: the chemically sensitive person with symptoms of hyperactivity or ADD, who is already having difficulty coping, who exists on a diet deficient in needed vitamins and minerals, but filled with petroleum-based food additives, may have a very hard time controlling destructive impulses. If he is already close to irrational behavior, it may not take more than some additive-filled snack foods to put him over the edge.

Surely, many factors combine to lead to violent behavior in some individuals. But to exclude the effects of foods, food additives and environmental chemicals is to throw away some important pieces of the puzzle, and in solving a puzzle, all of the pieces count.

The symptoms of violent behavior can be seen early in many children; Walt is a good example.

Walt's Story -- Dr. Jekyll and Mr Hyde

Lisa watched her child experience violent behavior as a result of synthetic food additives.

As he was exposed to more additives, his episodes of anger became more violent. He would suddenly strike out, screaming, hitting people and objects, breaking toys, furniture, or anything available. One memorable day, at the age of 18 months, Walt broke the windows in his room and tore the wallpaper off the wall.

Lisa had begun to suspect that the violent episodes were related to food. When they went to their favorite fast food restaurant she gave him the orange drink (artificially colored and flavored) in preference to the soda with caffeine. He would go into the restaurant calm, well behaved and agreeable. Then an hour or two afterward he would be out of control and not return to normal behavior for three days.

Walt was three when Lisa came across Dr. Feingold's book, *Why Your Child is Hyperactive*. She began following the diet and saw some dramatic changes in her son. Visits to the doctor's office had always been a disaster. (Walt liked to take the scale apart, tear off down the hall, etc.) In their first post-Feingold doctor's visit, the three-year-old sat patiently, and asked "Mommy, would you count with me?"

During an illness the doctor insisted Walt needed to take an artificially colored medicine. After Lisa gave him the pink antibiotic he began screaming uncontrollably, banging his head on the wall, throwing toys, etc. She called the doctor, who was astonished at the violence he heard over the phone. After that Lisa had his support using the diet.

During the years he has been on the Feingold Program, Walt has been able to enjoy all the activities his friends do. He has gone to scout camp and on camp-outs, to church camp; he plays soccer and the saxophone. Walt has become a proficient label reader and educates the adults he comes in contact with. He avoids nitrites, MSG, and aspartame (NutraSweetTM, EqualTM) which result in a "horrible, blinding headache."

Today he is an honor student in junior high school.

Young and violent

The response to juvenile crime -- looking for answers in all the wrong places.

Following a particularly violent summer in 1993, the Colorado legislature met in special session to create laws designed to attempt to stem the tide of juvenile crime. More prisons for teens and tougher gun control were proposed. There was no mention of funds allocated to determine possible causes of those crimes, no investigation of biochemical factors that may play a part in the violent behaviors.

Meanwhile, in another part of the country, researchers were reporting some startling findings. William Walsh, Ph.D., of the Carl Pfeiffer Treatment Center in Naperville, IL found there are measurable physiological differences between the normal population and those who have committed serious crimes. An autopsy of one mass killer showed that he had very high levels of lead, which may have been the result of frequent exposure to firearms, inhaling the lead vapor which is given off when a gun is fired. He had been a champion sharpshooter.

Another convicted criminal, James Humerty, who opened fire on the customers in a McDonald's, had extraordinarily high levels of cadmium, a lethal substance. His exposure to cadmium had apparently come from his profession as a welder. (He had resigned his job, explaining that the welding fumes were "making him crazy.")

Abnormally low levels of minerals are also associated with criminal acts. Charles Manson's copper level was found to be astonishingly low. Dr. Carl Pfeiffer, whose work has served as the model for the Treatment Center, reported success helping children with hyperactivity, learning disabilities and attention deficit disorder. Dr. Walsh and his colleagues have continued this work, along with their interest in the causes of criminal behavior.

Addressing the Well Mind Association in 1991, Dr. Walsh noted, "The answer to crime prevention is not in bigger prisons and more stringent penalties but in identifying children and intervening biochemically before their lives are ruined. Allergies are often an aggravating factor, sometimes the only factor. Sugar and yellow and red food dyes hit kids hard. Eventually we'll learn all about what needs to be known in the prevention of crime."

Dr. Walsh and his colleagues are endeavoring to demonstrate their success in controlled, double blind studies, and until this happens it will be difficult to have an impact on the approach to crime and behavior disorders.

Recently FAUS was contacted by a treatment center for juvenile offenders. The Association can provide information on clinical successes by Feingold and others who have seen success in this area: Reed, Schoenthaler, and Schauss, to name a few. We can provide studies demonstrating the connection between food additives and hyperactivity. But the work showing the connection between crime and chemicals in food and in the environment has not been published in mainstream medical journals.

Without this type of documentation, the treatment center would not consider something as simple as a switch in the brands of food served. This translates to more time lost, more criminal acts and more victims or crimes that probably didn't have to happen.

Dim prospects

A study published in *Archives of General Psychiatry* (Vol. 50, July 1993, pp. 565-567) documents the poor prospects of young adults who had been diagnosed hyperactive.

The study followed ninety-one males for more than a decade and found that now, in their mid-twenties, these men have had a significantly higher incidence of antisocial personality disorder (18% vs. 2%) and drug abuse (16% vs. 4%) compared to their peers who had not been diagnosed ADHD (attention deficit hyperactivity disorder). In addition, the ADHD subjects were less successful in school and in their jobs.

The article, authored by Mannuzza, Klein, Bessler, Mallow and LaPadula, only serves to confirm what Feingold parents have long known -- had they not found help for their children, the prospects for their child's future would have been dim.

Crime Times - This is a publication on the biochemical causes of criminal behavior. For information contact *Crime Times*, 1106 N. Gilbert Rd., Suite 2132, Mesa AZ 85203.

Dr. Feingold's Recommendations

In 1981, Dr. Feingold addressed the New York State Assembly Standing Committee on Child Care. He focused his attention on juvenile delinquency:

"It is not necessary to cite statistics to support the contention that juvenile delinquency, vandalism, violence, assault and crime in general show a persistent rise in prevalence.... Every procedure for correction of behavior has not been successful, while every modality for rehabilitation of delinquency and adult criminals has failed. Since all these procedures have been structured on psychosocial factors, we must look elsewhere for the answers, and that answer is to be found in the biosciences, which include genetics, molecular genetics, pharmacogenetics, behavioral toxicology, behavioral teratology, immunology, immunochemistry, allergy, endocrinology, with a focus on nutrition, which encompasses all these areas."

"Huffing"

The practice of children and teens sniffing fumes from common household products is increasing dramatically, with devastating results.

Some of the effects of the practice known as 'huffing' simulate a learning disorder. After repeated abuse, a child can suffer permanent damage to the brain, nerves, lungs, kidneys, liver and bones. Hearing and coordination can be impaired, and the child may have difficulty with basic learning skills, according to Neil Rosenbery, a neurologist with the International Institute for Inhalant Abuse. The Institute was established by the Chemical Specialties Manufacturers Association.

Sniffing the fumes will provide a "high" of short duration by causing the heart to beat irregularly and interfering with breathing. Some individuals can tolerate these effects for awhile, but for others the first exposure is fatal.

The New England Journal of Medicine calls inhalant abuse a problem of epidemic proportions.

The National Institute on Drug Abuse estimated the incidence in 1975 at 10 percent of high school seniors, which increased to 17 percent in 1992. Children as young as five have been found huffing. The Institute estimates more than 60 American children died in 1993 after sniffing such products. But researchers writing in the *New England Journal of Medicine* in 1990 believe the number is higher, since inhalant abuse is not generally considered when a child's death is investigated.

Because the products that produce the "high" are legal, they are easily obtained, and stores report brisk sales on Friday nights.

Some of the products which are used and can result in damage include: aerosol sprays, glues, nail polish remover, lighter fluid, gasoline, butane and propane gases, freon, paint thinner, magic markers and nitrous oxide canisters -- called "whippets."

"Snorting"

Ritalin use as a recreational drug can be fatal

Members who combine stimulant medication and diet management need to be aware of the increasing abuse of Ritalin among teens. If this drug is present in your home, please keep close tabs on it.

A 19-year-old Roanoke, VA high school student died after snorting Ritalin at a party. This practice has become widespread within the past few years, and the drug is seen as a socially acceptable substitute for cocaine.

Young people generally assume it is relatively harmless, and are known to use it in school bathrooms, or even during class. But the practice is anything but harmless; breathing in the crushed pills causes the drug to be directly absorbed into the bloodstream. The practice of snorting Ritalin and drinking alcohol greatly intensifies the effect. It triggers a burst of energy and rapid speech, increases blood pressure, causes the heart rate to speed up, and can trigger seizures, hallucinations and cardiac arrest.

Some of the attractions of getting high on Ritalin are: the ease of obtaining it, the low price, and the fact that the effects last for about two hours. Some teens take pills from a sibling's prescription; others buy it from peers who resist taking it for ADD. The going rate is $3 to $5 apiece.

It's easier for a teenager to obtain the drug than it is to buy beer. Many teens are under the impression that the drug is safe to use recreationally since they see it prescribed for young children.

"I Want to Help!"

Once you experience the exciting improvement in your child, you may want to reach out to others who are still going through the difficulties (hell) you previously knew.

There are many ways you can help, and your choice depends on how much time you can offer, as well as your personal preferences. Some Feingold volunteers would sooner face a firing squad than give a workshop, while others of us can't get our mug in front of an audience often enough. Some of us enjoy writing while others like phoning.

The Feingold Association can provide everything from brochures to bumper stickers, as well as literature for professionals of all disciplines. There are press releases ready to go which need only to be sent to a newspaper. Of, if you like to write letters to newspaper and magazine editors, these are a terrific way to reach out and let others know about the help available. A single letter from a mom has led to more than one television show, with thousands of families helped as a result.

Perhaps a second copy of this book could be used to loan out to friends, or you may want to donate one to your child's school, your library, church or club. Contact Pear Tree Press for information on how to purchase additional copies at the wholesale price.

"Why Won't They Even Try the Diet?"

Your child's response to the Feingold Program has been spectacular. Teachers, neighbors and relatives are impressed, but the one person you can't wait to tell is your friend who has also been looking for a way to help her child. To your astonishment, she is not interested, even after she sees the change in your child.

Why a concerned parent would be reluctant to try something as simple and risk-free as diet is a puzzle we've never really understood. We have even asked enthusiastic new members who resisted the program for many months themselves, but they are not able to explain.

An obvious reason -- that the parent believes it will require a lot of cooking and doesn't want to do this -- is sometimes not the factor at all. Occasionally we encounter a mom who is disinterested despite the fact that she loves to cook, and makes many dishes from scratch.

What's going on? While we don't have any clear answers, there are a variety of possibilities. A panel of supportive professionals who addressed our 1990 conference in Towson, MD suggested some of these. [Note: This article is for your consideration; we are not suggesting that anyone "play therapist" or use this article to confront another person.]

The exhausted parent

Some people have tried and failed at so many approaches in helping their child, they are afraid of yet another failure and the disappointment it will bring. Even if she is interested in trying diet management, the mom may be under such stress that the idea of taking on another responsibility could be more than she can face.

In some cases, a mom is advised to not use the diet because it will create more stress for her. When she realizes that simply buying the microwave popcorn in the blue box instead of the red box will mean she avoids synthetic additives, she sees how little change might be needed.

The sad thing is that these moms are already working hard to help their kids. It's just that what they're doing isn't working very well.

It's hard to change

Change is uncomfortable, and most of us resist it. It may actually feel more comfortable to stay with the familiarity of the problems than to experience the discomfort of change -- even if it is a change for the better.

Even if she is willing to change, her spouse may not be. In fact he may be more "hyper" than her child.

She may be using food -- such as candy -- as a reward, and be reluctant to have to change, even if it means only a change to a different brand of candy.

The "bad mother"

Moms of ADD and ADHD kids have generally been given the message that they're doing something wrong. Now she gets the message that the food she gives her family is pretty bad stuff and it may be more guilt than she can handle. It's not the consumer's fault that BHT is hidden in so many things, that the fault lies with the industry and the government agencies whose job it is to regulate them; the mom whose kid has problems has become very good at believing *everything* is her fault.

Help from a prescription

For many distraught parents, the diagnosis of ADD/ADHD is a profound relief. This may be their first indication that the child's problems are not their fault. When the person giving them this comforting information, the first person who really understands what they have been going through, goes on to assure them that medication is the only answer, it carries a lot of clout. To reject the advice to use medication then is seen as risking loss of the comforting support of the professional and/or the parent group that advocates it.

If the medicine brings about any improvement at all, parents are understandably reluctant to consider discontinuing it, even if the side effects are considerable. The parent probably does not realize that there is good reason to avoid certain food additives, whether the child is on medicine or not.

Who's in charge?

Similarly, she may be reluctant to question authority of any kind. If her doctor says diet is ineffective and he is wrong, does this mean other authority figures might also be wrong about what they have taught her?

Food has many meanings

Ask anyone battling obesity, food has meanings on many levels; it is a lot more than just the stuff that makes and repairs cells. Food is part of our earliest experience in life and is intertwined with memories and mores. For most people, some foods evoke familiarity and comfort. One mom who learned that she would have to switch from the chocolate chips in the yellow bag to the unfamiliar brown bag was genuinely upset. What memories must have been tied to that bright colored bag!

Food is personal

And it's incredibly subjective. Here again, a parent may feel she is being asked to make too big a change, particularly if she receives misinformation about what the Feingold Program really is.

The well educated parent

The parent who has a degree in one of the sciences may be as resistant as one who simply believes what she has been taught in childhood. The parent who conducts her own research on ADD and ADHD will find many negative references to diet management, but is not likely to understand that most of this information is faulty and comes from special interests.

Money and credentials

When a parent is raised with phrases such as "you get what you pay for," it's hard to accept that a Feingold membership could be more effective than $150/hour therapy. And if they are unaware of Dr. Feingold's impressive credentials, it's easy to perceive the program as an invention of parents. The parent's authority then pales in comparison to that of the doctor/therapist/teacher, etc.

What is the parent's philosophy of life?

She may have been raised to believe that we have no power to influence our lives. If we have a child with problems, it's supposed to be that way; it's what we deserve.

The newsletter of the support group of South Africa addressed this: "...some people make their own decisions about what they want to achieve in life, decide how they are going to do it, use whatever tools they deem necessary and set about reaching for their dreams.... They are in control of their own life and are said to have an 'internal locus of control.'

"By contrast, people with an 'external locus of control' are controlled by circumstances beyond them. These are people who feel they cannot alter an unpleasant situation because they don't have the power to do so."

The reluctant Feingolder

One mom told us, "I had received the big package filled with information and hope for my little preschooler. Reading through it was encouraging -- other parents had faced this issue and found solutions; I knew that we would be able to be one of the successes as well. But there the package sat, and new issues of *Pure Facts* came. I read them, then added them to the stack of solutions that I somehow couldn't begin to use.

Then an unexpected phone call jolted me out of my comfortable procrastination. A friend of a friend had learned that we were members of the Feingold Association; she asked me how we were doing on the Program. I fibbed that everything was going well...how could I explain my hesitation when I didn't understand it myself?

My wonderful husband came up with the answer that seemed to make the most sense to me. He said that just as the alcoholic needs to grieve the loss of his "best friend," I needed to grieve the loss of some favorite foods and the memories connected with them. He was right! Warm recollections so often are imbued with the scent and taste of a food, a food I was convinced I could no longer enjoy. Oh no! Will I be eating only gray tasteless things?! I knew better than that, but still hung on to old memories. The times my friends and I sat together talking over a cup of hazelnut coffee was an especially treasured recollection.

That was last year and this year we are another Feingold success. My daughter's response has been all I had hoped for. It's hard to believe I could have waited so long to begin enjoying our additive-free lifestyle. There's plenty to eat, and *none* of it is gray! And I've ordered some all-natural coffee flavorings, so I'll be enjoying our new, calm life, and my fond memories, while I sip a cup of natural hazelnut coffee.

SCIENTIFIC STUDIES

Foods and additives are common causes of the attention deficit hyperactive disorder in children

Marvin Boris, MD and Francine S. Mandel, PhD
Annals of Allergy, Vol. 72, May 1994, pages 462-468

This double blind, placebo-controlled study is the most supportive to date; 73% of the ADHD children responded to an elimination diet and symptoms returned when they were challenged with foods/additives.

The May 1994, issue of *Annals of Allergy* contains the results of the most dramatic study to date on the effect of foods and food additives on ADHD children. Researchers Marvin Boris, MD, and Francine Mandel, PhD, selected the first 26 children referred to the allergy practice who met the criteria for a diagnosis of ADHD. The children ranged from age 4 to 11, with the average age of seven-and-a-half.

Substances eliminated: The children were tested in their own homes, during a break from school. The first phase lasted for two weeks, and eliminated dairy, wheat, corn, yeast, soy, citrus, egg, chocolate, peanuts -- foods not restricted on the Feingold diet -- as well as artificial colors and preservatives. The investigators did not remove artificial flavorings or salicylates.

Ratings: Parents filled out a questionnaire (Connors Parent Rating Scale) before the start of the elimination diet, and at the end of it two weeks later.

Testing the foods/additives: The second phase of the program lasted for one month. During this time parents added back one of the eliminated foods/additives at a time every two days. If the child reacted to any of the items, it was removed and later reintroduced and tested to confirm that it had triggered the reaction. All of the 19 children who had responded were sensitive to several foods and/or chemicals. The parents were asked to identify which food/additive produced the worst reaction, and this was used as the challenge during the double blind test period.

Double blind challenge: The term "double blind" refers to a method of testing where neither the subject nor the researcher know whether the challenge contains the substance being tested, or a "placebo." A placebo looks just like the item tested, but contains an inactive ingredient.

The children whose worst reaction was to a food were tested with 5 grams (about 1 teaspoon) of the food in a powdered form. When dye triggered the worst reaction the challenge dose was 100mg. The dyes used in the challenge materials were: Red 40 (40%), Yellow 5 (28%), Yellow 6 (25%) and small quantities of other red and green dyes.

"Dietary factors may play a significant role in the etiology of the majority of children with ADHD"

Milk was the food used as a challenge for five of the children; food dyes were given to four, corn was used for three children and wheat for two. One child's worst offender was soy, while for another it was oranges.

The researchers were able to successfully disguise the foods/dyes used as a challenge in apple cranberry sauce (a salicylate) and in lentil soup (which may contain salicylate).

Test period: The challenging took place over a seven-day period (a very short time by Feingold standards, since a single reaction can last 3 to 4 days). Three of the children dropped out of the study and that left sixteen.

Parents were asked to rate their children for the following symptoms:

impulsiveness
tearfulness
restlessness
destructiveness
incomplete tasks
distractibility
moodiness
frustration tolerance
activity level
tendency to disturb other children

Results: The parents used the Conners Parent Rating Scale to measure the above characteristics on each of the seven testing days. The difference in the behavioral ratings was very significant. Before any dietary changes were introduced the mean score was a high one of 25, indicating many behavioral problems. With the offending foods/dyes removed the scores dropped to just over 8. When they were challenged, the scores rose to 18 -- a dramatic jump from the low of 8, but still below the pre-diet rating of 25.

In other words, the effect of diet on the behaviors of these children was dramatic, and could be objectively measured.

Allergies: Boris and Mandel were impressed with the role of allergies in ADD and ADHD. Not only were some foods major culprits, but of the 26 children originally slated for inclusion in the study, 18 of them had allergic symptoms (asthma, skin problems, stuffy nose, hives) and showed a positive reaction to skin tests for environmental allergens such as ragweed, dogs, grasses, etc. The allergic children were found to be more likely to respond to such an elimination diet than non-allergic children.

Conclusions: The authors point out the serious limitations of early studies on diet and hyperactivity. Most were 'single agent elimination' tests. Rather than remove all of the offending additives/salicylates, most of the studies focused on one (sometimes two) agents, eliminating them and then challenging with them. The more recent studies by Egger (1985) and Kaplan (1989) were 'multiple agent elimination diets,' which means they initially removed many potential offenders.

Boris and Mandel write: "In summary this DBPCFC (double blind placebo controlled food challenge) study supports the role of dietary factors in ADHD. Through a simple elimination diet symptoms can be controlled. Atopic (allergic) children with ADHD had a significantly more beneficial response to the elimination diet than nonatopic (non-allergic) children.

"Challenge tests after a broad elimination diet can aid in the identification of precipitating factors. It would also be important to determine whether dietary control affects any of the metabolic dysfunctions observed in ADHD.

"Elimination of the causes of ADHD is preferable to the pharmacologic therapy of this condition."

Editorial comments: This well controlled, objectively measured test of diet and the symptoms generally called ADD and ADHD is heartily welcomed. Nevertheless, Feingold families can't help wondering 1) Why were artificial flavorings and salicylates not eliminated? 2) How much more successful would the test have been if a current Foodlist had been utilized to remove all the hidden sources of BHA, BHT and TBHQ? 3) If a more generous amount of time had been allotted, would the success rate have climbed above the 73% reported? Repeated challenges during a one-week period are far too much for a sensitive child.
These are small complaints, however, in view of the success of this important work.

Synthetic food coloring and behavior; A dose response effect in a double-blind, placebo-controlled, repeated-measures study

Katherine S. Rowe, MBBS, MPH, Dip Ed, FRACP
Kenneth J. Rowe, BA, MSc
From the Department of Pediatrics, University of Melbourne, Royal Children's Hospital, and the Centre for Applied Educational Research, University of Melbourne, Parkville, Victoria, Australia.
The Journal of Pediatrics, November, 1994

The purpose of the Rowe study was to determine if a synthetic food dye could trigger behavioral reactions in children identified as "hyperactive." Those behaviors believed to be triggered by the dye were: irritability, sleep disturbances, restlessness, aggression and reduced attention span.

Parents of 34 children had reported these characteristics in their children, and believed that they were triggered by synthetic food dyes. A group of 20 children who did not have these behaviors participated in the study as "controls."

The first group of children had been following a diet free of synthetic dyes for at least three months, and as a result their parents had seen a significant improvement in behavior. The controls followed a similar regimen for six weeks prior to the study.

Tartrazine (Yellow No. 5) was the only dye tested. The doses used were: 1, 2, 5, 10, 20 and 50 mg. During a 21-day period, each child consumed these amounts at different times. The dye was administered double blind. (At the time of the study neither the family nor the researchers knew when the dye was being given.) It was hidden in capsules and in packaged orange juice. Two to three days were allowed between challenges with the dye.

Of the 34 children identified as sensitive to dyes, 22 of them had clear reactions to the challenges. Two of the 20 children in the control group also had behavioral reactions. When they reacted to the dye, the younger children had "constant crying, tantrums, irritability, restlessness, and severe sleep disturbance," and were described as "disruptive, easily distracted and excited, high as a kite, and out of control." The older children became whiny and unhappy, irritable, aimlessly active, and lacked self-control.

All of the children who reacted had a history of allergies and suffered from conditions such as asthma, eczema and rhinitis. Most of the sensitive children had close relatives with a history of migraine headaches.

CONCLUSION

The authors note, "This study demonstrated a functional relation between the ingestion of a synthetic food color (tartrazine) and behavioral change in 24 atopic (allergic) children, aged 2 to 14 years, with marked reactions being observed at all six dosage levels of dye challenge."

Surprisingly, the parents were able to identify a reaction to the smallest dose of *only 1-mg* of yellow dye! While the small doses -- up to 10 mg -- appeared to have a profound effect, the disturbed behavior did not last very long. Above 10 mg of tartrazine reactions tended to last more than 24 hours, suggesting a dose-related response.

Reliability of parental reports was confirmed in this study, as it has been in previous studies by Carter et al.

The Rowe study and the Feingold Program

The Feingold Program is very different from the Rowe study -- a test that removed only dyes and challenged with a single one. Nevertheless, the results are dramatic and very supportive. Using controlled scientific methods, the childrens' behavior was found to be directly related to the ingestion of a petroleum-based dye. One could not attribute the reactions to psychological factors. Critics cannot say that a subject "was all boy," "was going through a phase," "had poor parenting," "watched too much TV," or needed stimulant medicine to address some hypothetical brain disorder.

In an earlier study by Egger et al (*The Lancet,* March 9, 1985), 79 percent of the hyperactive children tested reacted to Yellow 5 and to the preservative benzoic acid.

Adverse reactions to tartrazine -- the name for the notorious Yellow No. 5 -- were first reported in medical journals decades ago. This dye is widely acknowledged to trigger reactions such as asthma and hives, and now its effect on children's behavior is indisputable. Does this mean we can expect to see a change in the diagnosis and treatment of ADD or ADHD? Will this affect the foods served to schoolchildren? Will the Food and Drug Administration reconsider its judgment that this petrochemical is a "safe and suitable" food additive? Probably not.

Effects of a few foods diet in attention deficit disorder

C M Carter, M Urbanowicz, R Hemsley, L Mantilla, S Strobel, P J Graham, E Taylor

***Archives of Diseases in Childhood*, 1993;69:564-568**

This British study has yielded some very positive data on the connection between diet and behavior/learning.

The children who participated in the study all met DSM III criteria for attention deficit disorder and were between ages 3 and 12, with an average range of IQ scores. Prior to the start of the study, the children were given extensive assessment tests.

For a period of three to four weeks, the children were on a very restricted diet, generally consisting of: turkey, lamb, rice, potato, banana, pear, various vegetables, bottled water, sunflower oil and milk-free margarine. In some cases diets were adjusted to avoid suspect allergy foods or avoid those a child disliked.

Seventy-eight children completed the first part of the study. The parents of 59 of the children reported a worthwhile improvement in behavior; 17 reported no improvement; and 2 were said to become worse. This represents:

Improved: 76%
No change: 22%
Worse: 3%

The 59 children who responded were then challenged with various foods and some food additives. Additive-containing foods were found to be the worst offenders (70% reacted).

Chocolate was the second most often reported culprit (64%). [We assume the researchers used chocolate free of the synthetic additive vanillin.] Cow's milk also provoked reactions in 64%, followed by orange (57%), cow's cheese (45%), wheat (45%), other fruits (36%), tomato (22%), and egg (18%).

The additives used consisted of a blend of ten dyes, only 4 of which are used in foods in the US, benzoic acid and sodium metabisulphite. [These preservatives are not routinely eliminated on the Feingold Program. Those which we do remove -- BHA, BHT and TBHQ -- are restricted in England.]

The amount of additives given to the children was quite small, the upper limit of the dyes being 26 mg per day.

Despite the small quantity of dyes in the challenge, they had a significant effect. The authors write, "When food colours were suspected, we asked parents to give their children colour capsules. Sixteen agreed to do this. Three children were not affected, two had behavioural problems and physical symptoms, eight had behavioural problems only, and three had physical symptoms only."

Of the sixteen children who were challenged with 26 mg or less of food dyes, thirteen had adverse reactions.

There are many differences between this study and the Feingold Program; but while it cannot be seen as a test of our program, it offers some valuable support. One of the conclusions the researchers emphasized was that parental observations should be taken seriously. They write: **"This trial indicates that diet can contribute to behaviour disorders in children and that this effect can be shown in a double blind, placebo controlled trial."**

They also state: **"The ways in which diet worked remain unclear. Toxic, pharmacological, or allergic mechanisms could be involved, and the physiological effects of different foods might induce changes in brain perfusion similar to those reported in attention deficit disorder by Lou et al. These results argue against the notion that the only mechanism involved is the 'placebo effect' of expectation and suggestion, and testing this was a main purpose of the study."**

Throughout the paper, the authors refer to the dietary regimen as difficult and restrictive. Unlike the Feingold Program, which permits a tremendous variety of foods even in Stage One, the Carter study did severely restrict food choices. They suggest that a study design limiting only the most likely offenders might be worth pursuing.

The authors believe that a study testing additives alone would not be of much benefit since so few children appeared to react to them alone. Considering the small amount and limited number of additives used in the challenges, this conclusion is understandable. The researcher's design allowed for a two week "wash-out" period between testing the active material and the placebo; this is a welcomed improvement over many of the old tests. They also improved on early studies by having the children evaluated daily.

Although the children in this study met the criteria for diagnosis with attention deficit disorder, and their scores improved on one of the learning tests, the major improvements were seen in their behavior. Parents noted the children exhibited fewer of these symptoms: restlessness, disturbing others, frequent crying, and temper outbursts. The authors suggest this indicates more of an effect on irritability than on "attention deficit."

Dr. Feingold did not place learning difficulties in a category separate from behavior problems, but felt that, for most of the children he helped, they were simply different characteristics of the same problem. While some children on the Feingold Program show an immediate improvement in their ability to attend and learn, many parents report that the child's behavior improves first, and schoolwork improves gradually.

Effect of Diet Treatment on Enuresis in Children with Migraine or Hyperkinetic Behavior

J. Egger, M.D., C.M. Carter, M.A., J.F. Soothill, M.D., J. Wilson, Ph.D., F.R.C.P.

***Clinical Pediatrics*, May 1992,**

This study is one of a series testing the effects of certain foods and food additives. It involved twenty-one children whose symptoms of hyperactivity or migraine had responded to a diet consisting of few foods. All of the 21 children also suffered from enuresis (bedwetting and daytime wetting). The researchers were able to identify offending foods and thereby enabled twelve of the twenty-one children to recover from the enuresis and four to improve. When the offending foods were reintroduced, the enuresis returned. Nine of the children who responded participated in a double-blind test and six of them reacted to the offending food, but none to the placebo.

Dietary Replacement in Preschool-Aged Hyperactive Boys

Bonnie J. Kaplan, PhD, Jane McNicol, RD, Richard A. Conte, PhD, and H.K. Moghadam, MD
from the Departments of Pediatrics and Psychology, University of Calgary, the Department of Dietetics, Alberta Children's Hospital, and the Learning Centre, Calgary, Alberta, Canada
Pediatrics, January 1989; 83:7-17.

This ambitious double blind, placebo-controlled study came closer to the Feingold Program than any previous test. It involved 24 preschool aged boys who had been diagnosed as hyperactive, and who exhibited various physical symptoms or sleep disorder.

All of the food was provided for the families during the 10 weeks the test lasted. Some items permitted on the Feingold Program were limited or removed, while others (particularly salicylates) were not removed.

Despite the discrepancies between this test and the Feingold Program, the results were impressive. The authors note, "According to the parental report, more than half of the subjects exhibited a reliable improvement in behavior and negligible placebo effects."

Results: Of the 24 boys, behavioral ratings indicated that 10 of them showed an improvement of 50%, and another 4 were "mild responders," with a behavioral improvement of 12%. The remaining 10 did not show a response. This yields figures of 42% responding and 16% mildly responding, for a combined figure of 58%.

Study design: Unlike many of the previous studies this was a "dietary replacement design" where all of the food eaten by the child and his family was supplied by the researchers.

Those studies that involved a "challenge" -- generally with synthetic dye -- produced enormous variations in data and in the interpretation of the data. Unfortunately, they were often interpreted as a test of the Feingold Program, resulting in a great deal of confusion.

Ages: The children ranged from 3-1/2 to 6 years of age. The decision to limit the subjects to young children was based on the findings of earlier researchers. In the Harley (1978) study, all ten of the preschool children responded to the Feingold diet. And in the Weiss (1979) study, the most dramatic responder was very young.

Non-food considerations: Some effort was made to minimize exposure to irritating substances, such as scented products, and chewable vitamins were free of the prohibited additives. The report did not indicate if any of the children were exposed to other common irritants (colored toothpaste, play dough, finger paint, etc.)

The double blind: The researchers appear to have been successful in preventing the parents from realizing that the focus of the study was food additives. This supports Feingold's conclusions that "placebo effect" or "parental expectations" were not responsible for the improved behavior.

Other design improvements were that none of the children were taking behavior-modifying medicine, and some allowance in the ratings was made when it was known that there had been an infraction.

Behavior ratings: Another improvement in the design of the Canadian study was that parents rated their children's behavior on a daily basis, rather than once weekly. Parents also observed their child for the presence or absence of nine physical symptoms: skin rashes, red cheeks, dry skin, stomach bloat or cramps, leg cramps, stuffy nose, headaches, ear aches, and bad breath.

The major physical improvement noted by parents was the child's breath (halitosis). There was also a lessening of sleep disturbances (difficulty in getting to sleep and frequency of awakening).

Funding: Funding was provided by national and provisional agencies. Unlike some of the studies carried out in the U.S., there was no involvement of food/chemical industry lobbies in the design, funding or implementation of the study.

Nutrition: Nutritional data collected during the study did not show a correlation between an improvement in nutrition leading to improved behavior.

Conclusion: The authors conclude: "Our research ... demonstrates a larger potential impact of diet than previously reported. These results suggest that pediatricians and other practitioners might consider dietary modifications worth trying, particularly in younger children."

Editorial comment: The Kaplan study came closest to a study of the Feingold Program of all those conducted to date. An important difference, however, is that for all but 4 of the children, natural salicylates were not removed. Feingold members have found the initial elimination of natural salicylates is often a critical factor in the diet's success.

Controlled trial of hyposensitisation in children with food-induced hyperkinetic syndrome

Joseph Egger, Adelheid Stolla, Leonard M. McEwen
The Lancet, Vol 339; May 9, 1992

This double-blind, placebo-controlled study demonstrates that foods and food additives can trigger "hyperactive" behavior in the majority of children diagnosed as hyperkinetic.

Symptoms of children in the study: Short attention span, distractible, impulsive, and poorly organized. Also restless or overactive, excitable, impulsive, disturbs other children, fails to complete tasks, constantly fidgeting, inattentive. easily frustrated, cries often and easily, mood changes quickly, explosive, unpredictable behavior.

Study design - first phase: 185 children were placed on a restricted diet for four weeks. The foods consumed were limited to: lamb, chicken, potatoes, rice, banana, pears, cabbage, sprouts, cauliflower, broccoli, celery, carrots and cucumber (the only salicylate included). The beverage provided was water. (The childrens' diet was supplemented with vitamins and minerals to ensure nutritional adequacy.)

Results: Of the 185 children participating, 116 demonstrated what both parents and teachers judged to be a significant improvement. By reintroducing foods, the researchers were able to identify those that provoked a behavioral reaction.

Second phase: Fifty-four of the children whose response was especially dramatic were invited to participate in a second phase, where they were given "enzyme-potentiating desensitization" injections. The purpose of the shots was to enable the children to consume the allergy foods without a hyperactive reaction.

The injections were developed for: dairy foods, eggs, fish and seafood, meats, grains, yeast, vegetables, fruits, and nuts. Injections were also given for chocolate, several food dyes, and the preservatives BHT and benzoic acid.

The effects of the injections lasted for a matter of months (and varied with the children.) When the effects wore off a new injection generally enabled an allergic child to again consume the food for a few months more. The authors express their belief that desensitization such as this should be used with caution, and only after extensive testing to identify the allergy foods.

Conclusion: The authors speculate, "Sensitisation to new foods may take place in hyperkinetic children treated by diet, either at the time of viral infection or as the result of excessive intake of a previously 'safe' food."

Editor's note: If a child is more vulnerable to developing an allergy -- or sensitivity -- to a substance "at the time of viral infection" could this mean that when medicine with added synthetic colors and flavors is given to a sick child he is being sensitized to these additives?

Viral infection: Dr. Feingold addressed the concept of how a viral infection could bring about a sensitivity in a person who had not previously been affected. In a 1981 letter to the Feingold Association of New York, he offered the following theoretical model: "The viral infection alters the nerve tissue to varying degrees in some individuals so that an individual who was tolerant to an environmental factor can no longer tolerate this agent. We observe this clinically not only in hyperactivity but also in seizures."

The Egger study and the Feingold Program: The Feingold Program deals with sensitivity to additives and salicylates, while the Egger study addressed allergic responses. But the results are significant for the understanding and treatment of both hyperactivity and attention deficit disorder (ADD).

During the first four weeks of the test, the researchers first placed all of the children on a very restricted diet -- one which makes the Feingold Program look like a breeze by comparison. During this period the children ate only two meats, two starches, two fruits and several vegetables, plus water. (The report emphasized that the diet was strictly monitored. Assuming this to be the case, it appears that the children's diets also excluded all synthetic dyes, artificial flavorings, BHA, BHT, TBHQ and all but one salicylate. This means that in addition to the allergy restrictions, the children were on the Feingold diet for four weeks. There is no mention of exposure to non-food products such as colored toothpaste, and no information about whether the supplements were free of dyes, flavorings or salicylates. But considering the care given to designing and implementing the diet, it seems safe to assume the supplements were at least uncolored and unflavored.)

Conclusion: Let's take another look at the results of the four-week elimination diet. Out of the 185 children, 116 improved significantly. This equals just under a 63% response -- a far cry from the 1%, 5% or 'small' response often attributed to diet management.

This study has many similarities to the earlier work by Egger et al (*The Lancet*, March 9, 1985). Both follow the careful protocol of a double-blind, placebo-controlled test, both were published in peer-review journals, and both reinforce the philosophy of the Feingold Association.

Review of the Studies Prior to 1988

The following is taken from *Social Skills and Learning Disabilities: Current issues and recommendations for future research* by Stephen J. Hazel and Jean Bragg Schumaker. This is a section of *Learning Disabilities: Proceedings of the National Conference,* edited by James F. Kavanagh and Tom J. Truss, Jr. (York Press, 1988, pp. 331-333)

"The possible relationship between sensitivities to environmental substances and behavior was initially brought to national attention by the late Benjamin F. Feingold, M.D. (1966, 1976, and 1981; Feingold, Suzer, and Fallman, 1968). On the basis of his clinical experience with over 1,200 cases, he claimed that children's hyperactivity and other manifested social and learning problems were related to sensitivities to certain substances in their diets. Specifically, Feingold focused his attention on the relationship between salicylates, artificial flavorings, and artificial colorings in foods and children's behavior. He designed a salicylate- and additive-free diet (known as the K-P [Kaiser Permanente] diet) to be used with hyperactive and learning disabled children, which he claimed produced dramatic improvement in the behavior of a large portion of these children.

"Following this widely publicized claim, a number of researchers investigated the relationship that he so strongly espoused. Connors, Goyette, Southwick, Lees, and Andrulonis (1976) were among the first to do a double-blind experiment with hyperkinetic children. Although they found some improvement in teacher's rating of the children's behavior when the children were given the controlled diet in an experimentally controlled manner, they reported no change in the parent's ratings. Since they found a significant order effect and only a few children actually showed improvement, the authors advised caution with regard to the interpretation of their results. This report, which was also widely publicized, convinced the public and many physicians that Feingold's claims were disproved. This work by Conners et al has recently been criticized for a variety of methodological flaws: inappropriate outcome measures, inadequate dosages of food dyes, the type of placebo used, the type of blood test used to determine allergies, the observation period after dosage delivery, and presenter bias (Rippere, 1983; Schauss, 1984). Such criticism is largely unknown to the public at large.

"Although a number of additional studies have focused on the effects of Feingold's K-P diet, very few meet even minimal standards of adequate research methodology (Wender, 1986). Of those that do, only one conducted by Swanson and Kinsbourne (1980) has shown adverse reactions in children to food dyes. After Swanson and Kinsbourne determined that the appropriate dosages of food dyes to be administered should be three to six times as strong as those used by Conners et al (1976) to more closely approximate the dietary intake of those substances, they used these larger dosages in a double-blind experiment with hyperkinetic children. The authors found adverse reactions in more than one-half of the children on a laboratory learning task. Nevertheless, this study has also been criticized for a number of flaws (Matter, 1983).

"Since the research in the area has been so flawed, it is impossible to draw firm conclusions from it. Some authors (for instance, Wender, 1986) have even suggested that further research on the K-P diet may be inappropriate since the diet itself is flawed in terms of screening out all salicylates. Another possible problem that may doom further research in the area is the possibility that a certain category of foods might not cause behavior problems in all hyperactive children. That is, a variety of different substances might cause these problems in individuals. Indeed, even combinations of particular substances may cause these problems.

"A few investigators have studied this possibility by challenging hyperactive children with a variety of foods and other environmental substances. O'Shea and Porter (1981), for example, challenged hyperkinetic children with intradermal and sublingual doses of a variety of foods (e.g., milk, corn, eggs, food dyes) and inhalants (dust, mold, and tree pollen) in a double-blind experiment. They found that a majority of the children exhibited behavioral changes related to such substances as food dyes (80 percent of the children) and milk (73 percent) and that smaller proportions of the group had adverse reactions to such foods as peanuts (47 percent), corn (40 percent), and chocolate (33 percent). Such data indicate that individual children's problems may be related to an individual pattern of sensitivities.

"This hypothesis has been pursued by a group of researchers at London's Institute of Child Health and Hospital for Sick Children. Using a carefully controlled research protocol, including a double-blind design, Egger, Carter, Wilson, Turner, and Soothill (1983) found a relationship between migraine, other physical symptoms (joint pain, abdominal pain), and behavioral and learning problems and ingestion of particular foods. They reported that most of the children had adverse reactions to several different foods. Using a similar research protocol, Egger, Carter, Graham, Gumley, and Soothill (1985) found a relationship between certain foods and hyperactive children's behavior. Although many of the children reacted to food dyes and preservatives, none of them were sensitive to these substances alone.

"Even though the research design of both of the Egger et al studies has been described as being 'too good to be true' (Podell, 1985, p. 120), the studies do provide impetus for additional work to determine the relationship of individual patterns of sensitivities to social behavior in children."

Problems with the Early Studies

There were many problems with the studies conducted in the 1970s. Generally, they bore little resemblance to the diet as it was actually being used by parents, and numerous mistakes were made by the researchers. But most of the studies yielded some very positive results, but critics and the industry consultants who wrote extensively of them overlooked these. In some cases, a researcher who first reported positive data later reversed himself and claimed his study demonstrated the opposite.

The following are researcher's quotes from their papers first printed in medical journals:

"The results of this study strongly suggest that a diet free of most natural salicylates, artificial flavors, and artificial colors reduced the perceived hyperactivity of some children suffering from hyperkinetic impulse disorder."
C. Keith Conners, Ph.D. et al
Pediatrics, Vol 58, no. 2, August 1976

"The results of this study offer data that a diet free of artificial flavors and colors results in a reduction of symptoms in some hyperactive children."
J. Ivan Williams, Ph.D. et al
Pediatrics, Vol. 16, No. 6, June 1978

"Our results suggest that the administration of food colorings may affect normal development, and they mandate a more critical evaluation of the effects of food colorings in both animals and children. Our results also suggest that hyperactivity should not be the sole factor investigated, and that measures of the effects of food coloring on cognitive function must be carefully evaluated in any future study."
Bennett A. Shaywitz, et al
Annals of Neurology, Vol. 4, No. 2, August 1978

Another early study: The 1976 Harley study at the University of Wisconsin, funded by the food industry lobby (the Nutrition Foundation) has been frequently referred to as negative despite the fact that:
13 of the 36 mothers
14 of the 30 fathers
6 of the 36 teachers
of the school-aged children rated them as improved on the diet.

Of the 10 preschool children tested, all 10 mothers and 4 of the 7 fathers rated the children's behavior as improved on the diet.

Study designs did not follow Feingold Program: In view of the many mistakes in the study designs, it is remarkable the children improved at all. The actual dietary habits of families involved in most of the research studies are very different from those of the typical Feingold Association member. Some of the more dramatic deviations are noted:

Feingold Program: "A successful response to the diet depends on 100% compliance" (*The Feingold Cookbook*, p.8)

Deviation: "The analysis of our data in terms of dietary infractions indicate the children made approximately one to two dietary infractions a week during our study" (letter from Dr. Harley, January 24, 1977).

Feingold Program: "Use only those foods listed in the Stage One Foodlist..." (*The Feingold Handbook*, p. 5).

Deviation: "Other food additives such as BHA, BHT, MSG, nitrites, nitrates, etc. were not given consideration in this study." (letter from Dr. Harley, June 4, 1976)

The Williams study did not eliminate salicylates, the children cheated, and they ingested synthetic dye each day in the form of colored pills!

Feingold Program: "The diet is usually not effective if the child is receiving behavior-modifying drugs" (*The Feingold Cookbook,* p. 9).

It can take an additional 30 to 40 days for a child to respond once behavior-modifying medication has been discontinued.

Deviation: None of the studies addressed this consideration, and the children in the Williams study received medication during half of the study.

Feingold Program: Parents beginning the Program are asked to keep a daily diary and to note behavior at least once a day.

Deviation: The children's behavior in the Harley study was rated only once a week, making the ratings very insensitive to variations.

Other problems with the early studies

The dosage of dye in the challenge material was typically 26 mg. Swanson & Kinsborne found that this was an error, and that the typical amount ingested by a child was between 76 and 150 mg.

One researcher (Dr. Williams) acknowledged that the children found the cookies (which contained the dye) to be very filling and often did not eat all of them.

Children who are well established on the diet frequently do not react to a challenge of synthetic additives or salicylates. Many report that unless they go back to consuming them on a regular basis, there is little or no reaction. This was overlooked in the Mattes study.

Nutritional criticism not supported

The FDA California study conducted by Dr. Bernard Weiss found that the Feingold diet was nutritionally satisfactory. A major criticism it has received is the temporary restriction of some salicylate fruits high in vitamin C. However, the allowed fruits and vegetables include many that are rich in vitamin C. A half grapefruit provides the entire RDA of vitamin C, and tropical fruits such as papaya and kiwi are excellent sources, rivaling oranges.

After a few weeks' elimination, most people are able to return some or all of the natural salicylates into their diet.

NIH Report

The National Institutes of Health evaluated the studies. Because there has been so much controversy surrounding the Feingold diet, it was the subject of a consensus development conference held in 1982 by the NIH. After reviewing all of the studies conducted to date, the NIH scientific panel concluded:

1. The Feingold diet is a valid option for the treatment of childhood hyperactivity.
2. While some children were clearly helped, the scientific studies did not support the clinical reports of 60 - 70% success.
3. But the studies were seriously flawed, and dealt almost exclusively with dyes, and thus were not a valid test of the Feingold diet.

In other words, they concluded there never has been a scientific test of the Feingold diet!

The NIH panel's conclusion was: "Controlled challenge studies have primarily involved the administration of food dyes to children, but have not included other food flavors or preservatives that are allegedly implicated in the causation of hyperactivity. Therefore, these controlled challenge studies do not appear to have addressed adequately the role of diet in hyperactivity."

Defined Diets and Childhood Hyperactivity, report of the scientific panel of the NIH Consensus Development Conference, January, 1982

Contact the Feingold Association for a bibliography of studies and journal articles relating to diet and hyperactivity/learning disabilities/ADD.

Feingold Association of the United States
P.O. Box 6550, Alexandria, VA 22306
U.S.A.

Common Additives

Although it's possible to be sensitive to anything, most food additives present no problem, even for the chemically sensitive individual. Here are some of the ones in common use.

Bold type = eliminated on the Feingold Program
* = natural salicylate
Bold italic = possible problem for those on the Feingold Program

Acetic acid - pH control
Acetone peroxide - maturing & bleaching
Adipic acid - pH control
Agar agar - thickener
Alginic acid - antifoaming agent
Alpha tocopherol - antioxidant, nutrient
Amalases - dough conditioners
Ammonium bicarbonate - alkali
Ammonium phosphate - leavening
Ammonium sulfate - leavening
Annatto extract - coloring
Artificial flavoring
Ascorbic acid - nutrient, antioxidant, preservative
Aspartame (NutraSweetTM, EqualTM) - synthetic sweetener
Autolyzed yeast - flavor enhancer, contains MSG

Benzoic acid - preservative
Benzoate of soda - preservative
Benzoyl peroxide - maturing & bleaching, dough conditioner
Beta-apo-8' carotenal - coloring
Beta carotene - coloring
BHA (butylated hydroxyanisole) - antioxidant preservative
BHT (butylated hydroxytoluene) - antioxidant preservative

Calcium alginate - stabilizer, thickener, texturizer
Calcium bromate - maturing & bleaching, dough conditioner
Calcium carbonate - neutralizer, alkali
Calcium caseinate - texturizer, flavor enhancer
Calcium chloride - firming agent
Calcium citrate - buffer, dough conditioner
Calcium disodium EDTA (see EDTA)
Calcium hexametaphosphate - sequestrant, texturizer, emulsifier
Calcium hydroxide - firming agent

Calcium lactate - preservative, buffer, yeast food
Calcium oxide - yeast food, dough conditioner
Calcium peroxide - bleach
Calcium phosphate - leavening, bleach, dough cond., texturizer
Calcium propionate - preservative (mold inhibitor)
Calcium silicate - anticaking
Calcium sorbate - preservative
Calcium stearate - anticaking
Calcium stearoly-2-lactylate - emulsifier, stabilizer, dough cond.
Calcium sulfate (plaster of Paris) - maturing/dough conditioner
Canthaxanthin - coloring
Caramel - coloring
Carboxymethyl cellulose thickener
Carbon dioxide - propellant, carbonation
Carob bean gum - stabilizer, thickener, texturizer
Carotene - coloring
Carrageenan - emulsifier, stabilizer, thickener, texturizer
Casein (milk protein) - texturizer
Cellulose - stabilizer, thickener, texturizer
Chlorine - bleach
Chlorophyll - coloring
Citric acid - preservative, antioxidant, pH control
Citrus Red No. 2 - synthetic coloring
Cochineal - coloring
Corn sweetener, corn syrup - sweetener
Cyclamate - synthetic sweetener

Dehydrated beets - coloring
Dextrin - crystallization inhibitor, thickener, antifoaming
Dextrose - sweetener, similar to corn syrup
Diglycerides - emulsifiers
Dimethylpolysiloxane - antifoaming
Dioctyl sodium sulfosuccinate, DSS – stabilizer, emulsifier
Dipotassium phosphate - sequestrant, buffer, emulsifier

EDTA (ethylenediamine-tetraacetic acid) - antioxidant
Erythorbic acid - antioxidant
Ethoxylated mono- and digylcerides - dough conditioners
Ethyl cellulose - binder, filler
Ethyl formate - mold inhibitor
Ethyl vanillin - synthetic (artificial) flavoring

FD&C colors - synthetic (artificial) coloring
Ferrous gluconate - flavor enhancer, sequestrant, buffer
Fructose - sweetener, similar to corn syrup

Fumaric acid - acidifier

Gelatin - stabilizer, thickener, texturizer
Glucose - sweetener, similar to corn syrup
Glutamates - flavor enhancers which contain MSG
Glutamic acid - flavor enhancer which contains MSG, salt substitute
Glycerine - humectant
* Grape skin extract - coloring
Guar gum - stabilizer, thickener, texturizer
Gum arabic - stabilizer, thickener, texturizer
Gum tragacanth - stabilizer, thickener

Heptylparaben - preservative
High flavored yeast - flavor enhancer, may contain MSG
High fructose corn syrup - sweetener
Hydrogen peroxide - maturing/bleaching, dough conditioner
Hydrogenated oil- emulsifier
Hydrolyzed oat flour - contains flavor enhancer, MSG
Hydrolyzed protein/vegetable/plant protein - flavor enhancer, , contains MSG

Invert sugar - sweetener
Iodine - nutrient
Iron-ammonium citrate - anti-caking
Iron oxide - coloring
Isopropyl citrate - antioxidant, sequestrant, acidifier

Lactic acid - pH control, preservative
Lactose (milk sugar) - sweetener
Lactyllic stearate - dough conditioner
Lecithin - emulsifier
Locust bean gum - stabilizer, thickener, texturizer

Magnesium carbonate - alkali, anticaking
Magnesium chloride - firming, color retention
Magnesium hydroxide - alkali
Magnesium silicate - anticaking
Malic acid - acidifier
Malt extract, *malt flavoring* - flavor enhancer, may contain MSG
Maltodextrin - texturizer, flavor enhancer
Mannitol - sweetener, anti-caking, stabilizer, thickener, texturizer
Methylparaben - preservative
Methyl silicone - antifoaming
Modified food starch - stabilizer, thickener, texturizer
Monoglycerides - emulsifier
Monoammonium glutamate - flavor enhancer, contains MSG

Monopotassium glutamate - flavor enhancer, contains MSG
MSG (monosodium glutamate) - flavor enhancer
Monosodium phosphate - emulsifier, humectant

Natural flavoring - may be flavor enhancer, may contain MSG or salicylate
Niacinamide - nutrient

Papain - tenderizer
* Paprika (and oleoresin) - flavor, coloring
Partially hydrogenated oil - emulsifier
Pectin - stabilizer, thickener, texturizer
Phosphates, Phosphoric acid - pH control
Plant protein extract - flavor enhancer, contains MSG
Polydextrose (dextrose, sorbitol & citric acid) - filler, sweetener, like corn syrup
Polysorbates - emulsifiers
Potassium alginate - stabilizer, thickener, texturizer
Potassium bicarbonate - leavening
Potassium bisulfite - preservative
Potassium bromate - maturing/bleaching, dough conditioner
Potassium iodide - nutrient
Potassium metabisulfite - preservative
Potassium propionate, sorbate - preservatives
Potassium sulfite - preservative, antioxidant
Propionic acid - preservative
Propyl gallate - antioxidant
Propylene glycol - stabilizer, thickener, texturizer, humectant
Propylparaben - preservative

Riboflavin - nutrient, coloring

Saccharin - synthetic (artificial) sweetener
Saffron - coloring
Silicon dioxide - anti-caking
Sodium acetate - pH control
Sodium acid pyrophosphate - buffer, leavening
Sodium alginate - stabilizer, thickener, texturizer
Sodium aluminum sulfate - leavening
Sodium ascorbate - antioxidant preservative
Sodium benzoate - preservative
Sodium bicarbonate - leavening
Sodium bisulfite - preservative
Sodium carbonate - neutralizer
Sodium caseinate - flavor enhancer, contains MSG
Sodium citrate - pH control
Sodium erythrobate - preservative

Sodium hexametaphosphate - emulsifier, stabilizer, thickener
Sodium metabisulfite - preservative
Sodium metaphosphate - dough conditioner
Sodium nitrite, nitrate - preservative
Sodium potassium tartrate - emulsifier, acidifier
Sodium propionate - mold inhibitor
Sodium pyrophosphate - thickener, emulsifier
Sodium sorbate - preservative
Sodium stearyl fumarate - maturing/bleaching, dough conditioner
Sodium sulfite - preservative
Sorbic acid - preservative
Sorbitan monostearate - emulsifier
Sorbitol - humectant, sweetener
Soy isolates - filler
Soybean extract - flavor enhancer, may contain MSG
Stearic acid - fatty acid
Stearoyls - dough conditioners, emulsifiers
Sucrose (table sugar, brown sugar) - sweetener
Sulfites - preservatives
Sulfur dioxide - preservative
Sulfuric acid - acidifier, buffer

Tartaric acid - pH control
Tartrazine - FD&C Yellow No. 5, synthetic (artificial) coloring
TBHQ (tertiary butyl hydroquinone) - antioxidant
Textured soy protein - flavor enhancer, contains MSG
Thiamine - nutrient
Thiamine hydrochloride, mononitrite - nutrient
Titanium dioxide - coloring
Tocopherols (vitamin E) - nutrient, antioxidant
Torula yeast - flavor enhancer, may contain MSG
Tragacanth gum - stabilizer, thickener, texturizer
Tricalcium phosphate - anticaking
Tumeric (oleoresin) - flavoring, coloring

Vanilla - flavoring
Vanillin - artificial flavoring
Vitamin C (ascorbic acid) - nutrient, preservative, antioxidant
Vitamin E (tocopherols) - nutrient, antioxidant

Xanthan gum - thickener, stabilizer
Xylitol - sweetener

Yeast extract - flavor enhancer, contains MSG
Yellow prussiate of soda - anti-caking

Sources of Vitamin C

Here is a listing of the vitamin C content of a typical serving of fruits and vegetables. "Natural salicylates" are listed in bold type.

FRUITS
Guava - 242
Papaya - 118
Orange - 90
Strawberries - 88
Grapefruit juice - 78
Kiwi - 75
Watermelon - 63
Mango - 57
Lemon - 53
Grapefruit - 48
Lime - 37
Kumquat - 36
Tangerine - 35
Raspberries - 33
Cantaloupe - 33
Honeydew - 32
Pineapple juice - 23
Star fruit - 21
Pineapple - 17
Cherries - 15
Banana - 15
Avocado - 14
Rhubarb - 12
Nectarine - 10
Peach - 8
Pear - 8
Apricot nectar - 7 1/2
Apple - 5
Pumpkin - 5
Plum - 4
Pomegranate - 4
Grapes - 3
Cranberry sauce - 2 1/2
Apple juice - 2 1/2
Figs - 2
Raisins - less than 1/2
Grape juice - 0
Coconut, dried - 0
Dates - 0

VEGETABLES
Chili pepper, raw - 242
Broccoli, raw - 113
Broccoli, cooked - 90
Brussels sprouts - 87
Cauliflower, raw - 78
Sweet red pepper - 64
Kale - 62
Cauliflower, cooked - 55
Spinach, raw - 51
Cabbage, raw - 47
Collards - 46
Jalapeno pepper, raw - 44
Sweet potato - 44
Summer squash, raw - 44
Tomato - 35
Cabbage, cooked - 33
Green pepper - 32
Asparagus - 26
Onion, scallions - 25
Spinach, cooked - 25
Peas - 20
Potato, baked - 20
Lettuce, Romaine - 18
Radishes - 13
Onion, raw - 10
Yams - 9
Beans, Lima - 9
Corn - 9
Artichoke - 8
Beans, green - 8
Lettuce, iceberg - 8
Carrot - 8
Cucumber or Pickle - 6
Bean sprouts - 6
Chives - 6
Beets - 5
Bamboo shoots - 4
Mushrooms - 3
Celery - 2

A

A-1 Sauce · 158
Abbott Laboratories · 107
Accent · 72, 238
Additives – listing · 381
Adults · 261
Agriculture, Department of · 159
Airlines · 234
Alberta Children's Hospital · 371
Alcohol · 108, 134
Allergic irritability syndrome · 348
Allergies · 48, 200, 326, 344, 365
Allergy vs. sensitivity 345
Almonds · 17, 160
Aloe Vera · 269
Alternative Therapy Network · 340
Amaranth · 244, 330
American Academy of Pediatrics Committee on Drugs · 144, 286
American Medical Association · 15, 280
Ammonia · 146
Amusement parks · 240
Annals of Allergy · 67, 346, 348, 363
Annatto · 273, 381
Antibiotics · 325
Antifungal drugs · 199
Antioxidants · 67
Apples & apple juice · 84
Aranow, Dr. Ruth · 67
Archives of Diseases in Childhood · 195, 309, 368
Archives of General Psychiatry · 356
Arsenic · 61
Arthritis · 282
Artificial coloring · 57
Artificial flavorings · 64
Aspartame · 74
Asperger's syndrome 193
Asphalt and tar · 180
Aspirin · 84, 265, 329, 330
Asthma · 284
Auditory enhancement · 292, 293
Australia · 247, 366
Autism · 289

B

Baba, Dr. Jeffery · 75
Baby · 10, 250
Baby food pear juice · 28
Baby vitamins · 253
Balloons · 155
Barrier cloth · 269
Beasley, M.D., Joseph · 349
Bedwetting, enuresis · 307
Beef Stew, Easy · 53
Bellinger, Dr. David · 259
Benzoate · 79, 87, 159, 244, 330
Berthold-Bond, Annie · 268
BHA, BHT, TBHQ · 67, 68
Biblical foods · 230
Bio Integral Resource Center · 270
Birmingham University · 302
Blaylock, Dr Russell · 74
Blue No. 2 · 61, 286, 330
Blueberries · 79, 158
Bluestone, Dr. Charles · 325, 326
Boris, Marvin, M.D. · 363
Brain · 195
Breakfast · 49, 98, 232, 239, 245
Breslow, M.D., Michael · 82
British Medical Journal · 325
Brown U School/Medicine · 193, 281, 341
Browning, Dr. George · 325
Bruun, M.D., Ruth · 341
Bufferin · 91
Bug-killer · 62
Bunday, Sally · 201
Bunny Cake · 149
Bureau of Alcohol, Tobacco & Firearms · 108
Business Week · 186
Butter · 99, 115, 246

C

Caffeine · 82, 83
Cakes · 160
Calcium propionate · 93, 244
Calendar, School Year · 162
Camps · 231
Cancer · 68, 350, 351
Candy and Sugar · 46, 94, 104, 176
Cantekin, Ph.D., Erdem I. · 325, 326
Caramel Corn · 157
Carl Pfeiffer Treatment Ctr · 315, 343, 355
Carlton, Richard, M.D. · 140
Carmoisine · 244, 330
Carnival · 155
Carpeting · 268
Carter, C. M. · 195, 200, 367, 368, 370, 377

Cereals · 97
Certified Color Manufacturers Assoc · 59
Cheese · 98
Chemical Injury Information Network · 270
Chicken broth · 74
Childhood Depression · 265, 310
Chinese food · 70, 73, 237
Chlorine bleach · 382
Chocolate · 83, 95, 243, 368
Cholesterol · 115
Church · 227
CIBA Geigy · 335
Cleaning products · 180, 268
Clinical Pediatrics · 310, 370
Coffee · 17, 82, 83, 98
Cola drinks · 83, 102
Coleman, Dr. Arthur – MSG · 73
College · 248
Comings, M.D., David · 281, 342
Committee on Labor and Human Res · 75
Compounding pharmacists · 143
Consumer Beware · 65, 67
Conte, PhD, Richard · 371
Cooking · 110
Corn sweetener, corn syrup · 70, 93, 106
Cosmetic, Toiletries and Fragrances Association · 59
Cosmetics · 246, 268, 272
Coulombe, Dr. Roger · 75
Council for Exceptional Children · 224
Cranberries · 79, 158
Creamy Frosting · 150
Crib death · 338
Crime Times · 356
Crook, William, M.D. · 348
Cyclamate · 107

D

D&C dyes · 62
Dad won't cooperate · 122
Dairy products · 116
Dasun Company · 180
Defeat Autism Now · 306
Defined Diets and Childhood Hyperactivity-NIH conference · 6, 380
Delaney Clause · 59, 61
Denmark · 243
Dentist · 146
Department of Agriculture · 159
Depression · 265, 310, 313
Developmental Delay Resources · 320
Diaper pail deodorizers · 254
Diet Diary · 55
Dietary Replacement in Preschool-Aged Hyperactive Boys · 371
Dietitians · 173
Dilantin · 144
Disinfectant sprays · 254
Disney World · 240, 241
Divorce & Feingold Diet · 124
Doctors · 138
Donuts · 99
Dried fruits · 175
Dry cleaning · 268
Drug schedules 207
Duke University · 302

E

Ear infections · 324
Easter · 149
Easy Beef Stew · 53
Echinacea · 146
Education · 186, 187
Edward and the K.I.S.S. Plan 187
Egger, Joseph · 104, 195, 200, 310, 330, 367, 370, 373, 374, 375, 377
Elimination diet · 365
Elsas, Dr. Louis · 75, 77
Enuresis · 307, 310, 370
Environmental Protection Agency · 60, 271
Enzymes · 197, 302
Essential Update, The · 72
Eugenol · 278
Europe · 201, 242
Eustachian tube · 326
Exceptional Children · 217, 224
Excitotoxins, the Taste that Kills · 74
Eye shadow · 274
Eye-muscle disorders · 327

F

Fairfax County · 185
Fast food restaurants · 153, 236
FDA Consumer · 82, 274, 281, 286
Fighting for Tony · 290
First Four Days of Feingold · 1, 27
Flavorings, synthetic · 64
Fluoride · 147
Foam insulation · 268
Food additives - what they are made from? · 56
Food and Drug Administration (FDA) · 57, 76, 273, 278, 279, 286, 338, 350

Food dyes · 25, 57
Formaldehyde · 254
Fragile X syndrome · 295
Fragrance-free · 274
Fragrances · 268, 270, 278
France · 201, 242, 243
Freed, Jay, M.D. · 140
Fresh Fields Markets · 94, 267
Fresh pineapple · 87
Frosting, Creamy · 150
Fructose · 70
Fumes · 276

G

Gas appliances · 268
Glucose · 70
Glutamate, Glutamate Assoc. · 71
Gluten · 302
Grandparents · 125
Gravy · 158
Great Britain · 201, 242

H

Hair gel · 269
Halloween · 43, 90, 154
Hand lotion · 269
Happiness is a Choice · 291
Harley study · 371, 378, 379
Harvard Medical School Health Letter · 273, 286
Harvard School of Public Health · 139
Hazel, Stephen · 375
Headaches · 73
Health Hazards Evaluation Board · 72
Healthy Homes, Healthy Kids · 269
Heimlich, Mrs. Jane · 139
Heinz white vinegar · 101, 108
Helping Your Hyperactive/ADD Child · 169
Henkel · 68
Herbs · 146
High-fructose corn syrup · 70
Hives · 328
Hoffstein, Barbara, R.D. · 115, 252
Honey · 239
Hospital stay · 141 - 144
Hotels and motels · 269
Huffing · 357
Human Ecology Action League (HEAL) · 270, 278
Hunter, Beatrice Trum · 60, 65, 67, 71, 107
Hyperactive Children's Support Group · 201
Hypo-central vision · 293

I

Ice cream · 160
IEP · 170
Imitation vanilla · 64
In Bad Taste - The MSG Syndrome · 72
Inactive ingredients · 144
Indigo carmine · 330
Indoor pollution · 168
Integrated pest management (IPM) · 180
International Institute for Inhalant Abuse · 357
International Journal of Biosocial Research · 187
International Life Sciences Institute · 105
Introduction to Clinical Allergy · 86, 345, 346
IQ scores and additives · 78
Iraqi poisonings · 259

J

Janice Cottons · 269
Japanese restaurants - possible MSG · 73
Journal of Allergy & Clinical Immunology · 285, 329
Journal of Pediatrics · 140, 329, 366
Journal of the American Dietetic Association · 84
Journal of the American Medical Association · 85, 326
Junior high and high school · 43

K

Kaiser Permanente · 15, 328
Kaplan, Bonnie · 352, 365, 371
Kaufman, Barry Neil · 290
Kavanagh, James · 375
Kellogg Report · 139, 349
Kelly, Marguerite · 80
Kindergarten · 12
Kotsanis, C.A., M.D. · 291
K-P Diet · 15, 344

L

Lactitol · 107
Latitudes · 341
Lavin, Paul, Ph.D. · 140, 209, 214
Lead · 61, 259
Learning Disabilities - Proceedings of the National Conference · 375
Levitan, Dr. Herbert · 59, 200
Lipstick · 274
Logan, M.D., Ivan S., M.D. · 334
Love is not a lollypop · 117, 148
Lunch · 232
Lysine · 146

M

Mahalik, Dr. Michael · 75
Mail order companies · 167
Mandel, PhD, Francine · 363, 365
Mann, Dr. John · 314
Margarine · 100
Mary Jo's Story · 38
Matalon, Dr. Reuben · 75
McCormick & Co · 64
McEwen, Leonard · 373
McNicol, RD, Jane · 371
Mebane, Andrew H., M.D. · 82
Medical bracelet · 91
Mercury · 57, 61
Methyl mercury · 259
Metzenbaum, Sen. Howard · 75, 77
Migraine headaches · 8, 310, 370
Milk · 101, 326, 364
Mobile homes · 268
Moghadam, MD, H. K. · 371
Moneret-Vautrin · 346
Moth balls · 269
Mother-in-law · 126
Mrs. Dash's Steak Sauce · 158
MSG, Latin American restaurants · 70
Musk · 278

N

Nail polish remover · 274, 275
Narcolepsy · 336
National Academy for Child Development · 293
National Center for Environmental Health Strategies · 270
National Institute on Drug Abuse · 357
National Institutes of Health · 216, 381
Needleman, Herbert · 259
Neurotransmitters · 196
New clothing · 269
New England Journal of Med. · 70, 73, 78, 105, 259, 260, 285, 286, 357
New York City's public schools · 187
New York State Assembly Standing Committee on Child Care · 357
Next Generation · 32
NIH Consensus Development Conference · 216, 380
Nitrites · 80, 228
NonScents · 180
Norepinephrine · 196
Nursery school · 170
NutraSweet, FDA approval · 76
NutraSweet · 74, 105, 355
Nutrition Foundation · 378
Nuts · 160
Nystagmus · 328

O

Office machinery · 269
Oil of Wintergreen · 17
Olive oil · 238
Olives · 18
Olney, M.D., Dr. John W. · 74
Option Institute · 291
Orange No. 17 · 61
Orenstein, Neil S., M.D. · 348
Otitis media · 325

P

Paint 269, 276
Para amino benzoic acid (PABA) · 154
Parenting the Overactive Child, Alternatives to Drug Therapy · 140
Particle board · 269
Peanut butter cups · 28, 96
Pear juice · 49
Pediatrics · 144, 260, 286, 329, 338, 342, 371, 377
Perfume · 181, 277
Perfumed diapers and pre-moistened wipettes · 254
Pesticides · 270
Pharmacists · 143
Phenols · 196

Phosphates · 81
Pineapple · 18, 87
Pizza Cheese · 98
Placebo effect · 131
Pommery, John C., M.D. · 314
Portland State University · 315
Potpourri · 182
Preschool · 170
Printing ink · 270
Product Information Committee, FAUS · 69, 109
Public Citizen Health Research Group · 59, 60, 287
Pumpkin pie · 159
Pumpkins · 156

R

Raisins and grapes · 89
Randolph, Dr. Theron · 345
Rapp, Doris, M.D. · 348
Reaction · 185, 334
Reading difficulties 203
Reagan, President Ronald · 60
Red dye · 62
Reitz, Syte, Ph.D. · 224, 226
Relish tray · 159
Resources for the highly chemically-sensitive · 270
Restaurants · 236
Rhus tox · 146
Rimland, Dr. Bernard · 297, 306
Rogers, Sheila · 340
Rosenberry, Neil · 357
Rowe, Katherine and Kenneth · 329, 366,

S

Salicylates · 31, 35, 84, 333
Saving money on food · 114
Scary Night sheet cake · 154
Scented products · 128, 182, 254, 270
Schauss, Alexander · 356, 376
Schoenthaler, Stephen · 187, 356
School · 169, 179, 187, 351
School Year Calendar · 162
Schumaker, Jean Bragg · 375
Schwartz, M.D., George · 72
Science News · 62
Seasonal notes · 168
Seizure disorders · 332
Senate, hearings on MSG · 75
Serotonin · 281, 303, 314
Sesame Place · 242
Shaywitz, Bennett · 378
Shish Kebab · 54
Shrimp 52, 100
Sinaiko, Robert, M.D. · 195
Sleep apnea · 336, 338
Sleep disorders & salicylates · 338
Sleep disturbances · 258, 335, 338
SmithKline Beecham · 326
Smoke · 270
Smoking · 326
Sniffing fumes · 357
Snorting · 358
Social skills · 190
Sodium benzoate · 79
Sodium metabisulphite · 330
Sodium phosphate · 81, 157
Solving the Puzzle of Your Hard to Raise Child · 348
Son Rise · 290
Sorbitol · 244
Sound of a Miracle · 293
Soy sauce · 158
St. Patrick's Day · 149
Stage Two · 19, 103, 108, 109, 158, 159
Stehli, Annabel · 293
Stelazine · 318
Stimulant medication, long term effects · 208, 224
Stolla, Adelheid · 373
Strabismus · 327
Study designs · 378
Stuffing · 158
Sucanat · 107
Sudden infant death syndrome (SIDS) · 338
Sugars · 49, 103
Sulfate · 305
Sulfites · 89, 108, 285
Sulfur · 305, 385
Summer school 203
Summertime · 154
Sunday school · 229
Sundrops candies · 42
Sunset Yellow · 330
Supermarket lunch · 235
Supramaniam · 329
Surimi · 100
Swanson & Kinsborne · 379
Swanson, Dr. James · 217, 224, 260, 376, 379
Sweden · 243, 346
Sweet potatoes · 159
Swift, M.A., Jerry · 349, 351
Swiss chocolate · 96, 243

Switzerland · 242, 243
Symptoms often helped · 19
Synagogue · 227

T

Tartrazine (Yellow dye No. 5) · 244, 330, 366,
Taylor, John, Ph.D. · 169, 170,
Tea · 79, 83, 107
Tegretol · 333, 334, 335
Tests for food allergy · 345
Thanksgiving · 157, 228
That Kid Who Drives You Crazy! -- for teachers · 183
The Essential Update · 72
The Human Ecologist · 273, 278, 279
The Impossible Child · 348
The Lancet · 195, 200, 285, 329, 330, 367, 373, 375
Thorazine · 318
Thyroid problems & red dye · 60
Tics · 340-343
Time magazine ·201
Titanium dioxide · 385
Toothpaste · 27, 147
Tourette syndrome · 36, 80, 81, 207, 208, 281, 340 - 343
Tourette Syndrome and Human Behavior · 281, 340, 341, 342
Traveling in France · 245
Truss, Jr., Tom J. · 375
Twinkies defense · 353
Tylenol · 143

U

Uh-huh factor · 191
United Kingdom · 201, 243, 247
Univ of North Carolina · 302, 306
Univ of Wisconsin · 378
University of Iowa · 105
University of North Carolina · 302, 306
University of Wisconsin · 378

V

Vacation · 234
Vaccinium family of plants · 159
Valentine's Day · 148, 149
Vanilla · 64, 65, 66
Vanillin · 64
Vegetables · 159
Verrett, M. Jacqueline, Ph.D. · 78
Video tape · 162
Vinegar · 107
Violent Behavior · 352
Viral infection · 374
Vitamin C · 91
Vitamin E for burns · 146
Vodka · 109

W

Walsh, Ph.D., William · 355, 356
Waring, Dr. Rosemary · 302, 303, 306
Washington University · 74,
Water · 28, 270
Watermelon · 153, 154
Weiss (1979) study · 371
Weiss, Bernard, Ph.D. · 251, 258, 371, 379
Well Mind Association · 355
Whipped cream · 103, 159
Why Your Child is Hyperactive · 8, 16, 299, 329
Wiley, Dr. Harvey · 70
Wilkenfeld, Irene · 179, 182
Williams, J. Ivan · 377, 378, 379
Wine · 108, 227
Winter, Ruth · 68
Wolraich · 105
Wurtman, Dr. Richard · 75, 78, 79
Wyden, Ron, Congressman · 273
Wysong Medical Corporation · 68

Y

Yeast extract · 385
Yellow dye · 159, 329, 331, 366

Membership in the Feingold® Association provides:

Foodlist & Shopping Guide – Thousands of brand name products available in the United States, researched by the Feingold Association and free of the unwanted additives. All types of foods are listed, including prepared foods, snacks, mixes, candy, cookies, sodas, toothpaste, and other food items. Foodlists are provided for various regions of the U.S.

The Feingold Handbook - The most current information on the use of diet to help children and adults with attention deficit disorder (ADD) with or without hyperactivity, chemical-sensitivity, and salicylate-sensitivity. A practical step-by-step guide based on the successful experience of thousands of members.

Medication List - To help you find prescription and over-the-counter medicines free of the additives eliminated on the Feingold Program. (USA products)

Recipes & Two-Week Menu Plan - Meal ideas and easy-to-follow recipes are designed to go along with the Foodlist and help you through your first few weeks on the Program.

Pure Facts - The newsletter will keep you updated on the changes in brand name foods -- which to add to your Foodlist and which to remove.

Articles describing new developments in helping children and adults show you how to deal with issues from finding educational help to gaining cooperation from your mother-in-law. Your membership provides 10 issues a year.

You will also receive:

✓ FAUS Counseling Line -- staffed by parents who are experienced in the Program and available to answer questions and give support.

✓ Salicylate/Aspirin Sensitivity program for extreme salicylate sensitivity

✓ Gluten/Casein-free diet information and resources

✓ List of mail order resources for hard-to-find products

1 (800) 321-3287 * www.feingold.org

Outside the USA, write to: Feingold Association of the United States

P.O. Box 6550, Alexandria, VA 22306 USA